FREE Study Skills D

MW00845751

Dear Customer,

Thank you for your purchase from Mometrix! We consider it an honor and a privilege that you have purchased our product and we want to ensure your satisfaction.

As a way of showing our appreciation and to help us better serve you, we have developed a Study Skills DVD that we would like to give you for <u>FREE</u>. This DVD covers our *best practices* for getting ready for your exam, from how to use our study materials to how to best prepare for the day of the test.

All that we ask is that you email us with feedback that would describe your experience so far with our product. Good, bad, or indifferent, we want to know what you think!

To get your FREE Study Skills DVD, email <u>freedvd@mometrix.com</u> with *FREE STUDY SKILLS DVD* in the subject line and the following information in the body of the email:

- The name of the product you purchased.
- Your product rating on a scale of 1-5, with 5 being the highest rating.
- Your feedback. It can be long, short, or anything in between. We just want to know your impressions and experience so far with our product. (Good feedback might include how our study material met your needs and ways we might be able to make it even better. You could highlight features that you found helpful or features that you think we should add.)
- Your full name and shipping address where you would like us to send your free DVD.

If you have any questions or concerns, please don't hesitate to contact me directly.

Thanks again!

Sincerely,

Jay Willis
Vice President
<u>jay.willis@mometrix.com</u>
1-800-673-8175

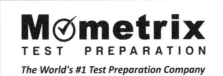

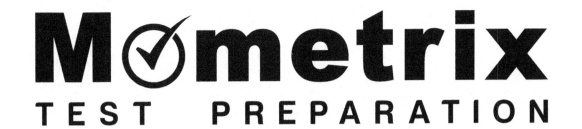

Family Nurse Practitioner

Certification Review

Nurse Practitioner Certification Examination Secrets Study Guide

Full-Length Practice Test

Step-by-Step Review
Video Tutorials

3rd Edition

Written and edited by Mometrix Test Prep

Printed in the United States of America

This paper meets the requirements of ANSI/NISO Z39.48-1992 (Permanence of Paper).

Mometrix offers volume discount pricing to institutions. For more information or a price quote, please contact our sales department at sales@mometrix.com or 888-248-1219.

Mometrix Media LLC is not affiliated with or endorsed by any official testing organization. All organizational and test names are trademarks of their respective owners.

Paperback
ISBN 13: 978-1-5167-1273-1
ISBN 10: 1-5167-1273-0

DEAR FUTURE EXAM SUCCESS STORY

First of all, **THANK YOU** for purchasing Mometrix study materials!

Second, congratulations! You are one of the few determined test-takers who are committed to doing whatever it takes to excel on your exam. **You have come to the right place.** We developed these study materials with one goal in mind: to deliver you the information you need in a format that's concise and easy to use.

In addition to optimizing your guide for the content of the test, we've outlined our recommended steps for breaking down the preparation process into small, attainable goals so you can make sure you stay on track.

We've also analyzed the entire test-taking process, identifying the most common pitfalls and showing how you can overcome them and be ready for any curveball the test throws you.

Standardized testing is one of the biggest obstacles on your road to success, which only increases the importance of doing well in the high-pressure, high-stakes environment of test day. Your results on this test could have a significant impact on your future, and this guide provides the information and practical advice to help you achieve your full potential on test day.

Your success is our success

We would love to hear from you! If you would like to share the story of your exam success or if you have any questions or comments in regard to our products, please contact us at **800-673-8175** or **support@mometrix.com**.

Thanks again for your business and we wish you continued success!

Sincerely,
The Mometrix Test Preparation Team

Need more help? Check out our flashcards at:
http://mometrixflashcards.com/NP

Table of Contents

Introduction

Thank you for purchasing this resource! You have made the choice to prepare yourself for a test that could have a huge impact on your future, and this guide is designed to help you be fully ready for test day. Obviously, it's important to have a solid understanding of the test material, but you also need to be prepared for the unique environment and stressors of the test, so that you can perform to the best of your abilities.

For this purpose, the first section that appears in this guide is the **Secret Keys**. We've devoted countless hours to meticulously researching what works and what doesn't, and we've boiled down our findings to the five most impactful steps you can take to improve your performance on the test. We start at the beginning with study planning and move through the preparation process, all the way to the testing strategies that will help you get the most out of what you know when you're finally sitting in front of the test.

We recommend that you start preparing for your test as far in advance as possible. However, if you've bought this guide as a last-minute study resource and only have a few days before your test, we recommend that you skip over the first two Secret Keys since they address a long-term study plan.

If you struggle with **test anxiety**, we strongly encourage you to check out our recommendations for how you can overcome it. Test anxiety is a formidable foe, but it can be beaten, and we want to make sure you have the tools you need to defeat it.

1

Secret Key #1 – Plan Big, Study Small

There's a lot riding on your performance. If you want to ace this test, you're going to need to keep your skills sharp and the material fresh in your mind. You need a plan that lets you review everything you need to know while still fitting in your schedule. We'll break this strategy down into three categories.

Information Organization

Start with the information you already have: the official test outline. From this, you can make a complete list of all the concepts you need to cover before the test. Organize these concepts into groups that can be studied together, and create a list of any related vocabulary you need to learn so you can brush up on any difficult terms. You'll want to keep this vocabulary list handy once you actually start studying since you may need to add to it along the way.

Time Management

Once you have your set of study concepts, decide how to spread them out over the time you have left before the test. Break your study plan into small, clear goals so you have a manageable task for each day and know exactly what you're doing. Then just focus on one small step at a time. When you manage your time this way, you don't need to spend hours at a time studying. Studying a small block of content for a short period each day helps you retain information better and avoid stressing over how much you have left to do. You can relax knowing that you have a plan to cover everything in time. In order for this strategy to be effective though, you have to start studying early and stick to your schedule. Avoid the exhaustion and futility that comes from last-minute cramming!

Study Environment

The environment you study in has a big impact on your learning. Studying in a coffee shop, while probably more enjoyable, is not likely to be as fruitful as studying in a quiet room. It's important to keep distractions to a minimum. You're only planning to study for a short block of time, so make the most of it. Don't pause to check your phone or get up to find a snack. It's also important to **avoid multitasking**. Research has consistently shown that multitasking will make your studying dramatically less effective. Your study area should also be comfortable and well-lit so you don't have the distraction of straining your eyes or sitting on an uncomfortable chair.

The time of day you study is also important. You want to be rested and alert. Don't wait until just before bedtime. Study when you'll be most likely to comprehend and remember. Even better, if you know what time of day your test will be, set that time aside for study. That way your brain will be used to working on that subject at that specific time and you'll have a better chance of recalling information.

Finally, it can be helpful to team up with others who are studying for the same test. Your actual studying should be done in as isolated an environment as possible, but the work of organizing the information and setting up the study plan can be divided up. In between study sessions, you can discuss with your teammates the concepts that you're all studying and quiz each other on the details. Just be sure that your teammates are as serious about the test as you are. If you find that your study time is being replaced with social time, you might need to find a new team.

Secret Key #2 – Make Your Studying Count

You're devoting a lot of time and effort to preparing for this test, so you want to be absolutely certain it will pay off. This means doing more than just reading the content and hoping you can remember it on test day. It's important to make every minute of study count. There are two main areas you can focus on to make your studying count:

Retention

It doesn't matter how much time you study if you can't remember the material. You need to make sure you are retaining the concepts. To check your retention of the information you're learning, try recalling it at later times with minimal prompting. Try carrying around flashcards and glance at one or two from time to time or ask a friend who's also studying for the test to quiz you.

To enhance your retention, look for ways to put the information into practice so that you can apply it rather than simply recalling it. If you're using the information in practical ways, it will be much easier to remember. Similarly, it helps to solidify a concept in your mind if you're not only reading it to yourself but also explaining it to someone else. Ask a friend to let you teach them about a concept you're a little shaky on (or speak aloud to an imaginary audience if necessary). As you try to summarize, define, give examples, and answer your friend's questions, you'll understand the concepts better and they will stay with you longer. Finally, step back for a big picture view and ask yourself how each piece of information fits with the whole subject. When you link the different concepts together and see them working together as a whole, it's easier to remember the individual components.

Finally, practice showing your work on any multi-step problems, even if you're just studying. Writing out each step you take to solve a problem will help solidify the process in your mind, and you'll be more likely to remember it during the test.

Modality

Modality simply refers to the means or method by which you study. Choosing a study modality that fits your own individual learning style is crucial. No two people learn best in exactly the same way, so it's important to know your strengths and use them to your advantage.

For example, if you learn best by visualization, focus on visualizing a concept in your mind and draw an image or a diagram. Try color-coding your notes, illustrating them, or creating symbols that will trigger your mind to recall a learned concept. If you learn best by hearing or discussing information, find a study partner who learns the same way or read aloud to yourself. Think about how to put the information in your own words. Imagine that you are giving a lecture on the topic and record yourself so you can listen to it later.

For any learning style, flashcards can be helpful. Organize the information so you can take advantage of spare moments to review. Underline key words or phrases. Use different colors for different categories. Mnemonic devices (such as creating a short list in which every item starts with the same letter) can also help with retention. Find what works best for you and use it to store the information in your mind most effectively and easily.

Secret Key #3 – Practice the Right Way

Your success on test day depends not only on how many hours you put into preparing, but also on whether you prepared the right way. It's good to check along the way to see if your studying is paying off. One of the most effective ways to do this is by taking practice tests to evaluate your progress. Practice tests are useful because they show exactly where you need to improve. Every time you take a practice test, pay special attention to these three groups of questions:

- The questions you got wrong
- The questions you had to guess on, even if you guessed right
- The questions you found difficult or slow to work through

This will show you exactly what your weak areas are, and where you need to devote more study time. Ask yourself why each of these questions gave you trouble. Was it because you didn't understand the material? Was it because you didn't remember the vocabulary? Do you need more repetitions on this type of question to build speed and confidence? Dig into those questions and figure out how you can strengthen your weak areas as you go back to review the material.

Additionally, many practice tests have a section explaining the answer choices. It can be tempting to read the explanation and think that you now have a good understanding of the concept. However, an explanation likely only covers part of the question's broader context. Even if the explanation makes sense, **go back and investigate** every concept related to the question until you're positive you have a thorough understanding.

As you go along, keep in mind that the practice test is just that: practice. Memorizing these questions and answers will not be very helpful on the actual test because it is unlikely to have any of the same exact questions. If you only know the right answers to the sample questions, you won't be prepared for the real thing. **Study the concepts** until you understand them fully, and then you'll be able to answer any question that shows up on the test.

It's important to wait on the practice tests until you're ready. If you take a test on your first day of study, you may be overwhelmed by the amount of material covered and how much you need to learn. Work up to it gradually.

On test day, you'll need to be prepared for answering questions, managing your time, and using the test-taking strategies you've learned. It's a lot to balance, like a mental marathon that will have a big impact on your future. Like training for a marathon, you'll need to start slowly and work your way up. When test day arrives, you'll be ready.

Start with the strategies you've read in the first two Secret Keys—plan your course and study in the way that works best for you. If you have time, consider using multiple study resources to get different approaches to the same concepts. It can be helpful to see difficult concepts from more than one angle. Then find a good source for practice tests. Many times, the test website will suggest potential study resources or provide sample tests.

Practice Test Strategy

If you're able to find at least three practice tests, we recommend this strategy:

UNTIMED AND OPEN-BOOK PRACTICE

Take the first test with no time constraints and with your notes and study guide handy. Take your time and focus on applying the strategies you've learned.

TIMED AND OPEN-BOOK PRACTICE

Take the second practice test open-book as well, but set a timer and practice pacing yourself to finish in time.

TIMED AND CLOSED-BOOK PRACTICE

Take any other practice tests as if it were test day. Set a timer and put away your study materials. Sit at a table or desk in a quiet room, imagine yourself at the testing center, and answer questions as quickly and accurately as possible.

Keep repeating timed and closed-book tests on a regular basis until you run out of practice tests or it's time for the actual test. Your mind will be ready for the schedule and stress of test day, and you'll be able to focus on recalling the material you've learned.

Secret Key #4 – Pace Yourself

Once you're fully prepared for the material on the test, your biggest challenge on test day will be managing your time. Just knowing that the clock is ticking can make you panic even if you have plenty of time left. Work on pacing yourself so you can build confidence against the time constraints of the exam. Pacing is a difficult skill to master, especially in a high-pressure environment, so **practice is vital**.

Set time expectations for your pace based on how much time is available. For example, if a section has 60 questions and the time limit is 30 minutes, you know you have to average 30 seconds or less per question in order to answer them all. Although 30 seconds is the hard limit, set 25 seconds per question as your goal, so you reserve extra time to spend on harder questions. When you budget extra time for the harder questions, you no longer have any reason to stress when those questions take longer to answer.

Don't let this time expectation distract you from working through the test at a calm, steady pace, but keep it in mind so you don't spend too much time on any one question. Recognize that taking extra time on one question you don't understand may keep you from answering two that you do understand later in the test. If your time limit for a question is up and you're still not sure of the answer, mark it and move on, and come back to it later if the time and the test format allow. If the testing format doesn't allow you to return to earlier questions, just make an educated guess; then put it out of your mind and move on.

On the easier questions, be careful not to rush. It may seem wise to hurry through them so you have more time for the challenging ones, but it's not worth missing one if you know the concept and just didn't take the time to read the question fully. Work efficiently but make sure you understand the question and have looked at all of the answer choices, since more than one may seem right at first.

Even if you're paying attention to the time, you may find yourself a little behind at some point. You should speed up to get back on track, but do so wisely. Don't panic; just take a few seconds less on each question until you're caught up. Don't guess without thinking, but do look through the answer choices and eliminate any you know are wrong. If you can get down to two choices, it is often worthwhile to guess from those. Once you've chosen an answer, move on and don't dwell on any that you skipped or had to hurry through. If a question was taking too long, chances are it was one of the harder ones, so you weren't as likely to get it right anyway.

On the other hand, if you find yourself getting ahead of schedule, it may be beneficial to slow down a little. The more quickly you work, the more likely you are to make a careless mistake that will affect your score. You've budgeted time for each question, so don't be afraid to spend that time. Practice an efficient but careful pace to get the most out of the time you have.

6

Secret Key #5 – Have a Plan for Guessing

When you're taking the test, you may find yourself stuck on a question. Some of the answer choices seem better than others, but you don't see the one answer choice that is obviously correct. What do you do?

The scenario described above is very common, yet most test takers have not effectively prepared for it. Developing and practicing a plan for guessing may be one of the single most effective uses of your time as you get ready for the exam.

In developing your plan for guessing, there are three questions to address:

- When should you start the guessing process?
- How should you narrow down the choices?
- Which answer should you choose?

When to Start the Guessing Process

Unless your plan for guessing is to select C every time (which, despite its merits, is not what we recommend), you need to leave yourself enough time to apply your answer elimination strategies. Since you have a limited amount of time for each question, that means that if you're going to give yourself the best shot at guessing correctly, you have to decide quickly whether or not you will guess.

Of course, the best-case scenario is that you don't have to guess at all, so first, see if you can answer the question based on your knowledge of the subject and basic reasoning skills. Focus on the key words in the question and try to jog your memory of related topics. Give yourself a chance to bring the knowledge to mind, but once you realize that you don't have (or you can't access) the knowledge you need to answer the question, it's time to start the guessing process.

It's almost always better to start the guessing process too early than too late. It only takes a few seconds to remember something and answer the question from knowledge. Carefully eliminating wrong answer choices takes longer. Plus, going through the process of eliminating answer choices can actually help jog your memory.

Summary: Start the guessing process as soon as you decide that you can't answer the question based on your knowledge.

How to Narrow Down the Choices

The next chapter in this book (**Test-Taking Strategies**) includes a wide range of strategies for how to approach questions and how to look for answer choices to eliminate. You will definitely want to read those carefully, practice them, and figure out which ones work best for you. Here though, we're going to address a mindset rather than a particular strategy.

Your chances of guessing an answer correctly depend on how many options you are choosing from.

How many choices you have	How likely you are to guess correctly
5	20%
4	25%
3	33%
2	50%
1	100%

You can see from this chart just how valuable it is to be able to eliminate incorrect answers and make an educated guess, but there are two things that many test takers do that cause them to miss out on the benefits of guessing:

- Accidentally eliminating the correct answer
- Selecting an answer based on an impression

We'll look at the first one here, and the second one in the next section.

To avoid accidentally eliminating the correct answer, we recommend a thought exercise called **the $5 challenge**. In this challenge, you only eliminate an answer choice from contention if you are willing to bet $5 on it being wrong. Why $5? Five dollars is a small but not insignificant amount of money. It's an amount you could afford to lose but wouldn't want to throw away. And while losing $5 once might not hurt too much, doing it twenty times will set you back $100. In the same way, each small decision you make—eliminating a choice here, guessing on a question there—won't by itself impact your score very much, but when you put them all together, they can make a big difference. By holding each answer choice elimination decision to a higher standard, you can reduce the risk of accidentally eliminating the correct answer.

The $5 challenge can also be applied in a positive sense: If you are willing to bet $5 that an answer choice *is* correct, go ahead and mark it as correct.

Summary: Only eliminate an answer choice if you are willing to bet $5 that it is wrong.

Which Answer to Choose

You're taking the test. You've run into a hard question and decided you'll have to guess. You've eliminated all the answer choices you're willing to bet $5 on. Now you have to pick an answer. Why do we even need to talk about this? Why can't you just pick whichever one you feel like when the time comes?

The answer to these questions is that if you don't come into the test with a plan, you'll rely on your impression to select an answer choice, and if you do that, you risk falling into a trap. The test writers know that everyone who takes their test will be guessing on some of the questions, so they intentionally write wrong answer choices to seem plausible. You still have to pick an answer though, and if the wrong answer choices are designed to look right, how can you ever be sure that you're not falling for their trap? The best solution we've found to this dilemma is to take the decision out of your hands entirely. Here is the process we recommend:

ONCE YOU'VE ELIMINATED ANY CHOICES THAT YOU ARE CONFIDENT (WILLING TO BET $5) ARE WRONG, SELECT THE FIRST REMAINING CHOICE AS YOUR ANSWER.

Whether you choose to select the first remaining choice, the second, or the last, the important thing is that you use some preselected standard. Using this approach guarantees that you will not be enticed into selecting an answer choice that looks right, because you are not basing your decision on how the answer choices look.

This is not meant to make you question your knowledge. Instead, it is to help you recognize the difference between your knowledge and your impressions. There's a huge difference between thinking an answer is right because of what you know, and thinking an answer is right because it looks or sounds like it should be right.

Summary: To ensure that your selection is appropriately random, make a predetermined selection from among all answer choices you have not eliminated.

Test-Taking Strategies

This section contains a list of test-taking strategies that you may find helpful as you work through the test. By taking what you know and applying logical thought, you can maximize your chances of answering any question correctly!

It is very important to realize that every question is different and every person is different: no single strategy will work on every question, and no single strategy will work for every person. That's why we've included all of them here, so you can try them out and determine which ones work best for different types of questions and which ones work best for you.

Question Strategies

READ CAREFULLY

Read the question and answer choices carefully. Don't miss the question because you misread the terms. You have plenty of time to read each question thoroughly and make sure you understand what is being asked. Yet a happy medium must be attained, so don't waste too much time. You must read carefully, but efficiently.

CONTEXTUAL CLUES

Look for contextual clues. If the question includes a word you are not familiar with, look at the immediate context for some indication of what the word might mean. Contextual clues can often give you all the information you need to decipher the meaning of an unfamiliar word. Even if you can't determine the meaning, you may be able to narrow down the possibilities enough to make a solid guess at the answer to the question.

PREFIXES

If you're having trouble with a word in the question or answer choices, try dissecting it. Take advantage of every clue that the word might include. Prefixes and suffixes can be a huge help. Usually they allow you to determine a basic meaning. Pre- means before, post- means after, pro - is positive, de- is negative. From prefixes and suffixes, you can get an idea of the general meaning of the word and try to put it into context.

HEDGE WORDS

Watch out for critical hedge words, such as *likely, may, can, sometimes, often, almost, mostly, usually, generally, rarely,* and *sometimes.* Question writers insert these hedge phrases to cover every possibility. Often an answer choice will be wrong simply because it leaves no room for exception. Be on guard for answer choices that have definitive words such as *exactly* and *always.*

SWITCHBACK WORDS

Stay alert for *switchbacks.* These are the words and phrases frequently used to alert you to shifts in thought. The most common switchback words are *but, although,* and *however.* Others include *nevertheless, on the other hand, even though, while, in spite of, despite, regardless of.* Switchback words are important to catch because they can change the direction of the question or an answer choice.

FACE VALUE

When in doubt, use common sense. Accept the situation in the problem at face value. Don't read too much into it. These problems will not require you to make wild assumptions. If you have to go beyond creativity and warp time or space in order to have an answer choice fit the question, then you should move on and consider the other answer choices. These are normal problems rooted in reality. The applicable relationship or explanation may not be readily apparent, but it is there for you to figure out. Use your common sense to interpret anything that isn't clear.

Answer Choice Strategies

ANSWER SELECTION

The most thorough way to pick an answer choice is to identify and eliminate wrong answers until only one is left, then confirm it is the correct answer. Sometimes an answer choice may immediately seem right, but be careful. The test writers will usually put more than one reasonable answer choice on each question, so take a second to read all of them and make sure that the other choices are not equally obvious. As long as you have time left, it is better to read every answer choice than to pick the first one that looks right without checking the others.

ANSWER CHOICE FAMILIES

An answer choice family consists of two (in rare cases, three) answer choices that are very similar in construction and cannot all be true at the same time. If you see two answer choices that are direct opposites or parallels, one of them is usually the correct answer. For instance, if one answer choice says that quantity x increases and another either says that quantity x decreases (opposite) or says that quantity y increases (parallel), then those answer choices would fall into the same family. An answer choice that doesn't match the construction of the answer choice family is more likely to be incorrect. Most questions will not have answer choice families, but when they do appear, you should be prepared to recognize them.

ELIMINATE ANSWERS

Eliminate answer choices as soon as you realize they are wrong, but make sure you consider all possibilities. If you are eliminating answer choices and realize that the last one you are left with is also wrong, don't panic. Start over and consider each choice again. There may be something you missed the first time that you will realize on the second pass.

AVOID FACT TRAPS

Don't be distracted by an answer choice that is factually true but doesn't answer the question. You are looking for the choice that answers the question. Stay focused on what the question is asking for so you don't accidentally pick an answer that is true but incorrect. Always go back to the question and make sure the answer choice you've selected actually answers the question and is not merely a true statement.

EXTREME STATEMENTS

In general, you should avoid answers that put forth extreme actions as standard practice or proclaim controversial ideas as established fact. An answer choice that states the "process should be used in certain situations, if…" is much more likely to be correct than one that states the "process should be discontinued completely." The first is a calm rational statement and doesn't even make a definitive, uncompromising stance, using a hedge word *if* to provide wiggle room, whereas the second choice is a radical idea and far more extreme.

BENCHMARK

As you read through the answer choices and you come across one that seems to answer the question well, mentally select that answer choice. This is not your final answer, but it's the one that will help you evaluate the other answer choices. The one that you selected is your benchmark or standard for judging each of the other answer choices. Every other answer choice must be compared to your benchmark. That choice is correct until proven otherwise by another answer choice beating it. If you find a better answer, then that one becomes your new benchmark. Once you've decided that no other choice answers the question as well as your benchmark, you have your final answer.

PREDICT THE ANSWER

Before you even start looking at the answer choices, it is often best to try to predict the answer. When you come up with the answer on your own, it is easier to avoid distractions and traps because you will know exactly what to look for. The right answer choice is unlikely to be word-for-word what you came up with, but it should be a close match. Even if you are confident that you have the right answer, you should still take the time to read each option before moving on.

General Strategies

TOUGH QUESTIONS

If you are stumped on a problem or it appears too hard or too difficult, don't waste time. Move on! Remember though, if you can quickly check for obviously incorrect answer choices, your chances of guessing correctly are greatly improved. Before you completely give up, at least try to knock out a couple of possible answers. Eliminate what you can and then guess at the remaining answer choices before moving on.

CHECK YOUR WORK

Since you will probably not know every term listed and the answer to every question, it is important that you get credit for the ones that you do know. Don't miss any questions through careless mistakes. If at all possible, try to take a second to look back over your answer selection and make sure you've selected the correct answer choice and haven't made a costly careless mistake (such as marking an answer choice that you didn't mean to mark). This quick double check should more than pay for itself in caught mistakes for the time it costs.

PACE YOURSELF

It's easy to be overwhelmed when you're looking at a page full of questions; your mind is confused and full of random thoughts, and the clock is ticking down faster than you would like. Calm down and maintain the pace that you have set for yourself. Especially as you get down to the last few minutes of the test, don't let the small numbers on the clock make you panic. As long as you are on track by monitoring your pace, you are guaranteed to have time for each question.

DON'T RUSH

It is very easy to make errors when you are in a hurry. Maintaining a fast pace in answering questions is pointless if it makes you miss questions that you would have gotten right otherwise. Test writers like to include distracting information and wrong answers that seem right. Taking a little extra time to avoid careless mistakes can make all the difference in your test score. Find a pace that allows you to be confident in the answers that you select.

12

KEEP MOVING

Panicking will not help you pass the test, so do your best to stay calm and keep moving. Taking deep breaths and going through the answer elimination steps you practiced can help to break through a stress barrier and keep your pace.

Final Notes

The combination of a solid foundation of content knowledge and the confidence that comes from practicing your plan for applying that knowledge is the key to maximizing your performance on test day. As your foundation of content knowledge is built up and strengthened, you'll find that the strategies included in this chapter become more and more effective in helping you quickly sift through the distractions and traps of the test to isolate the correct answer.

Now it's time to move on to the test content chapters of this book, but be sure to keep your goal in mind. As you read, think about how you will be able to apply this information on the test. If you've already seen sample questions for the test and you have an idea of the question format and style, try to come up with questions of your own that you can answer based on what you're reading. This will give you valuable practice applying your knowledge in the same ways you can expect to on test day.

Good luck and good studying!

Assessment

Health Promotion and Screening

PENDER'S HEALTH PROMOTION MODEL

Pender developed the **Health Promotion Model** in an effort to educate APRNs and other clinicians about the psychosocial aspects of health promotion behavior. Her model theorizes that an individual's tendency toward **health-promoting behavior** is affected by his or her previous behavior, as well as his or her inherited and acquired behavioral characteristics. The individual will commit to changing his or her behavior if he or she values the benefits gained from doing so; conversely, if the individual perceives barriers in achieving these benefits, commitment may waver, and behavior modification may be abandoned. An important barrier between current behavior and behavior modification is whether the individual believes that he or she actually can accomplish an effective change in behavior with expected results.

PROPOSED FACTORS

In the **Health Promotion Model**, Pender proposes a number of other factors that may influence an individual's **behavior modification**. For example, the HPM proposes that if the individual perceives/believes that he or she is able to effectively change his or her behavior, the individual will have fewer barriers in achieving the change or changes. When the individual perceives him or herself as being effective, he or she will likely develop a positive attitude toward the behavior, which will in turn increase the individual's level of commitment. An increase in the level of commitment, then, will result in more positive results over time. The HPM also theorizes that an individual will be more willing to commit to a behavior change if there is a significant other value or engagement in the modified behavior. Positive support from friends and family also increases the chance that the individual will remain committed.

ENVIRONMENTAL ASSESSMENT OF A HOME

Environmental assessments are very helpful when developing a care plan to provide for care and safety. Rooms should be assessed according to their function:

- **Entryway** should be free of obstacles and surfaces should be even. Handrails and/or ramps may be needed for those who are unsteady or wheelchair bound.
- **Stairs/steps** should have handrails, non-skid surfaces, and contrast markings for each step.
- **Living area** should be comfortable and furniture arranged for convenience. Chairs should be firm enough for people to stand from easily.
- **Bedrooms** should have a night light and phone near the bed. Bed should be positioned close to the nearest bathroom if possible and at the appropriate height for easy access and appropriate firmness.
- **Bathrooms** may need grab bars, hand-held shower, elevated toilet seat, and tub seat.
- **Kitchen** may need items moved for convenient access as well as a sturdy step stool. Unsafe equipment/tools should be removed.

ADDITIONAL ELEMENTS OF AN ENVIRONMENTAL ASSESSMENT

Some elements of an **environmental assessment** are not specific to rooms in the house but are general needs that must be met in order for people, especially the elderly or disabled, to remain safe:

- **Environmental hazards** such as piles of papers or junk on the floors, loose carpet or rugs, and cluttered pathways can cause falls and must be cleared, organized, or repaired.
- **Lighting** should be adequate enough for reading in all rooms and stairways.
- **Heat and air conditioning** must be adequate. The young and the elderly are especially susceptible to heat and cold injury.
- **Sanitation** should ensure that health hazards do not exist, such as from rotting food or infestations of cockroaches or rodents.
- **Animals** should be cared for adequately with access to food, water, toileting, and routine veterinary care.
- **Smoke/chemicals** in the environment may pose a hazard, such as exposure to cigarette smoking or cleaning materials.

METHODS OF ASSESSING ENVIRONMENTAL FACTORS

Environmental factors should be assessed within the **actual environment** if at all possible. If not, careful questioning and drawing of diagrams and approximate floor plans with the patient—or asking the patient to do drawings—can be useful, especially when showing the patient needed modifications. Family members may also assist with the assessment, providing useful information. Some patients, especially the elderly, may be reluctant to admit that the home is cluttered or that they are unable to maintain the home environment in a sanitary condition. Brochures and handouts about home safety and assistive devices should be provided to the patient as well as contact names and numbers for equipment needed in the home. A checklist should be compiled of all necessary changes or additions, with specific details, such as "Install 18-inch grab bar across from toilet." In some cases, a social worker or occupational therapist should visit the patient.

BENEFITS OF KNOWLEDGE OF EPIDEMIOLOGICAL PRACTICES

Epidemiology is important to nurse practitioners across all clinical settings. The nurse practitioner will treat a varied patient population during his or her career, and it is important to create a **plan of care** that is tailored to the patient; the patient's age, race, career, and religion all represent different populations to which he or she belongs, and may affect clinical course, treatment, and outcome. Armed with epidemiological knowledge about the patient, the nurse practitioner can create a clinical decision-making framework, an effective care plan, and the means to share this information with his or her peers to aid in the care of other patients.

COMPLETING A COMMUNITY HEALTH NEEDS ASSESSMENT AND IMPLEMENTING FINDINGS

There are a number of steps to completing a **community health needs assessment**:

1. Identify the **population/aggregate** to be assessed.
2. Determine the **information** that should be collected.
3. Select data collection **methods**.
4. Develop **tools**, such as questionnaires or interview questions, and data collection procedures.
5. **Train** data collectors.
6. Select a representative **sample** of the whole aggregate if necessary (depending on the type of study and the size of the aggregate).

16

7. Conduct the needs assessment.
8. **Analyze** the data and identify needs.

In order to **implement findings**, an action plan must be developed. First, a list of problems should be compiled and prioritized to determine which should receive the most focus. Then, the actions required for each problem in order to meet set goals and desired outcomes, those responsible for carrying out or supervising the action, and a timeline for completion should be determined.

Clinical Prevention

Clinical prevention refers to the practice of maintaining health and wellness and performing tasks that identify risk of disease at an early stage. Clinical prevention may involve **screening** for risk factors for certain illnesses. If risks are identified as a result, then further steps can be taken to manage these risks and possibly prevent the disease or illness from occurring. Examples of screenings that may be used as clinical prevention include screening colonoscopies, blood pressure screenings, or skin testing. Clinical prevention may also refer to activities that **stop a condition from developing**. Examples include child and adult immunizations or counseling to teach patients about practicing healthy behaviors. Clinical prevention services may be available through a variety of measures. In hospital settings, some preventive measures are performed as ordered by physicians but many are part of routine nursing practice. Alternatively, some preventive services are available in the community, allowing quick and easy access for the population to receive screenings.

Prevention Interventions

Interventions for prevention of certain diseases involve screening and various other practices to determine the level of risk. **Screening practices** may involve performing lab tests, measuring vital signs, or performing clinical procedures. An example of a screening test would be a blood test to check glucose levels among a group of people. Those with elevated levels may be at higher risk of insulin resistance. Further testing is required on those who showed elevated results. Some **prevention measures** involve giving medications that will prevent disease development. For example, administering the flu shot to a segment of the population can help to reduce the risk of influenza in the community. Evaluation of effectiveness of prevention measures is important to determine success. **Follow-up** with patient groups after screenings can determine if high-risk patients developed the diseases they were screened for. Community-wide regimens require tracking of cases through public health records. Follow-up, tracking, and recordkeeping are essential for adequate evaluation of effectiveness of interventions.

Consumer-Focused Health Care

Consumer-focused health care recognizes that the needs of the patient are central to delivery of care and that provision of care should try to match the expectations of the patient. With the Internet, patients have easy access to much more medical information than previously, and as patients become better informed, they expect a greater role in their own healthcare decisions and better-quality care at lower prices. A primary component of consumer-focused health care is **evaluating customer satisfaction** and **utilizing continuous quality improvement methods** to improve service. The needs of the patient are viewed holistically, so that all healthcare needs are met, ranging from housing to medical treatment. The nurse practitioner must be an advocate for the patient, assessing patients' expectations and implementing changes to assure that the needs are met. Because patients often fail to express their dissatisfaction directly to healthcare providers, the nurse should ask patients directly if they have concerns.

Copyright © Mometrix Media. You have been licensed one copy of this document for personal use only. Any other reproduction or redistribution is strictly prohibited. All rights reserved.

Approaches to Patient Care

In addition to the interdisciplinary team approach, there are several other **recognized approaches to patient care**. One of these approaches is the **independent medical management approach**, in which one clinician works alone (for the most part) with limited contact with and clinical input from other clinicians. Another approach is the **multidisciplinary care approach**, in which each health care worker involved in the patient care works independently of the others involved in the care of the patient; these health care workers do not collaborate, but rather each is assigned a specific task to perform. The third approach is **consultative**; in this case, the clinician assumes the majority of patient care, but may request consultations from other clinicians.

Population-Based Health Policy and Advocacy for Equitable Services

Population-based health policy focuses on the needs of a specific population, but this may be interpreted broadly as those in one community or more narrowly as those within a specific ethnic or socio-economic group within a larger community. Interventions are aimed at diseases or conditions that affect the selected population as a whole rather than focusing on individuals in the population. For example, a population-based health policy may aim to provide safe housing for the homeless population in a city.

As an **advocate for equitable services** for a population, the family nurse practitioner must be prepared with data to support the need for services. The family nurse practitioner should determine which individuals, agencies, or organizations have the ability to provide assistance and target them in various ways: providing information, gathering supporters, disseminating information via news media and community events, lobbying politicians, and organizing others to assist.

Family Systems Theory

Bowen's Family Systems Theory suggests that one must look at the person in terms of his/her **family unit** because the members of a family have different roles and behavioral patterns, so a change in one person's behavior will affect the others in the family. There are 8 interrelated concepts:

- **Triangle theory**: Two people comprise a basic unit, but when conflict occurs, a third person is drawn into the unit for stability with the resulting dynamic of 2 supporting one or 2 opposing one. This, in turn, draws in other triangles.
- **Self-differentiation**: People vary in need for external approval.
- **Nuclear family patterns**: marital conflict, 1 spouse dysfunctional, 1 or more children impaired, and emotional distance.
- **Projection within a family**: Problems (emotional) passed from parent to child.
- **Transmission (multigenerational)**: Small differences in transmission from parent to child.
- **Emotional isolation**: Reducing or eliminating family contact.
- **Sibling order**: Influence on behavior and development.
- **Emotional process (society)**: Results in regressive or progressive social movements.

> **Review Video: Bowen Family Systems**
> Visit mometrix.com/academy and enter code: 591496

TOOLS TO ENGAGE PATIENTS IN DISEASE MANAGEMENT

Tools that can be used to engage the patient in managing their disease include:

- **Coaching:** Assisting patients to obtain the information and confidence they need to participate actively in the management of their own healthcare. The coach works in collaboration with the patient to provide support in self-management as well as emotional support. The coach conducts follow-ups with the patient and helps the patient navigate the healthcare system.
- **Motivating**: Encouraging patients to change behavior by appealing to their own sense of motivation. Motivating may include the use of motivational interviewing, which focuses on establishing an empathetic relationship with the patient and utilizes open-ended (not "yes"/ "no") questions, affirmations (expression of empathy), reflective listening, and summary.
- **Negotiating**: Taking the time to deliberate with a patient to determine the best course of action. The family nurse practitioner should present the pros and cons of treatment and provide clear explanations as to why a particular treatment may be indicated, taking into consideration the needs, desires, and concerns of the patient.

Sexuality

CDC'S RECOMMENDATIONS FOR PREVENTION OF STDS

The **CDC** has developed 5 strategies to **prevent** and **control** the spread of **sexually transmitted diseases (STDs)**:

- **Educate** those at risk about how to make changes in sexual practices to prevent infection.
- **Identify** symptomatic and asymptomatic infected persons who might not seek diagnosis or treatment.
- **Diagnose** and treat those who are infected.
- **Prevent infection** of sex partners through evaluation, treatment, and counseling.
- Provide pre-exposure **vaccination** for those at risk.

Practitioners are advised of patients' **sexual histories** and to assess risk. The 5-P approach to questioning is advocated. Practitioners should ask about:

- **Partners**: Gender and number.
- **Pregnancy** prevention: Birth control.
- **Protection**: Methods used.
- **Practices**: Type of sexual practices (oral, anal, vaginal) and use of condoms.
- **Past history of STDs**: High-risk behavior (promiscuity, prostitution) and disease risk (human immunodeficiency virus [HIV]/ hepatitis).

CDC RECOMMENDATIONS FOR PREVENTION OF SPREADING STDS

The **CDC** recommends a number of specific preventive methods as part of the clinical guidelines for **prevention of sexually transmitted diseases (STDs)**:

- **Abstinence**/reduction in number of sex partners.
- Pre-exposure **vaccination**: All those evaluated for STDs should receive hepatitis B vaccination, and men who have sex with men (MSM) and illicit drug users should receive hepatitis A vaccination.

- **Male latex (or polyurethane) condoms** should be used for all sexual encounters with only water-based lubricants used with latex.
- **Female condoms** may be used if male condom cannot be used properly.
- Condoms and diaphragms should not be used with spermicides containing **nonoxynol-9 (N-9)**, and N-9 should not be used as a lubricant for anal sex.
- **Non-barrier contraceptive measures** provide no protection from STDs and must not be relied on to prevent disease.

EMERGENCY CONTRACEPTION

Female patients who have had unprotected sexual intercourse, consensual or rape, are at risk for pregnancy and may desire **emergency contraception**. Emergency contraception inhibits ovulation and prevents pregnancy rather than aborting a pregnancy. Because the medications contain hormones (such as ethinyl estradiol and norgestrel or levonorgestrel) in differing amounts, this treatment is contraindicated in those with a history of thromboembolia or severe migraine headaches with neurological symptoms. The criteria for administration of emergency contraception include:

- <72 hours since unprotected sexual intercourse.
- Negative pelvic exam.
- Negative pregnancy test.

The regimen involves taking a first dose of 1-20 pills (depending upon the brand and concentration of hormones) and then a second dose of 1-20 pills 12 hours later. A follow-up pregnancy test should be done if the person does not menstruate within 3 weeks as the failure rate is about 1.5%. Side effects include nausea (relieved by taking medication with meals or with an antiemetic), breast tenderness, and irregular bleeding.

CONTRACEPTIVE DEVICES

There are a number of **contraceptive devices** available to prevent pregnancy:

- **Male and female condoms**: They are more effective if used with spermicides, but nonoxynol-9 (N-9) should be avoided because it interferes with protection against sexually transmitted diseases. Patients should have instruction in proper use to avoid semen leaking from the condom. Condoms are 80-90% effective.
- **Intrauterine device**: IUDs are usually T-shaped and are inserted through the cervix into the uterus (with the attached string palpable at the cervical opening. IUDs prevent pregnancy by causing a local inflammatory response that prevents fertilization. Some are plastic, but ParaGard® is copper, which has antisperm effects and can be left in place for up to 10 years. Adverse effects of IUDs include abnormal bleeding, discharge, or infection. Mirena® releases levonorgestrel (synthetic progestin) and can be left in place for 5 years. It can be used with smokers, but there may be some side effects because of the hormone: acne, increased facial hair, and thickening of cervical mucosa. IUDs are 95-99% effective.

- **Diaphragm**: This round device has a flexible supporting ring and a dome-like latex cup (requiring latex allergy assessment). The concave surface (facing the cervix) is coated with spermicide before the diaphragm is inserted. The diaphragm is fitted to the individual using sized fitting rings during a pelvic exam so it seats properly below cervix and is held in place by vaginal muscles. Diaphragms range in size from 50-90 mm. They should not be placed more than 2 hours prior to intercourse because spermicide loses effectiveness. Diaphragms are left in place for at least 6 hours after intercourse (but not more than 12 hours). Each act of intercourse requires additional insertion of spermicide vaginally. The diaphragm should be washed with soap and water after use and inspected under bright light for tears or holes prior to each use. They are 85-95% effective if used properly. Changes in weight or pregnancy can alter size requirements, so diaphragms should be refitted when either of these has occurred.
- **Cervical cap**: This latex cap is smaller than the diaphragm (22-35 mm) and more cone-shaped, and it fits about the cervix rather than below it. Like the diaphragm, it is used with spermicide. It may cause cervical irritation, so women may need Pap smears more frequently (every 3 months), but it has the advantage of being able to stay in place for up to 48 hours, but leaving it in for long periods increases the risk of vaginitis and toxic shock syndrome. Cervical caps do not require additional spermicide for each act of intercourse and are 85-95% effective.
- **Contraceptive sponges**: These are donut-shaped spongy barrier devices that are impregnated with nonoxynol-9 (N-9), so they are 85-95% effective but do not protect against sexually transmitted diseases (STDs). Sponges have a concave central indentation on one side that fits over cervix to act as a barrier. The outside has a string for easy removal. The sponge is left in place for 6 hours after intercourse but not >30 hours.

NATURAL CONTRACEPTIVE PRACTICES

There are **natural contraceptive practices**, but they are less effective than other methods:

- **Coitus interruptus**: This requires withdrawing the penis from the vagina prior to ejaculation. It is a frequently used method of birth control, especially among teenagers, but it is completely unreliable, as sperm may leak prior to ejaculation.
- **Rhythm methods**: Using rhythm methods requires determining when the woman ovulates and abstinence from sex during the fertile phase, but pregnancy rates are about 40%; so, this method is only advised if couples are very disciplined, monitor their cycles carefully, and are willing to abstain from sex for long periods during each cycle. This method is often used because of religious restrictions against artificial birth control. Ovulation detection kits (such as Ovulindex®) are available over the counter. They detect the enzyme guaiacol peroxidase in cervical mucosa. This indicates ovulation will occur in about 6 days. These kits, however, are more reliable for those attempting to become pregnant than to avoid pregnancy.

Screening and Social Determinants of Health

HEALTH SCREENING

Health screening is broad screening for conditions that are very likely to occur and diseases that are likely to kill if they are not identified. The assessment should be trustworthy using proper techniques and proper follow-up. The assessment needs to be sensitive, with a true positive outcome when the outcome is positive, and it should be particular, with a true negative for someone that does not have the condition.

BIRTH TO 10-YEAR POPULATION

The US Preventive Services Task Force issued a list of screening tests that are recommended for the **birth to 10-year** population; these screening tests were determined to be of importance based on the risks associated with this age group. Recommended basic screening includes **height and weight** measurements, which can be compared to published age-specific height and weight charts to determine whether the child is in an acceptable range. **Blood pressure** testing is also recommended. **Vision** testing is advised for children over the age of 3 (though it may be necessary in younger children if serious vision problems are suspected). In addition to these screening tests, a number of tests are recommended for all children soon after birth; these include hemoglobinopathy screening, phenylalanine level, and thyroid hormone levels (thyroxine and thyroid-stimulating hormone).

SCREENING PROCEDURES FOR CHILDREN THROUGHOUT CHILDHOOD

Additional screening procedures are available for children, including extensive laboratory testing that may be indicated if there is cause for concern that a child may have a disorder.

- **Genetic disorders**: Screening is usually done at birth according to state guidelines, and then may be indicated if there is concern that a child has a disorder that requires treatment.
- **Hearing**: Testing is usually done with newborns, between 3-8 years and then every 2-3 years until age 18.
- **Fasting blood sugar**: Done every 2 years for those at risk.
- **Head circumference**: Measurement is done at birth, 1 year, and 2 years.
- **Dental screening**: Bottle-fed babies may require earlier screening, as they often fall asleep with the bottle in their mouths, leading to infant caries. Dental screening is done periodically throughout childhood, especially after the new teeth come in to evaluate for malocclusion or other problems.
- **Alcohol/drug use**: Screening may be done periodically for children between 11-18 years, especially if they are at risk.
- **Developmental screening**: There are a number of screening tests that are available and can be used if a child appears to have a developmental delay or abnormality. Screening tests must be age-appropriate. The tests are not diagnostic, but can help to confirm developmental abnormalities. Tests may assess motor skills, language, and cognitive ability.

11 TO 24-YEAR AGE POPULATION

For the **11 to 24-year** age population, the US Preventive Services Task Force recommends continued **height and weight** measurements, in addition to continued **blood pressure** readings. A **Papanicolaou test** (Pap smear) is recommended for sexually active females; if the sexual history is unknown or questionable, Pap smears should be performed for women 18 years of age and older. Sexually active individuals within this age group should also be screened for chlamydia. **Immunization records** should be verified in children older than 12 years of age; if the immunization history is not available, a rubella titer should be ordered.

25 TO 64-YEAR AGE POPULATION

Height, weight, and blood pressure measurements are again recommended as part of the screening process. Yearly total **blood cholesterol** testing is recommended as well, beginning at age 25 for men, and at age 45 for women. For sexually active women, a **Papanicolaou test** is recommended at least every 3 years; those with previously abnormal Pap smears may be advised to have this test done yearly or twice yearly, depending on the situation. Starting at the age of 50, both men and women should have yearly **fecal occult blood testing**, as well as a **sigmoidoscopy**. Yearly breast examination and mammogram is advised for women beginning at age 50 as well. Women of childbearing age should be questioned about their vaccination history; if the history of rubella vaccination is unclear or unknown, a rubella titer should be drawn.

ADULTS

Adults should have the following screenings:

- Blood pressure (2 years apart).
- Cholesterol (5 years apart).
- Dental (yearly).
- ECG (over 40, yearly when there are cardiac risks).
- Pap smear (female over 18, 3 years apart following two fine outcomes and no risks).
- Self breast exam (over 20, monthly).
- Clinical breast exam (over 40, yearly; 20-39 3 years apart).
- Mammogram (over 40, yearly; some say 1-2 years apart).
- Colorectal screen (over 50, yearly).
- Prostate-specific antigen (men over 50, yearly).
- Glaucoma (over 40, yearly when there are risks).
- Hearing (if patient has a lot of contact with noise).
- Chest x-ray (not advised).
- Thyroid palpation (20-39, 3 years apart; 40 and up, yearly).
- Urinalysis (debatable).
- Hgb/Hct (debatable).
- Health education and promotion (every time patient is seen).

POPULATION OLDER THAN 65 YEARS OF AGE

For adults **older than 65 years** of age, there are, of course, the all-important **blood pressure, height, and weight** measurements. Yearly **fecal occult blood testing** and **sigmoidoscopy** are also part of the screening process in this population. For women aged 65 to 69, yearly **mammograms** and clinical **breast exams** are also advised. **Papanicolaou testing** may or may not be necessary; this is dependent on whether past results have been consistently normal or not. If previous tests have been consistently normal, the Pap smear may be discontinued after the age of 65 (assuming that the patient is not engaging in risky sexual behavior). Adults 65 years of age and older should also have yearly **vision and hearing** testing as well.

PREGNANT WOMEN DURING THEIR FIRST VISIT

The list of screening tests recommended for a **pregnant woman's first visit to a clinician** is somewhat lengthy. **Blood pressure** and **weight** measurements should be taken, of course. The pregnant woman's **hemoglobin** and **hematocrit** should be tested to make sure that she is not anemic, and that her baby is not being starved of oxygen and vital nutrients. A hepatitis B surface antigen test should be done to make sure that the mother has been immunized. An RPR/VRDL test should be done to detect syphilis, and if the woman is younger than 25 years of age, a chlamydia screen should also be done. Blood typing and antibody screening are also important, as well as rubella titers. Tests that may be offered, but are not required, include HIV, amniocentesis, and hemoglobinopathy screening.

PREGNANT WOMEN DURING FOLLOW-UP VISITS

When the pregnant woman is seen for a **follow-up** visit, blood pressure should be measured. It is important to measure the **blood pressure** at every visit, and to keep a close eye on it; pregnancy-induced hypertension (or preeclampsia) is a serious complication. A **urine specimen** should also be collected between 12 and 16 weeks; the urine should be cultured to determine whether bacteria are present. During follow-up visits, **amniocentesis** may again be offered to the mother; she is not required to consent to this procedure, which can identify genetic abnormalities in the fetus. **Serum alpha-fetoprotein testing** may also be offered; high levels of the protein have been associated with an increased risk of neural tube defects such as spina bifida. These tests are generally recommended for women older than 35 years of age, as advanced maternal age is a risk factor for certain genetic diseases.

ADMINISTRATION OF THE NIHSS

The **NIHSS** is administered with careful attention to directions. The examiner should record the answers and avoid coaching or repeating requests although demonstration may be used with aphasic patients. The scale comprises 11 sections, with scores for each section ranging from 0 (normal) to 2-4:

- **Level of consciousness**: response to noxious stimulation (0-3), request for age and age (0-2), request to open and close eyes, grip and release unaffected hand (0-2).
- **Best gaze**: Horizontal eye movement (0-2).
- **Visual**: Visual fields (0-3).
- **Facial palsy**: Symmetry when patient shows teeth, raises eyebrows, and closes eyes (0-3).
- **Motor, arm**: Drift while arm extended with palms down (0-4).
- **Motor, leg**: Leg drift at 30° while patient supine (0-4).
- **Limb ataxia**: Finger-nose and heel-shin (0-2).
- **Sensory**: Grimace or withdrawal from pinprick (0-2).
- **Best language**: Describes action of pictures (0-3).
- **Dysarthria**: Reads or describes words on list (0-2).
- **Distinction and inattention**: Visual spatial neglect (0-2).

SCREENING FOR SCOLIOSIS

Scoliosis is the lateral curvature ≥11° of the spine, usually occurring (in 2-3% of adolescents) during the period between 10-15 when the child goes through a growth spurt, so screening should be done at least twice during this period. Scoliosis is more common in girls than boys. Screening includes:

- Child stands upright and **shoulders, waist, and hips** are assessed.
- **Adams forward bending test**, in which the child bends over at the waist (as in toe touching) and the screener observes the hips to determine if there is a difference in height.
- **Scoliometer** measures the curvature of the spine in the thoracic and lumbar area when the child bends over.
- **Moire topography** uses a grating positioned near the child so it casts shadows that show contour lines.
- **X-rays** confirm positive screenings.

Positive findings may include one shoulder lower than another, uneven waistline, prominence of shoulder blade(s), one hip higher than another, or lateral leaning when upright.

PRE-PARTICIPATION CARDIOVASCULAR SCREENING FOR COMPETITIVE ATHLETES (HIGH SCHOOL AND COLLEGE)

Sudden death in athletes <35 years usually relates to **congenital or acquired cardiovascular disorders**. The most common causes of sudden death are hypertrophic cardiomyopathy and coronary artery abnormalities. Sudden death in athletes >35 is usually attributed to

24

atherosclerotic coronary disease. The American Heart Association **pre-participation cardiovascular screening** includes:

- **Medical history**: The athlete must be questioned about chest pain on exertion, episodes of syncope, dyspnea on exertion, history of heart murmur, and hypertension.
- **Family history**: A complete cardiac history of the family should be obtained, focusing on deaths or disability related to heart disease <50 and any known cardiac conditions.
- **Physical examination**: This must include auscultation of the heart with the athlete supine and standing and with Valsalva maneuver, palpation of femoral pulses, examination for physical indications of Marfan syndrome, and bilateral brachial artery blood pressure (with athlete sitting).

BRONCHOPROVOCATION TESTS

A **bronchoprovocation test** is done when a patient has symptoms of bronchoconstriction but the pulmonary function tests are normal. It is used to determine the presence of **hyperactive airways**. It is sometimes done before occupational exposure or to assess occupational exposure. For 8 hours prior to testing, patients should refrain from using any bronchodilating agents, including caffeine and nicotine. Maintenance medications, with the exception of steroids, should also be withheld for a period of 48 hours. The patient inhales a substance to provoke bronchoconstriction, usually methacholine or histamine and then pulmonary function testing (flow volume loop) is done to assess the response of the airways. The test is positive if there is a 10% drop in the FEV_1. A bronchodilator is administered following the test to reverse bronchospasm.

COMMON SITES TO SCREEN FOR DIABETIC FOOT ULCERS

Most **diabetic ulcers** are on the foot, ranging from the toes to the heels. Ulcers may first appear as laceration, blisters, or punctures, and the wound is usually circular with well-defined edges. There is often callus in the periwound tissue.

Common sites:

- **Toes**: The toes are frequent sites for ulcers because of the potential for trauma. The interphalangeal joints often have limited flexibility that causes pressure and friction. The dorsal toes may have hammertoes from injuries or improperly fitted shoes that are easily injured. Distal toes may suffer injury from poor perfusion, heat, or short footwear.
- **Metatarsal heads** may have poor flexibility, increasing pressure.
- **Bunions** may erode because of deformities or narrow footwear.
- **Midfoot** may suffer injury from trauma or Charcot's fracture.
- **Heels** are susceptible to unrelieved pressure, often related to prolonged periods of bed rest.

ABI EXAMINATION
PROCEDURE

The **ABI (ankle-brachial index) examination** is done to evaluate peripheral arterial disease of the lower extremities.

1. Apply BP cuff to one arm, palpate brachial pulse, and place conductivity gel over the artery.
2. Place the tip of a Doppler device at a 45-degree angle into the gel at the brachial artery and listen for the pulse sound.
3. Inflate the cuff until the pulse sound ceases and then inflate 20 mm Hg above that point.
4. Release air and listen for the return of the pulse sound. This reading is the brachial systolic pressure.

5. Repeat the procedure on the other arm, and use the higher reading for calculations.
6. Repeat the same procedure on each ankle with the cuff applied above the malleoli and the gel over the posterior tibial pulse to obtain the ankle systolic pressure.
7. Divide the ankle systolic pressure by the brachial systolic pressure to obtain the ABI.

Sometimes, readings are taken both before and after 5 minutes of walking on a treadmill.

INTERPRETING RESULTS

Once the **ABI examination** is completed, the ankle systolic pressure must be divided by the brachial systolic pressure. Ideally, the BP at the ankle should be equal to that of the arm or slightly higher. With **peripheral arterial disease**, the ankle pressure falls, affecting the ABI. Additionally, some conditions that cause calcification of arteries, such as diabetes, can cause a false elevation.

Calculation is simple; if the ankle systolic pressure is 90 and the brachial systolic pressure is 120: $90 \div 120 = 0.75$

The **degree** of disease relates to the score:

- > 1.3: Abnormally high, may indicate calcification of vessel wall
- 1 to 1.3: Normal reading, asymptomatic
- < 0.95: Indicates narrowing of one or more leg blood vessels
- < 0.8: Moderate, often associated with intermittent claudication during exercise
- ≤ 0.6 to 0.8: Borderline perfusion
- < 0.5 to 0.75: Severe disease, ischemia
- < 0.5: Pain even at rest, limb threatened
- < 0.25: Critical, limb-threatening condition

NYLON MONOFILAMENT TEST

A simple test for neuropathy, commonly used to determine risk of ulcers in diabetic patients, is the **nylon monofilament test**, which is available in kits:

- Describe the procedure to the patient and ask the patient to indicate when the pressure of the monofilament is felt.
- Grasp a length of #10 monofilament in the instrument provided.
- Touch the monofilament against the bottom of the foot and then press the monofilament into the foot until the line buckles.
- Test the great, 3rd, and 5th toes.
- Test the left, medial, and right areas of the ball of the foot
- Test the right and left of the arch.
- Test the middle of the heel.

The test is evaluated according to how many of the 10 test sites the patient is able to detect. If the patient fails to detect the monofilament at fewer than 4 sites, this is indicative of decreased sensation and increased risk.

DIAGNOSTIC SCREENING TESTS FOR CAUSES OF HYPERTENSION

Screening tests to identify common **causes of hypertension** include:

- **Estimated glomerular filtration rate (GFR)**: Chronic kidney disease, such as chronic glomerulonephritis polycystic kidney disease, and hypertensive nephrosclerosis.
- **CT angiography**: Coarctation of the aorta.
- **Dexamethasone suppression test**: Cushing's syndrome and excess glucocorticoid states (as from steroid therapy).
- **Drug screening**: Drug-induced.
- 24-hour urine for metanephrine and normetanephrine: Pheochromocytoma.
- 24-hour urine aldosterone or measures of other mineralocorticoids: Primary aldosteronism.
- Doppler flow study, magnetic resonance angiography (MRA): Renovascular hypertension.
- Sleep study with O_2 saturation: Sleep apnea.
- Thyroid-stimulating hormone (TSH) and serum parathyroid hormone (PTH): Thyroid or parathyroid disease.

ISSUES THAT IMPACT ACCESS TO CARE

POVERTY

There are a number of issues that impact **access to care**, but **poverty** is one of the most significant and can affect care in many ways:

- Parents may not have **health insurance** and may not qualify for state medical assistance or may not be aware that they are eligible, so they do not take their children for routine medical visits.
- Practitioners may not accept **state medical assistance payments** because of low reimbursement rates, leaving parents with few options.
- Employers may not allow parents to take **time off from work** during the times that most practices are open to provide care, or the parents cannot afford to lose income, so most medical care is provided by emergency departments when a crisis arises.
- Parents may lack **automobiles** or have insufficient funds for or access to public transportation to take a child to medical visits, especially in more rural areas.

LANGUAGE BARRIERS

Language barriers often compromise patient's access to care and compliance with treatment, especially if the family are non-English speaking or have poor English skills. If the nurse practitioner's practice draws from a minority population, then the nurse should consider proactive steps to resolving the issue of language barriers, such as hiring bilingual staff, taking language classes, providing translated materials, such as treatment guidelines and pamphlets, or symbol-based signs. Many practices depend on family members, often children, to translate, but this is not a good solution as children often lack the maturity to assume this responsibility and may also lack the vocabulary or understanding to translate effectively, leading to serious misunderstandings. Interpreters should have training in **medical vocabulary**. In some cases, volunteer translators can be trained. Another solution is to pool translation resources among a number of practices so that costs are manageable.

DRUG COSTS AND TREATMENT COST-EFFECTIVENESS

The nurse practitioner is able to order drugs and treatments, but doing so without considering **costs** of medications and cost-effectiveness of treatments often leads to **noncompliance** on the part of children/parents because they cannot afford treatment; therefore, the nurse practitioner should determine if insurance will reimburse costs before prescribing, and this often involves discussing these issues with families while understanding that some families may be reluctant to admit that they cannot afford care. In many cases, more than one treatment option is open, and in that case, the least expensive option should be considered first. The nurse practitioner must **facilitate medical care** as well as order treatments. Newer medications are not necessarily better than older less expensive medications. For example, recent studies indicate that Glucophage® is just as effective as newer drugs for diabetes mellitus, Type II, and has fewer side effects.

PSYCHOLOGICAL, PHYSICAL, AND COGNITIVE BARRIERS TO SELF-CARE

The following are psychological barriers to self-care:

- **Emotional instability** may interfere with ability to learn and manage care.
- **Sexuality issues** may cause people to be anxious about body image, sexual dysfunction, and sexual activity. Homosexual patients may need special counseling, depending upon the disorder.

The following are physical barriers to self-care:

- **Vision impairment** requires that people wear glasses or any other modifiers in good light. Those who are legally blind need a tactile approach to teaching so that they can use their sense of touch.
- **Hearing impairment** requires a quiet environment or translator. Nurse should face patient to facilitate lip reading and use picture diagrams or videos.
- **Allergies** require people to try different systems to determine sensitivities or use modified systems.
- **Motor impairment** may necessitate simplified ostomy care and consultation with occupational therapist.

The following is a cognitive barrier to self-care:

- **Mental acuity** varies, and some may not be able to be independent in care or may need repeated step-by-step instruction over a prolonged period of time.

Comprehensive History and Physical Assessment

CONDUCTING PATIENT HISTORY SO THAT THE PATIENT IS COMFORTABLE AND SECURE

The **patient interview** is the first step in the process of treating a patient, and it is often where the most important information is obtained. Because it is such a crucial part of the overall assessment of the patient, it is important to make the patient feel **comfortable**. The FNP is not likely to get a great deal of information from a patient if they make a negative impression. If possible, conduct the interview in a quiet area. If this is not a possibility, remain calm and relaxed while interviewing the patient, and take time both when asking questions and listening to the answers. If the patient is given the impression that the NP is impatient or in a rush, he or she may become uncomfortable and hesitant to answer questions.

TAILORING THE INTERVIEW PROCESS FOR PEDIATRIC PATIENTS

Conducting a history and physical examination on a **pediatric patient** has its challenges; however, there are things that the nurse practitioner can do to make sure that the process is as smooth and painless as possible for everyone involved. In most cases, one or more of the child's family members will be present; this will help the child to feel comfortable, but the interviewer should also strive to make sure that the child is as relaxed as possible. Speaking slowly and directly to the child, making eye contact, and getting down to the child's level are all ways to help the child feel more comfortable. Ask only one question at a time, and allow the child and his or her guardians to ask questions throughout the interview. Ask the child some questions that are not related to his or her illness; this will help establish some rapport and trust with the child.

DOCUMENTATION OF HISTORY

INFANTS AND CHILDREN

The nurse practitioner is expected to demonstrate competency in assessment, including history, as part of identifying and managing health concerns in infants and children. Complete and accurate **documentation** of findings is an essential element of the plan of care. This may be done in the classic manner that begins with a complaint and includes health history, review of systems, nutrition, developmental status, family history, and socioeconomic factors that may impact the health issue. A problem-oriented history builds upon the classic history by focusing on developmental health problems, functional problems, and diseases, moving from subjective information (history) to objective (physical/laboratory data):

- **Developmental assessment** includes motor, speech, cognitive, social, and adaptive behaviors.
- **Functional assessment** includes issues related to basic health behavior patterns, such as diet, sleeping, coping, sexuality, and elimination.
- **Diseases** are those diagnoses according to the International Classification of Diseases, Clinical Modification, (ICD-10), and interventions are planned based on diagnosis.

ADOLESCENTS

While the essential elements of assessment and **history-taking for adolescents** are similar to those for infants and children, there are some differences because often the adolescent is providing, or in some cases withholding, information. Additionally, the risk factors associated with adolescence vary from those of infancy or earlier childhood. Assessment should include lifestyle information, such as whether the teenager has been homeless, engaged in high-risk sexual behavior, violence, tobacco use, or drug taking. Documenting nutrition, weight concerns, peer relationships, and coping mechanisms can help to identify health concerns. A complete history may require more than 1 visit. Successful assessment includes:

- **Listen** and show respect for the adolescent.
- **Question** adolescent/parent cause for concern.
- **Interview** both the adolescent and the parent(s) alone.
- Provide **questionnaires/surveys** in advance to parents, healthcare providers, and teachers and review those as part of the history.
- Observe **non-verbal behavior and interactions** among children and parents.

COMMUNICATION REGARDING SEXUAL HISTORY

When communicating regarding sexuality, the family nurse practitioner should be comfortable with their own **sexuality**, and maintain an **objective, nonjudgmental attitude**. Clearly specify the privacy of information that the patient can expect during and after the interview. Do not assume marital status or orientation. Ask open-ended questions, provide examples that illustrate an acceptance, and signify a "no-wrong-answer" attitude that gives the patient permission to speak freely. Use terms that the patient understands, and be clear in the use of terms. Clarify any terms the patient uses that might be ambiguous.

29

AGE-RELATED SKIN CHARACTERISTICS

Age is an important consideration when evaluating the skin because the characteristics of the **skin change as people age**:

- The skin of **premature infants** is especially friable, allowing for transepidermal water loss and evaporative heat loss.
- An **infant**'s skin is thinner than an adult's because, while the epidermis is developed, the dermis layer is only about 60% of that of an adult and continues to develop after birth.
- During **adolescence**, the hair follicles activate and the thickness of the dermis decreases about 20% and epidermal turnover time increases, so healing slows.
- As people continue to **age**, Langerhans' cells decrease in number, making the skin more prone to cancer, and the inflammatory reactions decrease. The sweat glands, vascularity, and subcutaneous fat all decrease, interfering with thermoregulation and contributing to dryness and irritation of the skin. The epidermal-dermal junction flattens, resulting in skin prone to tearing. The elastin in the skin degrades with age and solar exposure. The thinning of the hypodermis can lead to pressure ulcers.

WOUND CLASSIFICATION

Wounds are classified according to the cause:

- **Vascular changes** can result in wounds that occur most commonly in the lower extremities, such as those that result from arterial insufficiency and ischemia, those that relate to changes in the lymphatic system, and those related to venous insufficiency.
- **Neuropathic changes** that occur with chronic diseases, such as diabetes, and chronic alcoholism can decrease sensation and circulation, resulting in ulcerations.
- **Shear, friction, and pressure**, especially over bony prominences such as the sacral area and heels, causes erosion of the tissue.
- **Trauma** often results in contaminated wounds.
- **Surgery** can involve wounds that are originally contaminated or originally clean, depending upon the type of surgery and the reason.
- **Inflammation and infection** may result in deteriorating wounds or fistulas.
- **Self-inflicted wounds** vary widely, from minor cuts to traumatic gunshot wounds.
- **Hypergranulation/keloid formation** can change the character of a wound and prevent adequate healing.

MODIFIED WAGNER ULCER CLASSIFICATION SYSTEM

The modified **Wagner Ulcer Classification System** divides foot ulcers into 6 grades, based on lesion depth, osteomyelitis or gangrene, infection, ischemia, and neuropathy:

1. At risk but no open ulcers.
2. Superficial ulcer, extending into subcutaneous tissue; superficial infection with or without cellulitis.
3. Full-thickness ulcer to tendon or joint with no abscess or osteomyelitis.
4. Full-thickness ulcer that may extend to bone with abscess, osteomyelitis, or sepsis of joint and may include deep plantar infections, abscesses, fascitis, or infections of tendon sheath.
5. Gangrene of area of foot but the rest of foot is salvageable.
6. Gangrene of entire foot, requiring amputation.

While this classification system is useful in predicting outcomes, it does not contain information about the size of the ulcer or the type of infection, so it should be only **one part of an assessment**, as more detailed information is needed to fully evaluate an ulcer.

NATIONAL PRESSURE ULCER ADVISORY PANEL STAGING FOR PRESSURE ULCERS

The National Pressure Ulcer Advisory Panel developed a staging system to ensure that definitions for pressure ulcers were standardized:

- **Stage I: Nonblanchable erythema** – Intact, reddened area that does not blanch. (Difficult to assess in darker skin). Area remains intact but the physical appearance is altered.
- **Stage II: Partial thickness** – Destruction of the epidermis and/or dermis. This type of injury may be an intact blister, ruptured blister, or an open ulcer if it has a pinkish or a reddish wound bed.
- **Stage III: Full thickness skin loss** – Epidermis and dermis have experienced loss and the injury now extends through to the subcutaneous fat tissue. Tunneling could be present. Muscle, tendons, and bones have not been injured.
- **Stage IV: Full thickness tissue loss** – Damage has progressed to bone, muscle, or tendons. There is often tunneling present, osteomyelitis is common, and the depth of the ulcer will vary by location.
- **Unstageable/Unclassified** – Injury is present and involves full thickness, but cannot be staged until slough is removed.
- **Suspected Deep Tissue Injury** – Discolored skin that is still intact but has been damaged. Suspect it is deeper than stage I, but the epidermis is still intact.

SAD CLASSIFICATION SYSTEM FOR LOWER-EXTREMITY NEUROPATHIC DISEASE

The **Size, Area, Depth (SAD) classification system** for lower-extremity neuropathic disease is one of many that builds upon the original or modified Wagner classification system and assigns a 0-3 grade based on 5 categories: area, depth, sepsis, arteriopathy, and denervation.

1. No pathology evident.
2. Ulcer is <10 mm², involving subcutaneous tissue with superficial slough or exudate, diminution or absence of pulses, and reduced sensation.
3. Ulcer is 10-20 mm², extending to tendon, joint, capsule, or periosteum with cellulitis, absence of pulses except for neuropathy dominant ulcers that have palpable pedal pulses.
4. Ulcer is >30 mm², extending to bones and/or joints, with osteomyelitis, gangrene, and Charcot's foot.

This, as most other classification systems, is useful but does not distinguish between those wounds that follow an **atypical pattern** or may be consistent with the grade in some areas and **inconsistent** in others.

INITIAL NUTRITIONAL ASSESSMENT

Nutritional assessment should be done within the first 24 hours of care for hospitalized patients and at first visit for others to ensure that nutritional requirements are met. The history and physical exam should include the following information about the **previous 3 months**:

- Changes in food intake, including number of meals eaten daily.
- Weight loss (or gain).
- Episodes of depression or stress that may relate to dietary intake.
- A sample of a usual daily menu should be developed. Additional screening should include:

- Daily number of protein, fruit, grain, and vegetable servings.
- Usual fluid intake, including type, amount, and frequency.
- Method of feeding, independent or assisted.
- Mobility.
- Mental status.
- Body mass index (BMI), midarm circumference, and calf circumference.
- Living status (independent or dependent).
- Prescription and non-prescription drugs.
- Pressure sores or other wounds or skin problems.

PHYSICAL ASSESSMENT FOR NUTRITIONAL DEFICIENCY

The physical assessment is an important part of nutritional assessment to determine **malnutrition** or problems with self-feeding:

- **Hair** may be dry and brittle or thinning.
- **Skin** may show poor turgor, ecchymosis, tears, pressure areas, ulcerations, abrasions, or other compromises.
- **Mouth** may show dry mucous membranes. Lips may have cheilosis, cracking at the corners, and scaly lips (riboflavin deficiency). Gums may be swollen or bleeding, teeth loose or needing care, or dentures poorly-fitting. Tongue may be inflamed, dry, cracked, or have sores.
- **Nails** may become brittle. Spoon shaped or pale nail bed indicates low iron.
- **Hands** may be crippled or arthritic, making eating difficult.
- **Vision** may be compromised so that people can't see to prepare food or have difficulty feeding themselves.
- **Mental status** may be impaired to the point that people can't understand diet instructions or prepare or eat meals.
- **Motor skills** may decrease, including hand-mouth coordination or ability to hold utensils.

NUTRITIONAL ASSESSMENT TOOLS

The MNA® (**Mini-Nutritional Assessment**) by Nestle Nutrition is designed for nutritional assessment of those over age 65 and is only valid for that population. It is a screening and assessment tool to determine the risk for malnutrition and comprises 15 questions about dietary habits and 4 measurements, including body mass index (BMI) using height and weight, mid-arm, and calf circumference.

The **Nutritional Screening Initiative**® is another tool for geriatric patients and screens for dietary information as well as social and environmental factors, such as whether the person eats alone, prepares meals, drinks alcohol, and has sufficient income.

The **Subjective Global Assessment**® assesses nutritional status by a thorough history and physical examination. The history assesses weight change, dietary intake, gastrointestinal symptoms and functional impairment. The results of this assessment tool are evaluated subjectively and scores assigned to determine if malnutrition risks are normal to severe.

TST, MAC, MAMC

PURPOSE

Triceps skinfold thickness (TST) evaluates fat stores, which often change slowly, so this is not a sensitive test for malnutrition, but it can be used to determine if fat is increasing while muscle mass

32

is decreasing. **Mid-arm circumference (MAC)** measures muscles, bones, and skin. **Mid-arm muscle circumference (MAMC)** measures lean body mass. These vary considerably between individuals so are more useful to track muscle wasting over time than for comparisons. The TST, MAC, and MAMC are recorded as a percentage of standard measurements, which are quantified for males and females.

<u>MALES</u>
TST = 12.5 mm
MAC = 29.9 cm
MAMC = 25.3 cm

<u>FEMALES</u>
TST = 16.5 mm
MAC = 28.5 cm
MAMC = 23.3 cm

To obtain the percentage, the measurement for each test is divided by the standard measurement. For example, a male's TST of 11.8 mm would be calculated as:

$$TST = \frac{11.8}{12.5} = 0.944 = 94.4\%$$

PROCEDURE

Triceps skinfold thickness is measured using special calipers. The midpoint between the axilla and elbow of the nondominant arm is measured and located and then the skin is grasped about 1 cm above the midpoint between the thumb and index finger by grasping at the edges of the arm and moving the finger and thumb inward until a firm fold of tissue is observed. The calipers are placed about this fold at the midpoint (right below the fingers) and squeezed for 3 seconds and then a measurement is taken to the nearest millimeter. Three readings are taken, with the average of the 3 used as the measurement.

Mid-arm circumference (MAC) measurement is obtained by measuring in centimeters at the midpoint between the axilla and elbow.

Mid-arm muscle circumference (MAMC) is calculated by multiplying the triceps skinfold thickness (in millimeters) by pi (~3.14), and subtracting the result from the midarm circumference with results in centimeters.

BMI

The **Body Mass Index (BMI)** formula is a measurement that uses height and weight as an indicator of obesity/malnutrition. This cannot be used alone to diagnose obesity because body types differ. Women often have more body fat than men. Tables are available to make calculations simple, but the BMI can be calculated manually using either metric or English units:

$$\text{BMI} = \frac{\text{Weight in kilograms}}{(\text{Height in meters})^2} = \frac{(\text{Weight in pounds}) \times 703}{(\text{Height in inches})^2}$$

Resulting scores for adults age 20 and over are interpreted according to this chart:

Below 18.5 = Underweight
18.5 − 24.9 = Normal weight
25.0 − 29.9 = Overweight

33

$$30 \text{ and above} = \text{Obese}$$

The BMI for those under age 20 uses age-sex specific charts provided by the CDC, containing a curved line that indicates percentiles. Criteria for obesity based on these charts and BMI for age <20 follow:

$$< \text{5th percentile} = \text{Underweight}$$
$$\text{85th}-< \text{95 percentile} = \text{At risk for overweight}$$
$$\geq \text{95th percentile} = \text{Overweight}$$

WHR

The **Waist Hip Ratio (WHR)** is the ratio of fat stored about the abdomen and the fat stored around the hips. This ratio is considered of increasing import because an increase in this ratio is associated with increased risk of heart disease, brain attacks, and diabetes mellitus. The formula:

$$\text{WHR} = \frac{\text{waist circumference}}{\text{hip circumference}}$$

The waist measurement is taken at the smallest circumference, usually slightly above the umbilicus, and the hip measurement at the widest part of the hips, usually about 7 inches below the waist.

The results of the calculation provide a score with risks according to gender:

- For males, WHR >1 = increased risk
- For females, WHR >0.85 = increased risk

Studies have indicated that people who carry more weight around their waists relative to their hips (apple-shaped) are more at risk for complications related to weight than those that carry more weight in their hips (pear-shaped).

MEASURING HEAD CIRCUMFERENCE TO ASSESS NUTRITION

Head circumference measurements are taken for children during the first 3 years. While there can be non-nutritional reasons for decreased growth of the head, it can also be a sign of severe **lack of nutrition** and may be associated with decreased linear growth as well. The procedure:

1. Use non-stretchable measuring tape.
2. Child should be standing or held in sitting position with head upright.
3. Place tape around head just above the eyebrows in the font and around the occipital area in the back.
4. Take at least 3 readings or more until 2 measurements are within 0.1 cm.
5. Use growth chart to determine if measurement is within normal limits.

The CDC provides **growth charts** for both head circumference and linear growth that are specific for gender, showing the percentile ranking of measurements. Evaluation depends upon various factors, including results of height and weight measurement, to determine if a child is undernourished although findings **below the 5th percentile** are usually cause for concern.

MATURITY ASSESSMENT

A **maturity assessment** should be part of the preparticipation examination for children and adolescents to determine their level of sexual, dental, and skeletal maturity:

- **Skeletal maturity** is usually assessed by measurements of the hand and wrist as well as weight/height for age. Skeletal maturity and chronological age may differ. For example, if the chronological age is 14.3 and the skeletal age is 15.5, this would be expressed as 15.5-14.3=SA+1.2. Another method is to divide the skeletal age by the chronological age: a score >1.0 equates with advanced skeletal maturity and <1 a delay in skeletal maturity.
- The most common assessment tool for **sexual maturity** is Tanner's 5 stages of assessment. This tool assesses maturity for both males and females, based on direct observation of breasts and genitals:
  - Females: breast development, onset of menses, and pubic hair distribution.
  - Males: Penis and testes development and pubic hair distribution.

ASSESSING HEARING DEFICITS IN INFANTS AND TODDLERS

Hearing deficits may be identified very early if careful observation of developmental characteristics in infants and children. Normal hearing responses include:

- **<3 months**: Positive Moro (startle) reflex to sound. Noise disturbs sleep, and reacts to sounds by opening eyes or blinking.
- **3-6 months**: Comforts at sound of parent's voice and tries to emulate sounds. Looks in the direction of sound.
- **6-12 months**: Begins to vocalize more with cooing and gurgling with different inflections. Responds to name and simple words and looks in the direction of sound.
- **12-18 months**: Begins first words at about 12-15 months and imitates sounds, follows vocal directions, and points to familiar items when asked.
- **18-24 months**: More verbal with about half of vocabulary understandable and knows about 20-50 words. Points to body parts or familiar objects when asked.

Risk Assessment

HOST RISK FACTORS

Host risk factors are those conditions or circumstances that put the host at increased risk of developing an infection. Host risk factors include the following:

- **Age**: Those who are very young or very old are often at increased risk. Infants may not have developed antibodies, and the elderly may have decreased immunity.
- **Disease**: Many diseases, such as diabetes and leukemia, increase the risk of infection.
- **Circulatory impairment**: Any decrease in perfusion to an area from disease or injury increases the chance of infection.
- **Medications**: Immunosuppressants and chemotherapy can reduce immunity. Improper use of antibiotics builds resistance.
- **Contact**: Close contact with the source of microorganisms increases the host risk factor.
- **Wounds and instrumentation**: Surgical wounds, ulcers, catheters, or any other thing that allows microorganisms easy access increases risk.
- **Absence of prophylactic antibiotics**: Antibiotics have proven to reduce risk of post-operative infections for some procedures, but guidelines for use are not always followed.

35

ASSESSING PATIENTS FOR EXPOSURE TO COMMUNICABLE DISEASES

Patient **exposure to communicable disease** can be difficult to assess as the person may not be aware of exposure or may be reluctant to discuss it because of privacy issues. Doing a careful and thorough **history and physical assessment** can provide information that suggests exposure. Questioning people about symptoms rather than diseases may elicit more information: "Have you had contact with anyone with a rash?" or "Have you experienced night sweats?" Exposure to a communicable disease can occur outside of the hospital as well as inside. Exposure to communicable disease can be endogenous (self-infection) or exogenous (cross-infection). **Endogenous infections**, for example, can result from the normal body flora or an area of infection (such as a boil) contaminating a surgical wound. **Exogenous infections** can occur by contact with someone who is infected, such as another patient or staff member, or by airborne particles. Both types of infection can occur in the hospital.

RISK FACTORS FOR URINARY INCONTINENCE

TYPES

Different types of **urinary incontinence** include:

- **Urge**: An urgency to urinate as soon as the bladder feels full, so person may urinate on the way to the toilet or in bed during the night. Diuretics may exacerbate urge incontinence.
- **Stress**: A sudden increase in bladder pressure from such things as coughing, laughing, or bending causes small amount of urinary leakage. It is common in people who are obese.
- **Overflow**: An overfull bladder causes dribbling of urine, usually in small amounts but the leakage can be almost constant.
- **Functional**: Incontinence caused by physical or mental impairment, such as dementia. May also be related to environmental barriers to urination, such as no accessible bathroom.
- **Reflex**: Loss of urine takes place without awareness of person because of fistula or bladder leak.
- **Mixed**: There may be more than 1 type of incontinence.
- **Induced**: Some surgical procedures (hysterectomy, prostatectomy, rectal surgery) can damage nerves or muscles that control urination.

MEDICAL RISK FACTORS

The following are medical conditions that are risk factors for **urinary incontinence**:

- **Pregnancy/childbirth**: Childbirth weakens the pelvic floor muscles and those of the urethral sphincter. Nerve damage and bladder prolapse can also occur, further contributing to incontinence.
- **Post-menopausal changes**: Loss of estrogen causes bladder and urethral tissues to weaken.
- **Hysterectomy**: The muscles and nerves in the urinary tract may be damaged by the procedure because the urinary tract is adjacent to the uterus.
- **Interstitial cystitis**: The inflammation sometimes causes incontinence.
- **Prostate enlargement**: Constriction of the urethra as the prostate enlarges can lead to urgency or overflow incontinence.
- **Prostate cancer**: May be caused directly by the cancer or may be a response to radiation or surgical removal of prostate.
- **Bladder cancer**: Dysuria and incontinence are common symptoms.

36

- **Neurological deficits**: Congenital or acquired neurological damage from injury or disease can result in inability to control urination.
- **Urinary tract obstruction**: An obstruction anywhere in the urinary tract can cause overflow incontinence.

NON-MEDICAL RISK FACTORS

Non-medical risk factors for **urinary incontinence** include:

- **Age**: Bladder and sphincter muscles loosen with age, so the older a person is, the more likely to have some type of urinary incontinence, stress or chronic.
- **Contributing diseases**: Kidney diseases, among others, may make an individual prone to develop urinary incontinence if the conditions are not well controlled.
- **Obesity**: Being overweight increases pressure on the bladder and the surrounding muscles, weakening them and causing stress incontinence. This is especially true for women.
- **Gender**: Women are more likely to suffer incontinence than men because of childbirth and menopausal changes. Also, the genitourinary anatomy of women with the vagina/bladder/urethra/rectum adjacent contributes to the danger of injury to the urinary system.
- **Smoking**: The chronic cough that many smokers develop can cause stress incontinence or can aggravate stress incontinence that is already present.
- **Sports**: High impact sports with vigorous activity, such as running, can put strong pressure on the bladder during those activities.

RISK FACTORS FOR FECAL INCONTINENCE

Common risk factors for **fecal incontinence** include:

- **Age**: Fecal incontinence is most common among people who are elderly and may suffer from other health problems, including urinary incontinence.
- **Sex**: Women suffer more from fecal incontinence than men because women often suffer damage to the sphincter after childbirth, especially as scar tissue forms after episiotomies or muscles weaken after multiple childbirths.
- **Neurological damage**: Congenital or acquired neurological defects are frequently associated with fecal incontinence. Additionally, people with chronic disorders, such as diabetes mellitus or multiple sclerosis may lose the ability to control defecation because of progressive neuropathy.
- **Dementia/Alzheimer's disease**: Late stage Alzheimer's disease is characterized by both fecal and urinary incontinence.
- **Physical disability**: Congenital or acquired physical disabilities may lead to fecal incontinence for many reasons. People confined to wheelchairs might find toilet access difficult. People may not be able to express the need to defecate. Others may not be able to physically manage toileting without assistance.

ASTHMA RISKS
RISK-REDUCTION THROUGH REDUCING EXPOSURE TO ALLERGENS

It is difficult if not impossible to control **asthma** without reducing or at best eliminating exposure to allergens. When this accomplished, asthma severity drastically decreases and quality of life increases for the patient:

- To control **animal dander**, it may be necessary to remove the pet from the home or at least from the patient's bedroom.
- **Air filters** placed over bedroom vents help to control air circulation.

37

- **Dust mites** can be controlled by encasing mattresses and pillowcases in allergen proof covers.
- Removing **carpet** is helpful to keep dust mites down.
- **Humidity** in the home should be less than 50%. Insect infestation should be controlled as well as mold and fungi.
- In extreme cases, one should limit **exposure to the outside environment**, especially during times of high pollen count or increased smog.

> **Review Video: <u>Asthma and Allergens</u>**
> Visit mometrix.com/academy and enter code: 799141

RISK FACTORS FOR DEATH

There are a number of risk factors associated with death from **status asthmaticus**. Many of the risk factors relate to poor management of asthma on an ongoing basis so that severe asthma attacks occur repeatedly:

- History of sudden, acute exacerbations of disease.
- Endotracheal intubation/ventilation for previous acute episodes of asthma.
- Prior hospitalization and treatment in intensive care for exacerbation.
- ≥ 2 hospitalizations for asthma in prior 12 months.
- ≥ 3 visits to the emergency department for asthma treatment in the prior 12 months.
- Overuse of inhaled β-adrenergic agonists (>2 canisters per month).
- Recent tapering and withdrawal of systemic corticosteroids.
- Cardiovascular comorbidity.
- Low economic status.
- Residence in urban area.

Economic status and place of residence probably reflect inadequate financial resources to bear the cost medical care and treatments, such as preventive medications.

RISKS FOR CARDIOVASCULAR DISEASE

The Joint National Committee on Prevention, Detection, Evaluation, and Treatment of High Blood Pressure identifies a number of **risks for cardiovascular disease**:

- **Hypertension**: >140/90 mm Hg.
- ↑ Resting heart rate and ↓ variability of heart rate; ≥83 at rest increases risk.
- **Age**: >55 in males and >65 in females.
- **Diabetes mellitus**: Associated with metabolic syndrome characterized by ↓ high-density lipoprotein (HDL), ↑triglycerides, and abdominal obesity.
- **Estimated glomerular filtration rate** (eGFR) <60 mL/min: chronic kidney disease.
- **Family history** of cardiovascular diseases: <55 years for men and <65 years for women.
- Microalbuminuria.
- **Obesity**: BMI ≥30 kg/m2 for men at ≥55 years and women at ≥65 years.
- Physical inactivity.
- **Use of tobacco**: Cigarettes cause more cardiovascular disease than other types of tobacco use.

CARDIOVASCULAR RISK REDUCTION IN CHILDREN

Some **children** are at increased risk of developing **cardiovascular disease**, such as coronary artery disease, including those with diabetes mellitus, Kawasaki disease, and familial hypercholesterolemia, which can cause severe coronary artery disease in <10 years. Screening children at risk should begin age 2 and include cholesterol levels to assess for an elevation of low-density lipoprotein (LDL):

- Total cholesterol <170 and LDL <110: Normal diet for age.
- Total cholesterol 170-199 and LDL 110-120: Borderline elevation.
- Total cholesterol >200 with LDL >130: Elevated.

Early dietary intervention to reduce cholesterol and prevent increase in LDL can significantly reduce morbidity and mortality. Dietary recommendations to reduce LDL include guidelines provided in the Therapeutic Lifestyle Changes diet by the American Heart Association (AHA; http://www.americanheart.org) for those at risk or with elevated cholesterol.

- <30% of diet from fat and <7% from saturated fat, >10% polyunsaturated fat, up to 15% monounsaturated fat.
- ≥55% carbohydrates.
- 15% protein.
- <200 mg dietary cholesterol per day.

AHA's RISK FACTORS FOR INFECTIVE ENDOCARDITIS

Infective endocarditis occurs when bacteria invade in **heart tissue or heart valves**, usually in those with preexisting heart disorders. The American Heart Association's (AHA) risk factors include:

- Prosthetic heart valves.
- Previous endocarditis.
- History of rheumatic fever or other disorder causing valve damage.
- Congenital heart defects (such as ventricular or atrial septal defects).
- Heart transplant recipients.
- Hypertrophic cardiomyopathy.

The AHA has modified its recommendations for administration of prophylactic antibiotics, as there is little evidence that dental and gastrointestinal (GI) procedures cause endocarditis. Prophylaxis is recommended for genitourinary (GU) and GI procedures but for dental procedures ONLY for those with prosthetic valves or other prosthetic material for heart repair, history of endocarditis, unrepaired congenital heart disease (cyanotic) or repaired congenital heart disease with residual abnormalities, and cardiac transplant recipients with valve abnormalities.

RISK FACTORS FOR LEAD

There are a number of risk factors for **lower extremity arterial disease (LEAD)**, also known as **peripheral arterial disease (PAD)**:

- **Smoking** is a primary cause of LEAD with diagnosis of disease 10 years earlier than non-smokers. It increases the rate of atherosclerosis, decreases high-density lipoprotein (HDL), increases blood pressure, and decreases clotting time.
- **Obesity** raises blood pressure, decreases HDL in cholesterol while raising cholesterol and triglycerides, and increases risk of circulatory disease, including heart attack.

- **Lack of exercise** decreases pain-free walking distance.
- **Hypertension** correlates with changes in the vessel walls that result in narrowing of blood vessels and decreased circulation.
- **Diabetes mellitus** causes increased plaque formation, decreased clotting time, increased blood viscosity, and hypertrophy of vasculature. Insulin resistance, related to Type 2 diabetes increases atherosclerosis. Arterial disease typically progresses faster with diabetes.
- **High blood cholesterol**, especially low-density lipoprotein (LDL) increase atherosclerosis and circulatory impairment.

RISK FACTORS FOR CVI

There are a number of risk factors for **chronic venous insufficiency (CVI)**, also known as **lower-extremity venous disease (LEVD)**, primarily those that result in valvular dysfunction or calf-muscle dysfunction:

- Those with **obesity** with Body Mass Index >25 are more likely to have pressure on pelvic veins, causing valvular dysfunction.
- **Intravenous drug use** into lower extremities may damage vessels.
- **Thrombosis/leg trauma** may damage vessels and valves.
- **Thrombophlebitis** may cause direct damage to valves.
- **Thrombophilic conditions**, such as protein C deficiency, decrease clotting time of venous blood, increasing risk of thrombosis.
- **Varicose veins** slow venous return.
- **Pregnancy**, especially multiple or close pregnancies increase pressure on pelvic veins.
- **Lack of exercise**/sedentary lifestyle with prolonged periods of sitting result in calf muscle dysfunction.
- **Smoking** causes vascular changes.
- Age and gender studies show that **older women** most commonly develop CVI.
- **Comorbid conditions**, such as arthritis or those that limit mobility, affect calf-muscle function.

RISK FACTORS FOR PELVIC ORGAN PROLAPSE

Pelvic organ prolapse occurs when pelvic floor muscles stretch and weaken and cannot support the pelvic organs. There are a number of different factors that contribute to this weakening:

- Trauma related to **pregnancy and childbirth** is the primary cause of pelvic organ prolapse because labor and birth causes stress on the pelvic muscles and ligaments, especially if forceps are used to facilitate vaginal delivery or an episiotomy is performed.
- **Previous pelvic surgery**, especially hysterectomy or bladder repair, may damage nerves and tissues, increasing risk for prolapse.
- **Obesity** exerts pressure on the pelvic floor muscles.
- **Chronic cough/strain**, as may occur with chronic obstructive pulmonary disease or long-term smoking, may weaken the pelvic structures over prolonged periods of time.
- **Heavy lifting** can cause damage to pelvic muscles.
- **Spinal cord damage** whether congenital or acquired may cause paralysis or atrophy of the pelvic muscles, thereby weakening the support.

RISK FACTORS FOR NEUROPATHIC/DIABETIC ULCERS

There are a number of risk factors for the development of **neuropathic/ diabetic ulcers**:

- **Sensory loss** can cause sores and ulcers to go undetected in early stages.
- **Vascular insufficiency**, especially peripheral artery disease occurs 4 times more frequently in diabetics.
- **Autonomic neuropathy** decreases sweating, leaving feet dry and more prone to cracks and sores.
- **Long-term diabetes mellitus** with poor glucose control causes severe damage to circulatory system.
- **Smoking** increases vascular damage and arterial insufficiency.
- **Deformities or lack of mobility** may increase risk of developing ulcers or having ulcers that are undetected.
- **Obesity** decreases circulation and interferes with control of diabetes. Between 80-90% of diabetics are overweight.
- **Male gender** increases risk.
- **Poor vision** may cause people to overlook dangers or prevent them from examining feet and skin.
- **Age** is associated with increase danger of ulcers.
- **Ethnic background** can determine genetic risks: Native Americans, Hispanic Americans, African Americans and Pacific Islanders.
- **Improperly fitted and non-supportive footwear** can cause ulcerations.

RISK FACTORS FOR PRESSURE ULCERS

The Centers for Medicare and Medicaid Services (CMS) established a list of common risk factors for **pressure ulcers**. Many people present with more than 1 risk factor. Assessment should include evaluation of risks for the following:

- Impairment or decreased **mobility or functional ability** that prevents a person from changing position.
- **Comorbid conditions** affecting circulation or metabolism, such as renal disease, diabetes, and thyroid disease
- **Drugs** that interfere with healing, such as corticosteroids.
- **Impaired circulation**, such as generalized atherosclerosis or arterial insufficiency of lower extremity, reducing tissue perfusion.
- Patient **refusal of care**, increasing risk (positioning, hygiene, nutrition, hydration, skin care).
- **Cognitive impairment** that prevents patient from reporting discomfort or cooperating with care.
- Fecal and/or urinary **contamination of skin**, usually related to incontinence.
- **Under nutrition** or frank malnutrition and/or dehydration.
- **Previous healed ulcers**. Healed ulcers that were Stage III or IV may deteriorate and break down again.

BRADEN SCALE FOR PREDICTING RISK OF DEVELOPING PRESSURE SORES

The **Braden scale** is a risk assessment tool that has been validated clinically as predictive of the risk of patients' developing pressure sores. The scale scores 6 different areas with 1-4 points.

1. Sensory perception
   a. Completely limited (unresponsive to pain or limited ability to feel)
   b. Very limited (responds to painful stimuli and moans)
   c. Slightly limited (responds to verbal commands but limited communication)
   d. No impairment
2. Moisture
   a. Moist constantly
   b. Very moist (linen change each shift)
   c. Occasionally moist (linen change each day)
   d. Rarely moist
3. Activity
   a. Bed bound
   b. Chair bound
   c. Walks occasionally (short distances)
   d. Walks frequently
4. Mobility
   a. Completely immobile
   b. Very limited (makes occasional slight position changes)
   c. Slightly limited (makes frequently slight position changes)
   d. No limitations

RISK FACTORS AND SYMPTOMS OF DIVERTICULAR DISEASE

The following are risk factors for **diverticular disease**:

- **Age**: Incidence increases with age, affecting over 50% of those over 60.
- **Nationality**: More common in developed countries, such as the United States, England, and Australia where diets lower in fiber and high in processed carbohydrates are common. Diverticular disease is rare in Asian countries. People in Western countries primarily have diverticular disease in the left colon while Asians tend to have diverticular disease in the right colon.
- **Socioeconomic**: More common among those with lower income.
- **Genetics**: Occurs in family clusters.

Diverticulosis symptoms (diverticula present but not inflamed):

- **Absent**: May have no symptoms at all.
- **Abdominal**: Cramping and distention.
- **Intestinal**: Constipation or diarrhea. Muscles spasms in colon.

Diverticulitis symptoms (diverticula inflamed):

- **Systemic**: Fever, chills
- **Gastrointestinal**: Nausea, vomiting, constipation, gastrointestinal (GI) bleeding, blood in stool, rectal bleeding.

- **Abdominal**: Mild to severe cramping, pain (especially in left lower quadrant), abdominal tenderness.
- **Urinary**: Dysuria may be present.

RISK FACTORS AND INDICATORS FOR MALNUTRITION

There are a number of risk factors for **malnutrition**:

- **Hypermetabolism** resulting from various diseases, such as AIDS, and trauma, stress, or infection.
- **Weight loss**, especially sudden or loss of 10% of normal weight over a 3-month period.
- **Low body weight** of <90% of ideal body weight for age or
- Low Body Mass Index (BMI) <18.5.
- **Immunosuppressive drugs** interfere with absorption of nutrients.
- **Malabsorption of nutrients** caused by diseases, such as chronic failure of kidneys or liver.
- **Changes in appetite** that decrease intake of nutrients.
- **Food intolerances** such as lactose intolerance, resulting from lack of enzymes needed to completely digest food so it can be absorbed into the blood stream from the small intestine.
- **Dietary restrictions** such as limiting of protein with kidney failure.
- **Functional limitations** such as inability to feed oneself.
- Lack of teeth or dentures limiting intake.
- **Alterations of taste or smell** that render food unpalatable.

ASSESSING HISTORY FOR GENETIC OR FAMILIAL RISKS

Assessing family history for **genetic or familial risks** is an important part of disease prevention because, in some cases, early identification and intervention may reduce future health risks. Creating a genogram with the family is helpful. A thorough history should be broad and include assessment of the following:

- Early onset disorders, such as cardiovascular disease, hypertension, or Alzheimer's disease.
- Progressive neurological or neuromuscular diseases.
- Diabetes mellitus.
- Mental illness, such as depression, bipolar disorder, and schizophrenia.
- Intellectual disability, including Trisomy 21 (Down syndrome).
- Any unusual disabilities or abnormalities, such as birth defects.

Once risk factors are determined, the question of **screening tests** arises. If there is a possibility that a child is a carrier, then screening is usually deferred until the child can give informed consent. Screening is done for adults or for children with parental permission when it is in the best interests of the child, allowing for appropriate care and intervention.

ETHNICITY AND INCREASED RISK OF GENETIC DISORDERS

Some ethnic groups have increased **risk for genetic disorders** with high carrier rates, ranging from 1:6-1:40. The nurse practitioner should be aware of these risks and observant for symptoms in the child. A careful maternal and paternal family history may provide information about occurrence of the disease in other family members. Some disorders are covered in routine neonatal screening, but others are not. In some cases, it may be appropriate to recommend testing to ensure that early diagnosis is made so that treatment can be initiated. The following groups are at increased risk for specific genetic disorders:

- **Ashkenazi Jews**: Canavan disease, Tay Sachs disease, cystic fibrosis, and familial dysautonomia.
- **African Americans**: Sickle cell disease (carrier rate 1:6-12), other hemoglobinopathy.
- European Caucasians: cystic fibrosis.
- **Mediterranean**: Beta thalassemia.
- **South Asian**: Beta Thalassemia.
- **Southeast Asian**: Alpha and Beta Thalassemia.

GENETIC PREDICTIVE TESTING

Genetic predictive testing identifies a person with a **genetic disorder** that may manifest at a later date (such as Huntington's disease) or with an **increased risk of developing a disease** (such as breast cancer). Referral for genetic testing may be advised for familial cancer, retinoblastoma, familial adenomatous polyposis (which can cause colon cancer), cystic fibrosis, Huntington's disease, and amyotrophic lateral sclerosis. Identifying those **at risk for developing cancer** is especially important so that close monitoring and/or preventive measure can be taken. Familial cancer accounts for about 5-10% of cancers. The BRCA1 breast cancer gene has been mapped to chromosome 17q and the gene for BRCA2 on chromosome 13q. People carrying the abnormal gene have an 80-90% chance of developing breast/ovarian cancer. These women should be counseled about their options and the importance of close monitoring and surgical options. Tests are not available for all diseases with a genetic component (diabetes, hypertension, pyloric stenosis, spina bifida, psychiatric disorders, and Alzheimer's disease), but more genes are being identified.

NEWBORN SCREENING FOR GENETIC DISORDERS

Screening of the newborn to detect **genetic diseases** varies somewhat from one state to another. Because about 1 in 200 newborns has chromosomal abnormalities, screening is an important tool although many birth defects are not genetic in origin, such as defects caused by maternal alcohol abuse or vitamin deficiency. Screening tests are available for the following:

- Biotinidase deficiency (autosomal recessive).
- Congenital adrenal hyperplasia (autosomal recessive).
- Congenital hearing loss (autosomal recessive, autosomal dominant, or mitochondrial).
- Congenital hypothyroidism (autosomal recessive or autosomal dominant).
- Cystic fibrosis (autosomal recessive).
- Galactosemia (autosomal recessive).
- Homocystinuria (autosomal recessive).
- Maple syrup urine disease (autosomal recessive).
- Medium-chain Acyl-CoA dehydrogenase (autosomal recessive).
- Phenylketonuria (autosomal recessive).
- Sickle cell disease (autosomal recessive).
- Tyrosinemia (2 types are autosomal recessive; third type is unclear).

RISK FACTORS FOR NEONATES ASSOCIATED WITH MATERNAL DISEASE/BEHAVIOR

There are a number of **maternal factors** that put the infant at increased risk:

- **Diabetes mellitus**: Both gestational and pre-existing diabetes put the infant at risk of stillbirth, hypoglycemia, and macrosomia (larger size than normal) as well as birth injury. Maternal pre-existing diabetes is also associated with birth defects, including abnormal development of the cardiovascular and gastrointestinal systems, neurological and spinal cord disorders, and urinary tract abnormalities.
- **Alcohol ingestion**: No safe amount of alcohol for pregnant women has been determined. Infants are at risk for fetal alcohol syndrome that may include facial abnormalities, intellectual disability, and behavioral problems.
- **Tobacco**: Tobacco use causes increased miscarriage, prematurity, and underweight infants.
- **Drug use**: Infants may be born addicted to drugs and go through withdrawal. They may suffer seizure disorders or neurological impairment with long-term learning disabilities.
- **Human immunodeficiency virus (HIV)/Hepatitis B**: Infectious diseases may be transmitted during pregnancy or delivery.

FETAL ALCOHOL SYNDROME

Fetal alcohol syndrome (FAS) is a syndrome of birth defects that develop as the result of maternal ingestion of alcohol. Despite campaigns to inform the public, women continue to drink during pregnancy, but no safe amount of alcohol ingestion has been determined. FAS includes:

- **Facial abnormalities**: Hypoplastic (underdeveloped) maxilla, micrognathia (undersized jaw), hypoplastic philtrum (groove beneath the nose), short palpebral fissures (eye slits between upper and lower lids).
- **Neurological deficits**: May include microcephaly, intellectual disability, and motor delay, hearing deficits. Learning disorders may include problems with visual-spatial and verbal learning, attention disorders, delayed reaction times.
- **Growth retardation**: Prenatal growth deficit persists with slow growth after birth.
- **Behavioral problems**: Irritability and hyperactivity. Poor judgment in behavior may relate to deficit in executive functions.
- Indication of brain damage without the associated physical abnormalities is referred to as **alcohol-related neurodevelopmental disorder** (ARND).

FETAL DRUG EXPOSURE

There are many **drugs** that can profoundly **affect the growing fetus**. Some are prescribed drugs, such as Accutane®, but the greatest number are illicit drugs, such as crack, heroin, or cocaine. Increasing numbers of children are born to addicted mothers. While each drug has specific effects, there are many that are common:

- **Premature birth and low birth weight** with infants who are small for gestational age (SGA).
- **Failure to thrive** often related to poor sucking and dysphagia.
- Increased risk of **congenital infectious disease** (human immunodeficiency virus [HIV], hepatitis, cytomegalovirus [CMV]).
- Increased risk of sudden infant death syndrome (SIDS).
- **Withdrawal symptoms** may manifest <72 hours after birth:
  o Tremors, excitability, seizures.
  o Vomiting, diarrhea, diaphoresis.

45

o   Dry, red, irritated skin.
- **Developmental and cognitive problems** that vary with age. Initial problems often subside within the first couple of years, but in a small number of children learning disabilities and behavioral problems persist.

INFANT WITHDRAWAL

Fetal exposure to drugs, such as opioids, methadone, cocaine, crack, and other recreational drugs, causes **withdrawal symptoms** in about 60% of infants. There are many variables, which include the type of drug, the extent of drug use, and the duration of maternal drug use. For example, children may have withdrawal symptoms within 48 hours for cocaine, heroin, and methamphetamine exposure, but there may be delays of up to 2-3 weeks for methadone. Short hospital stays after birth make it imperative that children at risk are identified so they can receive supportive treatment, particularly since they often feed poorly and can quickly become dehydrated and undernourished. Polydrug use makes it difficult to describe a typical profile of *symptoms*, but they usually include:

- Tremors.
- Irritability.
- Hypertonicity.
- High-pitched crying.
- Diarrhea.
- Dry skin.
- Seizures (in severe cases).

Treatment is supportive, but children with opiate exposure may be given decreasing doses of opiates, such as morphine elixir, with close monitoring until the child is weaned off of the medication.

FETAL NICOTINE/CARBON MONOXIDE EXPOSURE FROM MATERNAL SMOKING OR SECONDHAND SMOKE

About 25% of pregnant women in the United States continue to **smoke throughout pregnancy** and others are exposed to secondhand smoke, putting the fetus at risk for a number of abnormalities from exposure to nicotine and carbon monoxide:

- **Fetal growth retardation** with damage to neurotransmitters with decrease in number of cells with concomitant damage to peripheral autonomic nervous system.
- Vasoconstriction from nicotine and interference with oxygen transport caused by carbon monoxide can lead to **fetal hypoxia**.
- Vasoconstriction increased risk of spontaneous abortion, prematurity and low birth weight.
- Increased risk for perinatal death and sudden infant death syndrome (SIDS).
- **Cognitive deficiency and learning disorders**, such as auditory processing defects. Children of mothers who smoke have a 50% increase in idiopathic intellectual disability.
- **Increased cancer risk**, especially for acute lymphocytic leukemia and lymphoma.

SCREENING FOR HIGH-RISK SEXUAL BEHAVIOR IN ADOLESCENTS

High-risk sexual behavior in teenagers is often coupled with other health-risk behaviors, such as drinking and drug use. Teenagers are also having sex at younger ages. About 47% of high school seniors have had sex, with many beginning as young as 10-12 years. Risk factors include poverty, single-family homes, lack of supervision, and siblings or peers who are sexually active. Those who have sex before age 15 are especially vulnerable, often having multiple partners and unprotected

46

sex, leading to sexually transmitted diseases (STDs) and pregnancy. They are emotionally vulnerable and often can't deal effectively with relationships. **Intervention** should begin early with age-appropriate honest **sex education**. Abstinence education, while the ideal, has not been successful in changing the sexual behavior of teenagers, with studies showing that many of those signing pledges to remain virgins are already sexually active. Teenagers who are sexually active should be advised regarding the use of condoms, birth control, and protection from STDs in a nonjudgmental manner.

SCREENING FOR ALTERNATIVE LIFE-STYLE CHOICES IN ADOLESCENTS

As young people become sexually active, most are attracted to members of the opposite sex, but others face **alternative lifestyle choices**:

- **Gay and lesbian** (homosexual) teenagers are attracted to members of their own sex while **bisexual** teenagers are attracted to both sexes. Between 1-10% of teenagers identify themselves as homosexual, often feeling different from a very young age. These adolescents are at increased risk of violence, sexual abuse, depression, and harassment. They may not be accepted by their families or friends and sometimes become homeless. They are at risk for sexually transmitted diseases (STDs) and human immunodeficiency (HIV) and suffer from high rates of suicide.
- Some children are **transgender**, sometimes identifying from preschool age with the opposite sex and choosing to live in that role. They often suffer much prejudice because there is little understanding of transgender issues.

Intervention includes providing support and acceptance as well as practical assistance for housing, safe sex instruction, counselling, and support groups.

SIGNS OF NEGLECT

While some children may not be physically or sexually abused, they may suffer from profound **neglect** or lack of supervision that places them at risk. Indicators include:

- Appearing **dirty and unkempt**, sometimes with infestations of lice, and wearing ill-fitting, torn clothing, and worn shoes.
- Being **tired** and sleepy during the daytime.
- Having untended **medical or dental problems**, such as dental caries.
- **Missing appointments** and not receiving proper immunizations.
- Being **underweight** for stage of development.

Neglect can be difficult to assess, especially if the nurse practitioner is serving a homeless or very poor population. Home visits may be needed to ascertain if there is adequate food, clothing, or supervision, and this may be beyond the care provided by the nurse practitioner, so suspicions should be reported so that a social worker can assess the home environment.

ISSUES RELATED TO CHILD ABUSE AND REPORTING

About 5 million cases of suspected **child abuse** are reported in the United States each year. In accordance with the Child Abuse Prevention and Treatment and Adoption Act Amendments (1996) and the Model Child Protection Act, all states have instituted mandatory reporting of child abuse.

The nurse practitioner should be knowledgeable about the statutes in the state of practice, but medical personnel are **mandatory reporters** and must report the following:

- **Child abuse or neglect** that places the child in risk of harm (physical or emotional), death, or exploitation.
- **Sexual abuse** including rape, molestation, prostitution, incest, or coercion to engage in any type of sexually explicit behavior.

While some statutes mandate reporting of suspicion, others mandate more knowledge; however, there is **criminal and civil liability** involved if child abuse is not reported and most states provide immunity for reporters, so the best course is to report suspicions to child protective services or the police, according to the state requirements.

SIGNS OF PHYSICAL ABUSE IN CHILDREN

Children rarely admit to being abused and, in fact, deny it and attempt to protect the abusing parent, so the nurse practitioner must rely on physical and behavioral signs to determine if there is cause to **suspect abuse**:

- **Behavioral indicators**: The child may be overly compliant or fearful with obvious changes in demeanor when a parent/caregiver is present. Some children act out with aggression toward other children or animals. Children may become depressed or suicidal or present with sleeping or eating disorders. Behavior may become increasingly self-destructive as the child ages.
- **Physical indicators**: The type, location, and extent of injuries can raise suspicion of abuse. Head and facial injuries and bruising are common as are bite or burn marks. There may be hand prints or grab marks, unusual bruising, such as across the buttocks. Any bruising, swelling or tearing of the genital area or sexually transmitted diseases are cause for concern.

DOMESTIC VIOLENCE

According to guidelines of the Family Violence Prevention Fund, **assessment for domestic violence** should be done for all adolescent and adult patients, regardless of background or signs of abuse. While females are the most common victims, there are increasing reports of male victims of domestic violence, both in heterosexual and homosexual relationships. The person doing the assessment should be informed about domestic violence and be aware of risk factors and danger signs. The interview should be conducted in private (or with children <3 years old). The FNP's office, bathrooms, and examining rooms should have information about domestic violence posted prominently. Brochures and information should be available to give to patients. Patients may present with a variety of physical complaints, such as headache, pain, palpitations, numbness, or pelvic pain. They are often depressed and may appear suicidal and may be isolated from friends and family. Victims of domestic violence often exhibit fear of spouse/partner, and may report injury inconsistent with symptoms.

CHARACTERISTIC INJURIES

There are a number of **characteristic injuries** indicating domestic violence:

- Ruptured eardrum.
- Rectal/genital injury—burns, bites, trauma.
- Scrapes and bruises about the neck, face, head, trunk, arms.
- Cuts, bruises, and fractures of the face.

48

- The pattern of injuries is also often distinctive:
  - Bathing suit pattern—injuries on parts of body that are usually covered with clothing as the perpetrator abuses but hides evidence of abuse.
- Head and neck injuries (50%).
- Abusive injuries (rarely attributable to accidents) are common:
  - Bites, bruises, rope and cigarette burns, welts in the outline of weapons (belt marks).
- Bilateral injuries of arms/legs.

Defensive injuries are indicative of abuse:

- Back of the body injury from being attacked while crouched on the floor face down.
- Soles of the feet from kicking at perpetrator.
- Ulnar aspect of hand or palm from blocking blows.

IDENTIFYING VICTIMS OF DOMESTIC VIOLENCE

The Family Violence Prevent Fund has issued **guidelines for identifying victims of domestic violence**. There are 7 steps:

1. **Inquiry**: Nonjudgmental questioning should begin with asking if the person has ever been abused—physically, sexually, or psychologically.
2. **Interview**: The person may exhibit signs of anxiety or fear and may blame himself/herself or report that others believe he/she is abused. The person should be questioned if he/she is afraid for his/her life or for children.
3. **Question**: If the person reports abuse, it's critical to ask if the person is in immediate danger or if the abuser is on the premises. The interviewer should ask if the person has been threatened. The history and pattern of abuse should be questioned, and if children, whether the children are abused. Note: State laws vary, and in some states, it is mandatory to report if a child was present during an act of domestic violence as this is considered child abuse. The FNP must be aware of state laws regarding domestic and child abuse, and all nurses are mandatory reporters.
4. **Validate**: The interviewer should offer support and reassurance in a non-judgmental manner, telling the patient the abuse is not his/her fault.
5. **Give information**: While discussing facts about domestic violence and the tendency to escalate, the interviewer should provide brochures and information about safety planning. If the patient wants to file a complaint with the police, the interviewer should assist the person to place the call.
6. **Make referrals**: Information about state, local, and national organizations should be provided along with telephone numbers and contact numbers for domestic violence shelters.
7. **Document**: Record keeping should be legal, legible, and lengthy with complete report and description of any traumatic injuries resulting from domestic violence. A body map may be used to indicate sites of injury, especially if there are multiple bruises or injuries.

ELDER ABUSE

There are many different types of **elder abuse**: physical (such as hitting or improperly restraining), sexual, psychological, financial, and neglect. Elder abuse may be difficult to diagnose, especially if the person is cognitively impaired, but *symptoms* can include: fearfulness, disparities in reports of injuries between patient and caregiver, evidence of old or repeated injuries, poor hygiene and dental care, decubiti, malnutrition, undue concern with costs on caregiver's part, unsupportive

49

attitude of caregiver, and caregiver's reluctance or refusal to allow patient to communicate privately with the FNP. **Self-abuse** can also occur when patients are not able to adequately care for themselves. *Diagnosis* of elder abuse includes a careful history and physical exam, including directly questioning patient about abuse. *Treatment* includes attending to injuries or physical needs, and referral to adult protective services as indicated. **Reporting laws** regarding elder abuse vary somewhat from one state to another, but all states have laws regarding elder abuse and 42 require mandatory reporting by health workers.

ALCOHOL USE

CHILDREN/ADOLESCENTS

Alcohol is a significant problem in adolescence and even in younger children. It is the most commonly abused substance. Studies have shown that about 32% of young people drink and 20% are binge drinkers. While alcohol can impair development of almost all body systems in a growing child, it is of particular concern for the effects on the **neurological system and liver**. Additionally, because it interferes with impulse control, adolescents who drink are often involved in violence, abuse, and at-risk sexual behavior. Drinking should be expected if a child has memory problems, changes in behavior, poor academic progress, emotional lability, and physical changes, such as slurring of speech, general lethargy, or lack of coordination. *Intervention* includes teaching children from about age 9 about the dangers of drinking, identifying those who are drinking, identifying underlying problems, and providing programs to help teenagers stop drinking, such as counseling or Alcoholics Anonymous.

ADULTS

All patients should be **assessed for alcohol use** as part of the initial history and physical exam as well as at subsequent visits, especially if there are health indications (abnormal liver function tests, falls, insomnia) or social indications (family problems, divorce, job loss). There are numerous **self-assessment screening tools** that ask the patient a number of questions about the frequency and amount of drinking as well as questions such as if he/she drinks in the morning or alone, has been arrested because of drinking, has lost a job or missed work, feels depressed, drinks to gain confidence. The assessment tools have a scale indicator that suggests a problem with certain scores. The FNP should discuss the assessment and score with the patient and provide information about resources (such as Alcoholics Anonymous and alcohol rehabilitation programs) and health consequences of drinking to the patient.

DRUG USE IN CHILDREN AND ADOLESCENTS

Drug use continues to be a serious problem for children and teenagers, with some starting as young as 9 or 10, using a wide variety of drugs, including marijuana, crack, prescription drugs, cocaine, inhalants (such as glue and lighter fluid), hallucinogens, and steroids. Risk factors include aggressive behavior, poor social skills, and poor academic progress coupled with lack of parental supervision, poverty, and availability of drugs. Small children are often reacting to circumstances **within the family** while teenagers are responding to peer pressure from **outside the family**. Studies have shown that **early intervention** to teach children better self-control and coping skills is often more effective than trying to change behavior patterns that are established, so family-based programs often show positive results. Teenagers may need help with basic academic skills and social skills to improve communication. Methods of resisting drugs must be provided and reinforced. Drug recovery programs can be helpful but are often too expensive or not available for those who need them.

Signs of Substance Abuse

Many people with substance abuse (alcohol or drugs) are reluctant to disclose this information, but there are a number of indicators that are suggestive of **substance abuse:**

Physical signs of substance abuse are as follows:

- Needle tracks on arms or legs.
- Burns on fingers or lips.
- Pupils abnormally dilated or constricted, eyes watery.
- Slurring of speech, slow speech.
- Lack of coordination, instability of gait.
- Tremors.
- Sniffing repeatedly, nasal irritation.
- Persistent cough.
- Weight loss.
- Dysrhythmias.
- Pallor, puffiness of face.

The following are **other signs** of substance abuse:

- Odor of alcohol/marijuana on clothing or breath.
- Labile emotions, including mood swings, agitation, and anger.
- Inappropriate, impulsive, and/or risky behavior.
- Lying.
- Missing appointments.
- Difficulty concentrating/short term memory loss, disoriented/confused.
- Blackouts.
- Insomnia or excessive sleeping.
- Lack of personal hygiene.

Assessment and Prevention of Falls

Falls are extremely common in the elderly population and are a significant cause of physical and psychological injury. Risk factors for falls include age over 75, living alone, history of a previous fall, need for a cane or walker, and cognitive, visual or neurological impairment. Elderly patients should be questioned about falls at each visit. An important part of the history is an assessment of the **living situation** and **potential hazards** that may exist there. Patients should also be questioned about medications they are taking. **Medications** that can increase a patient's risk for falling include any drug that is sedating, cardiac and antihypertensive medications, and hypoglycemic drugs. A patient with a history of falling should have a detailed physical exam. Special attention should be given to orthostatic vital signs, joints, and neurological exam, including visual, hearing and nutritional status. The goals of intervention are aimed at reducing the risk of falling. Interventions include education, minimizing risk factors, correcting any underlying cause, and reducing hazards in the home.

Management of Bereavement

Bereavement occurs after the death of a family member, friend, or someone to whom a person identifies closely. It is a time of mourning and is part of the natural grieving process, but some people are not able to move past the grieving discuss process and may suffer signs related to depression, such as poor appetite, insomnia, and other symptoms, such as chest pain, that may

51

mimic physical illnesses. Some may enter a stage of denial or anger that interferes with their daily activities and work. People suffering bereavement may present with vague and varied complaints. A careful history is important. *Treatment* varies according to the needs of the individual. In some cases, selective serotonin reuptake inhibitors (SSRIs, such as Prozac® [fluoxetine]) may provide temporary relief, but the patient should be referred for psychological counselling, bereavement services, or psychiatric care, depending upon the severity of symptoms.

Functional Assessment

ASSESSING CURRENT AND HISTORICAL FUNCTIONAL ABILITIES

Functional abilities should be assessed in an active manner, with the person demonstrating the ability to sit, stand, get on and off of the toilet, walk, bend down, remove shoes, shirt or jacket, and then put them on again, listen, read, and answer questions. Ideally, this should be in the home environment, but careful questioning about distances and type of facilities in the home environment can help with approximating the type of activities required. The person can walk up and down a hallway, for example, to approximate walking from the car to the front door. A careful **history of functional ability** can pinpoint when and if changes occurred. Again, specific questioning guides people, "When did you begin to use a cane?" "How old were you when you stopped using the tub?" "What is the biggest problem with caring for yourself?" or "When did you have a hysterectomy/prostatectomy, and how has that changed your life?"

ASSESSING FUNCTIONAL STATUS

Functional status assessment concerns the ability to do self-care, self-maintenance, and engage in physical activities, but other factors may prevent those who should be able to function well from doing so:

- **Psychological function** assesses anxiety, worry, grief, and depression. Those with depression may be at increased risk of physical disability or may neglect self-care.
- **Social function** assesses support from family or friends, the need for a caregiver, financial resources, mistreatment or abuse, the ability to drive, and the presence of advance directives.
- **Sensory function** assesses presence of cataracts, glaucoma, myopia, presbyopia, astigmatism, macular degeneration, or eye disorders that make it difficult for people to read medication labels or do self-care. The need for audio materials or enlarged print should be assessed. Hearing is evaluated in both ears for hearing deficits and high and low frequency hearing loss as well as waxy buildup in the ear canals.

BASIC ACTIVITIES OF LIVING

Functional status relates to the ability of people, especially the elderly, to perform social roles free of limitations or disabilities. Assessment should include basic activities of daily living:

- **Toileting** assesses the ability to adequately control urination and fecal evacuation, noting dysuria, constipation, diarrhea, the presence and degree of incontinence as well as the use of protective materials.
- **Mobility** assesses the ability to transfer from bed to chair, to walk, to toilet, and to maintain balance, noting recent falls or the need for assistive devices.
- **Hygiene** assesses the ability to bathe, brush teeth, dress, and maintain basic standards of cleanliness both for the person and the environment.

- **Mental status** assesses thinking, understanding, and memory because, by age 90, about 50% of people have some dementia.
- **Nutrition** assesses basic dietary knowledge, the ability to prepare or obtain food, and adequate food and fluid intake.

ASPECTS OF THE HEALTH ASSESSMENT
WORK AND SURROUNDINGS, TALKING TO AN ADOLESCENT

As part of the health assessment, get an account of the patient's **work** and the **atmosphere** where they spend time. Find out what kind of job they have, prior jobs, any dangerous contact with anything at home or on the job, time in the military or in a war (when applicable), where the patient lives and how long they have lived there, whether the home is anywhere near a factory, shipyard, or another thing that could have harmful elements, and find out about leisure pursuits and any other possible contact with unsafe elements. If the patient is an adolescent, let them be the one to give the account, and let them know that except when the issue becomes significant or puts their life in danger, the account is private. A broadly used system for getting a medical history from an adolescent is **HEADSS**: Home, Education, Activities, Drugs, Sex, and Suicide. This model includes age-appropriate direction.

RELATIVE'S HEALTH ISSUES, ATHLETICS, AND PSYCHOSOCIAL FACTORS

Next, as part of the health assessment, talk about **relatives**, including how old they are, how mom and dad's health is or why they died, well-being of sisters and brothers, health of children, and any conditions that are hereditary. Discuss any **restrictions** from athletics, rapid heart rate or chest hurting upon physical activity, seizure, concussion, prior loss of consciousness, whether the patient can run for a half- mile (or higher), and whether the patient has both kidneys. Find out about the patient's **psychosocial factors**, including where he currently lives, what level of schooling he has finished (or what grade he is currently in if it is an adolescent, including how his grades are and how the school experience is going), faith (as it relates to well-being and medical attention), his point of view of a normal day, optimistic or pessimistic prospects for what is to come, stress and coping mechanisms, depression, anxiety, or thoughts of suicide. Teens and young adults should be asked straight out, as in, "Have you ever thought about ending your own life?" Ask about the social network.

HISTORY, CURRENT HEALTH PROBLEMS, PRIOR HEALTH ISSUES, AND INDIVIDUAL ROUTINES

Finally, to conclude the health assessment get an account of **prior health issues** to know what activities give the patient more of a chance of problems. These problem areas will require proper instruction for that patient. The health history should include demographics and biographical information. It should include an account of current health problems, including the **OPQRST assessment**:

> **O** = Onset
> **P** = Provocative/palliative (getting well or problem going downhill)
> **Q** = Quality/quantity
> **R** = Region/radiation
> **S** = Setting
> **T** = Timing

Find out about prior health issues, including how the patient feels they are generally doing, prior conditions or times in the hospital, harm or operations (including when, what the medical attention was, and what check-ups were done afterwards), emotional well-being, sexual well-being, allergies to food or drugs (and the particular problem that happens including needed medical attention for it

53

if there is any), drugs (prescribed and over-the-counter), immunizations (when and what), sleep routines, and prior assessments for any part of the body. Discuss individual routines, including the utilization of tobacco, alcohol, drugs, caffeine, nutrition, physical activity, hobbies, athletics, and contact sports.

EFFECTS OF AGING ON IMMUNITY

The **elderly** often have decreased antibody-mediated and cell-mediated **immune responses**, leaving them less able to combat infections. Additionally, many elderly people suffer from **malnutrition**, which further impairs cell-mediated immunity. If patients have functional impairment, they may be dependent on staff for toileting and turning, and if not done adequately, patients can develop decubiti, increasing the chance of wound infection. Patients may have medical illnesses, such as circulatory impairment of diabetes that make them prone to infection. Invasive devices, such as feeding tubes and urinary catheters are used frequently, and infection is a common complication. Patients may be too weak to breathe deeply or cough so they are unable to clear bacteria from the respiratory tract. Another problem faced by the elderly is that their inflammatory response to infection is often altered, so they may exhibit fever without other symptoms, or they may exhibit no fever in the presence of infection, so diagnosis can be difficult.

GENITOURINARY SYSTEM CHANGES RELATED TO AGING

Changes in the **genitourinary system** related to **aging** include:

- **Renal dysfunction**: 30-40% of functional nephrons are lost, decreasing kidney size and resulting in decreased ability to concentrate urine. The filtration rate decreases, making processing of excess fluids difficult. Excess potassium may be secreted, leading to dehydration.
- **Neurological degeneration**: Breaks in neural pathways interfere with messages sent to and from the brain so that sensations, such as a full bladder, may take longer to be perceived. The incomplete nerve pathways may result in bladder spasms from contractions of the detrusor muscle.
- **Muscular atrophy**: Bladder and sphincter muscles lose tone, resulting in shrinkage of the muscles and less effective ability to contract and relax, resulting in more frequent urination and incontinence. Pelvic floor and sphincter muscles may atrophy, resulting in incontinence.
- **Mechanical obstruction**: An enlarged prostate or prolapse of the uterus or bladder can create an obstruction that interferes with the ability to urinate.
- **Nocturnal urine production** increases, and this may result in nocturia and enuresis.

FACTORS THAT INFLUENCE PRESENTATION OF ILLNESS IN OLDER ADULTS

There are 3 major factors that influence how an illness will present in an older patient. These factors, either alone or in combination with one another, have the potential to make an ordinarily standard clinical presentation confusing for the clinician. The first of these factors is **underreporting of illness** or the symptoms associated with illness. There are a number of reasons that illnesses are not reported: the patient may fear hospitalization or institutionalization, or loss of control, or the patient may be convinced that there really is no problem. Another factor is the **pattern of distribution of illness**; this affects presentation because there are a number of diseases and problems that are prevalent among older adults, including congestive heart failure, arthritis, osteoporosis, and pneumonia. The last factor is an **altered response to illness**; this can make diagnosis and treatment very difficult because symptoms may be exaggerated by other problems, or they may be nonexistent.

Diagnosis

HEENT

FOREIGN BODIES IN THE EAR

Foreign bodies in the ear (most often in children) can be organic or inorganic materials or insects. Careful history should be done to determine the type of foreign body before attempting removal. Children may require conscious sedation or general anesthesia for deep insertions. Irrigations should not be done if tympanic membrane is ruptured or cannot be visualized. Procedure:

1. Examine ear to determine if tympanic membrane is intact.
2. Drown insects with 2% lidocaine solution and then suction.
3. Irrigate small non-organic particles with pulsatile flow aimed at wall of the canal.
4. Use cerumen loops, right-angle hooks, and/or alligator forceps to grasp and remove item.
5. Carefully examine the ear canal after removal of the item for lacerations or abrasions.
6. Topical antibiotic if extensive cutaneous abrasion or laceration or for organic material.

OTITIS MEDIA

Otitis media, inflammation of the **middle ear**, usually follows upper respiratory infections or allergic rhinitis. The eustachian tube swells and prevents the passage of air. Fluid from the mucous membranes pools in the middle ear, causing infection. Common pathogens include Streptococcus pneumoniae, Haemophilus influenzae, and Moraxella catarrhalis. Some genetic conditions, such as trisomy 21 and cleft palate may include abnormalities of the eustachian tube, increasing risk. There are 4 forms:

- **Acute**: 1-3 weeks with swelling, redness, and possible rupture of the tympanic membrane, fever, pain (ear pulling), and hearing loss.
- **Recurrent**: 3 episodes in 6 months or 4-6 in 12.
- **Bullous**: Acute infection with ear popping pressure in middle ear, pain, hearing loss, and bullae between layers of tympanic membrane, causing bulging.
- **Chronic**: Persists ≥3 months with thick retracted tympanic membrane, hearing loss, and drainage.

Treatment includes:

- 75-90% resolve spontaneously so antibiotics are withheld for 2-3 days.
- Amoxicillin for 7-10 days.
- Referral for tympanostomy and pressure-equalizing tubes (PET) for severe chronic or recurrent infections.

> **Review Video: Otitis Media**
> Visit mometrix.com/academy and enter code: 328778

OTITIS EXTERNA

Otitis externa (OE) is infection of the **external ear canal**, either bacterial or mycotic. Common pathogens include bacteria, Pseudomonas aeruginosa, Staphylococcus aureus, and fungi, Aspergillus and Candida. OE is often caused by chlorine in swimming pools killing normal flora and allowing other bacteria to multiply. Fungal infections may be associated with immune disorders, diabetes, and steroid use. *Symptoms* include:

- Pain, swelling, and exudate.
- Itching (pronounced with fungal infections).
- Red pustular lesions.
- Black spots over tympanic membrane (fungus).

Treatment includes:

- Irrigate ear with Burrows solution or saline to clean and remove debris, foreign objects.
- **Bacterial**: Antibiotic ear drops, such as ciprofloxacin and ofloxacin. If impetigo, flush with hydrogen peroxide 1:1 solution and apply Bactroban® twice daily for 5-7 days. Lance pointed furuncles.
- **Fungal**: Solution of 5% boric acid in ethanol, Clotrimazole-miconazole solution with/without steroid for 5-7 days.
- Analgesics as needed.

LABYRINTHITIS

Labyrinthitis is a viral or bacterial inflammation of the **inner ear**, and may occur secondary to bacterial otitis media. Viral labyrinthitis may be associated with mumps, rubella, rubeola, influenza, or other viral infections, such as upper respiratory infections. Because the labyrinth includes the vestibular system that is responsible for sensing head movement, labyrinthitis causes balance disorders. The condition often persists for 1-6 weeks with acute symptoms the first week and then decreasing symptoms. *Symptoms* include:

- Sudden onset of severe vertigo.
- Hearing loss and sometimes tinnitus.
- Nausea and vomiting.
- Panic attacks from severe anxiety related to symptoms.

Treatment includes:

- Bacterial:
  o IV antibiotics
  o Volume replacement.
  o Antiemetics, such as Phenergan® suppositories.
  o Vestibular suppressant (antihistamine): Meclizine (Antivert®)
  o Benzodiazepine or SSRI for anxiety.
  o Referral to surgeon for I&D if necessary.
- Viral:
  o Symptomatic as for bacterial (except for antibiotics).

MÉNIÈRE'S DISEASE

Ménière's disease occurs when a blockage in the **endolymphatic duct of the inner ear** causes dilation of the endolymphatic space and abnormal fluid balance, which causes pressure or rupture of the inner ear membrane. *Symptoms* include:

- Progressive fluctuating sensorineural hearing loss.
- Tinnitus.

- Pressure in the ear.
- Severe vertigo that lasts minutes to hours.
- Diaphoresis.
- Poor balance.
- Nausea and vomiting.

Diagnosis includes complete physical exam and evaluation of cranial nerves (tuning fork sounds may lateralize to unaffected ear), and assessment of hearing loss.

Treatment includes:

- Low Na diet.
- Vestibular suppressant (antihistamine): Meclizine (Antivert®).
- Benzodiazepine or SSRI for anxiety.
- Antiemetics, such as Phenergan® suppositories.
- Diuretics, such as hydrochlorothiazide.
- Referral for surgical repair for persistent vertigo, but this will not correct other symptoms.

SINUSITIS

Sinusitis is inflammation of the **nasal sinuses**, of which there are 2 maxillary, 2 frontal, and 1 sphenoidal, as ethmoidal air cells. Inflammation causes obstruction of drainage with resultant discomfort.

Symptoms include:

- Frontal and maxillary presents with pain over sinuses.
- Ethmoidal present with dull aching behind eye.
- Tenderness to palpation and percussion of sinuses.
- Mucosa of nasal cavity edematous and erythematous.
- Purulent exudate.

Diagnosis includes:

- Transillumination of sinus (diminished with inflammation).
- CT for those who are immunocompromised or if diagnosis is not clear.
- Careful examination to rule out spreading infection, especially with signs of fever, altered mental status, or unstable vital signs.

Treatment includes:

- Symptomatic relief with analgesia: topical decongestants, nasal irrigation.
- Antimicrobial therapy if symptoms persist at least 7 days or are severe (avoid routine use): amoxicillin or TMP/SMX.
- Steroid nasal spray twice daily.

FOREIGN BODIES IN THE NARES

Children may insert various organic and inorganic **foreign bodies in the nose**. In most cases, this is observed, but persistent unilateral obstruction of nose, foul discharge, or epistaxis is suggestive of foreign body. Small or uncooperative children may need to be restrained with conscious sedation or a papoose board.

The procedure is as follows:

- Vasoconstrictor/topical anesthetic applied: 1 mL of phenylephrine with 3 mL of 4% Xylocaine.
- Aerosolized racemic epinephrine may be used for decongestion, to loosen foreign body.
- Examine nares with speculum.

The following are **removal techniques**:

- Positive pressure: Blowing nose on command. For small children, block opposite nares and have caregiver blow puff of air in mouth, forcing item out of nares.
- Suction with catheter.
- Use alligator or bayonet forceps to grasp item.
- Pass a curette behind item, rotate, and the use to pull item out.
- Pass Fogarty vascular catheter past item, inflate balloon, pull catheter back out.

TMB

Temporomandibular disorder (TMB) is jaw pain caused by dysfunction of the **temporomandibular joint (TMJ)** and the supporting muscles and ligaments. It may be precipitated by injury, such as whiplash, or grinding or clenching of the teeth, stress, or arthritis.

Symptoms include:

- Clicking or popping noises on jaw movement.
- Limited jaw movement or "locked" jaw.
- Acute pain on chewing or moving jaw.
- Headaches and dizziness.
- Toothaches

Diagnosis includes:

- Complete dental exam with x-rays to rule out other disorders.
- MRI or CT may be needed.

Treatment usually begins conservatively:

- Ice pack to jaw area for 10 minutes followed by jaw stretching exercises and warm compress for 5 minutes 3 to 4 times daily.
- Avoidance of heavy chewing by eating soft foods and avoiding hard foods, such as raw carrots and nuts.
- NSAIDs to relieve pain and inflammation.
- Night mouth guard.
- Referral for dental treatments to improve bite as necessary.

Respiratory

CROUP AND ASL

Croup is not a disease in itself but rather a syndrome of disorders characterized by a distinctive, harsh, "barking" repetitive cough and hoarseness, resulting from inflammation in the area of the

larynx. Croup syndromes may affect all areas of the upper respiratory system. Because the larynx is very small in infants and small children, inflammation may become obstructive.

Acute spasmodic laryngitis (ASL) occurs in children from 3 months to 3 years and usually appears suddenly at night with severe cough, dyspnea, and restlessness that awakens the child. Fever is absent. The symptoms usually are not evident in the daytime but do tend to recur. ASL may be related to allergies.

Treatment includes:

- Usually cool humidifiers are used in the child's room, but acute attacks may be relieved by the warm steam of hot running water (such as a running shower) in a closed room. Some children may stop coughing if exposed to cold air.
- Occasionally corticosteroids may be used to reduce inflammation.

ACUTE EPIGLOTTITIS

Acute epiglottitis (supraglottitis) requires immediate medical attention as it can rapidly become obstructive. The onset is usually very sudden and often occurs suddenly during the night with a fever but not usually a cough. *Symptoms* include:

- **Tripod position**: Person sits upright, leaning forward with chin out, mouth open, and tongue protruding.
- **Agitation**: Person appears restless, tense, and agitated.
- **Drooling**: Excess secretions combined with pain or dysphagia and mouth open position cause drooling.
- **Voice**: Voice sounds thick and "froglike."
- **Cyanosis**: Color is usually pale and sallow initially progressing to frank cyanosis.
- **Throat**: Epiglottis bright red and swollen.

Diagnosis is by direct examination with nasopharyngoscopy.

Treatment: Because this condition can lead to acute respiratory failure and carries a risk of death, immediate treatment is necessary. Treatments include:

- **Antibiotics** for suspected bacterial infections or as indicated by epiglottal cultures.
- **Respiratory support**, which may require intubation or tracheostomy and mechanical ventilation (especially for viral infection).
- **Corticosteroids** are usually administered during intubation.

ACUTE LARYNGOTRACHEOBRONCHITIS

Acute laryngotracheobronchitis occurs in children from 3 months to 8 years (usually <5). It is a viral infection, usually caused by the human parainfluenza viruses, types 1, 2, and 3 and accounts for about 75% of the total cases. It usually follows an upper respiratory infection that slowly encompasses the **larynx**, resulting in swelling of the mucosa and a progressive onset of low-grade fever with characteristic "croupy" cough. Swelling can cause respiratory obstruction, resulting in acute respiratory acidosis and respiratory failure.

Treatment includes:

- **Cool humidified air** is usually best, but some respond to a warm steamy atmosphere or cool outside air.
- **Nebulized racemic epinephrine** may be used in the hospital setting, but it is very short acting and can have a rebound effect, so children should not be treated in the ER and released.
- **Oral and nebulized steroids** (dexamethasone, budesonide) have been shown in recent studies to provide relief, and are safe to use in the home.
- Intubation and ventilation as needed.

ACUTE TRACHEITIS

Acute tracheitis occurs in children from 1 month to 6 years and is usually caused by Staphylococcus aureus, with an increase in community-acquired MRSA (CA-MRSA), although Group A β-hemolytic Streptococci and H. Influenzae and other organisms are implicated. This disorder may present with symptoms similar to acute laryngotracheobronchitis, but often fails to respond to the same treatment and can result in airway obstruction and respiratory arrest, so diagnosis, referral, and treatment are critical. This condition is usually preceded by an upper respiratory infection with croupy cough and strider as well as a high fever. One difference between this and other forms of crop is the production of copious amounts of thick, purulent tracheal exudate, which are implicated in dyspnea and obstruction.

Treatment includes:

- **Intubation and mechanical ventilation** to ensure patency of airway. Tracheostomy may be necessary in some cases.
- **Antibiotic therapy** should include vancomycin if there are signs of multi-organ failure or increased incidence of CA-MRSA.

ACUTE BRONCHITIS

Acute bronchitis is an inflammation of the bronchial tree in which swelling and exudate cause a partial obstruction that prevents the lung from fully inflating. Causes include viruses (most common), bacteria, yeasts and fungi, and non-infectious things, such as smoke or air pollutants. In adults, the most common viral triggers are influenza virus, adenovirus, and respiratory syncytial virus (RSV). Symptoms vary depending but may include:

- Dyspnea and tachypnea.
- Cyanosis.
- Heavy productive moist or raspy cough.
- Sputum clear, white, yellow, green, or bloody.
- Localized crackling rales and expiratory high-pitched sibilant wheezes.
- Fever may or may not be present, but prolonged or high fever may indicate a bacterial infection.

Since most cases of acute bronchitis are caused by viruses and are self-limiting in 2-3 weeks, antibiotics are not helpful, but *treatment* may include:

- **Bronchial dilators** (albuterol) to improve air exchange.
- **Cough suppressant** and/or expectorants to relieve cough.

- **Antihistamines** for those with allergic triggers.
- **Antibiotics** for bacterial infections.

COPD
PRIMARY COMPONENTS

Chronic obstructive lung disease (COPD) is a disease that causes limitations in airflow and may include both emphysema and chronic bronchitis, or more often a combination. While asthma (an abnormal condition of the airway) is now considered a different disorder, it often occurs with COPD and has similar symptoms although they may vary more than COPD. In the United States, COPD is the 4th leading cause of death. The primary components to COPD include:

- Progressive airflow limitation.
- Inflammatory response that causes a narrowing of the peripheral airways and thickening of the vessel walls of the pulmonary vasculature.

While **smoking** is the most common cause of COPD, other risk factors include air pollution, occupational exposure to pollutants, history of repeated respiratory infections, and heredity. The changes that occur in COPD are generally irreversible and treatment aims at preventing complications and slowing deterioration.

STAGES

Functional dyspnea, body mass index (BMI), and spirometry are used to assess the **stages of COPD**. Spirometry measures used are the ratio of forced expiratory volume in the 1st second of expiration (FEV_1) after full inhalation to total forced vital capacity (FVC). Normal lung function decreases after age 35; so normal values are adjusted for height, weight, gender, and age:

- **Stage I (mild):** Minimal dyspnea with/without cough and sputum. FEV_1 is $\geq$80% of predicted rate and FEV_1: FVC = <70%.
- **Stage 2 (moderate):** Moderate to severe chronic exertional dyspnea with/without cough and sputum. FEV_1 is 50-80% of predicted rate and FEV_1: FVC = <70%.
- **Stage 3 (severe):** As stage 2 but repeated episodes with increased exertional dyspnea and condition impacting quality of life. FEV_1 is 30-50% of predicted rate and FEV_1: FVC = <70%.
- **Stage 4 (very severe):** Severe dyspnea and life-threatening episodes that severely impact quality of life. FEV_1 is 30% of predicted rate or <50% with chronic respiratory failure and FEV_1: FVC = <70%.

MANAGEMENT

COPD is not reversible, so management aims at slowing progressing, relieving symptoms, and improving quality of life:

- **Smoking cessation** is the primary means to slow progression and may require smoking cessation support in the form of classes or medications, such as Zyban®, nicotine patches or gum, clonidine, or nortriptyline.
- **Bronchodilators**, such as albuterol (Ventolin®) and salmeterol (Serevent), relieve bronchospasm and airway obstruction.
- **Corticosteroids**, both inhaled (Pulmicort®, Vanceril®) and oral (prednisone) may improve symptoms but are used most for associated asthma.
- **Oxygen therapy** may be long term continuous or used during exertion.
- **Bullectomy** (for bullous emphysema) to remove bullae (enlarged airspaces that do not ventilate).

- **Lung volume reduction surgery** may be done if involvement in lung is limited; however, mortality rates are high.
- **Lung transplantation** is a definitive high-risk option.
- **Pulmonary rehabilitation** includes breathing exercises, muscle training, activity pacing, and modification of activities.

CHRONIC BRONCHITIS

Chronic bronchitis is a pulmonary airway disease characterized by severe cough with sputum production for at least 2 consecutive years. Irritation of the airways (often from smoke or pollutants) causes an inflammatory response, increasing the number of mucus-secreting glands and goblet cells while ciliary function decreases so that the extra mucus plugs the airways. Additionally, the bronchial walls thicken and alveoli near the inflamed bronchioles become fibrotic, and alveolar macrophages cannot function properly, increasing susceptibility to infections. Chronic bronchitis is most common in those >45 and occurs twice as frequently in women as men. *Symptoms* include:

- Persistent cough with increasing sputum.
- Dyspnea.
- Frequent respiratory infections.

Treatment includes:

- Bronchodilators.
- Long term continuous oxygen therapy or supplemental oxygen during exercise may be needed.
- Pulmonary rehabilitation to improve exercise and breathing.
- Antibiotics during infections.
- Corticosteroids may be used for acute episodes.

EMPHYSEMA

Emphysema, the primary component of **COPD**, is characterized by abnormal distention of air spaces at the ends of the terminal bronchioles, with destruction of alveolar walls so that there is less and less gaseous exchange and increasing dead space with resultant hypoxemia and hypercapnia and respiratory acidosis. The capillary bed is damaged as well, increasing pulmonary blood flow and raising pressure in the right atrium (cor pulmonale) and pulmonary artery, leading to cardiac failure. Complications include respiratory insufficiency and failure. There are 2 primary types of emphysema (and both forms may be present):

- **Centrilobular** (the most common form) involves the central portion of the respiratory lobule, sparing distal alveoli and usually affects the upper lobes. Typical symptoms include abnormal ventilation-perfusion ratios, hypoxemia, hypercapnia, and polycythemia with right-sided heart failure.
- **Panlobular** involves enlargement of all air spaces, including the bronchiole, alveolar duct, and alveoli, but there is minimal inflammatory disease. Typical symptoms include hyperextended rigid barrel chest, marked dyspnea, weight loss, and active expiration.

ASTHMA/STATUS ASTHMATICUS

Status asthmaticus is a severe acute attack of **asthma** that does not respond to conventional treatment. An acute attack of asthma is precipitated by some stimulus, such as an antigen that triggers an allergic response, resulting in an inflammatory cascade that causes edema of the mucous membranes (swollen airway), contraction of smooth muscles (bronchospasm), increased mucus production (cough and obstruction), and hyperinflation of airways (decreased ventilation and shunting). Mast cells and T lymphocytes produce cytokines, which continue the inflammatory response through increased blood flow coupled with vasoconstriction and bronchoconstriction, resulting in fluid leakage from the vasculature. Epithelial cells and cilia are destroyed, exposing nerves and causing hypersensitivity. Sympathetic nervous system receptors in the bronchi stimulate bronchodilation. The 3 primary symptoms of asthma are cough, wheezing, and dyspnea. In cough-variant asthma, a severe cough may be the only symptom, at least initially.

SYMPTOMS OF STATUS ASTHMATICUS

The person with **status asthmaticus** will often present in acute distress, non-responsive to inhaled bronchodilators:

- Airway obstruction.
- Sternal and intercostal retractions.
- Tachypnea and dyspnea.
- Increasing cyanosis.
- Forced prolonged expirations.
- Cardiac decompensation with ↑ left ventricular afterload and increased pulmonary edema resulting from alveolar-capillary permeability. Hypoxia may trigger and ↑ in pulmonary vascular resistance with ↑ right ventricular afterload.
- Pulsus paradoxus (decreased pulse on inspiration and increased on expiration) with extra beats on inspiration detected through auscultation but not detected radially. Blood pressure normally decreases slightly during inspiration, but this response is exaggerated. Pulsus paradoxus indicates increasing severity of asthma.
- Hypoxemia (with impending respiratory failure).
- Hypocapnia followed by hypercapnia (with impending respiratory failure).
- Metabolic acidosis.

INDICATIONS FOR MECHANICAL VENTILATION FOR STATUS ASTHMATICUS

Mechanical ventilation should be avoided, if possible, because of the danger of increased bronchospasm as well as barotrauma and decreased circulation. Aggressive medical management with β-adrenergic agonists, corticosteroids, and anticholinergics should be tried prior to ventilation. However, there are some absolute indications for the use of intubation and ventilation:

- Cardiac and/or pulmonary arrest.
- Markedly depressed mental status (obtundation).
- Severe hypoxia and/or apnea.
- Bradycardia

There are a number of other indications that are evaluated on an individual basis and may be an indication for **ventilation**.

- Exhaustion/ muscle fatigue from exertion of trying to breathe.
- Sharply diminished breath sounds and no audible wheezing.
- Pulse paradoxus >20-40 mm Hg. If pulse paradoxus is absent, this is an indication of imminent respiratory arrest. PaO2 <70 mm Hg on 100% oxygen.
- Deteriorating mental status.
- Dysphonia.
- Central cyanosis.

- ↑ Hypercapnia.
- Metabolic/respiratory acidosis; pH <7.20.

PLEURAL EFFUSION

Pleural effusion is the collection of fluid in the area between the **visceral and parietal pleurae**. The fluid may be high protein exudates from pleural irritation (such as from neoplasms, infections, pulmonary embolism, empyema, uremia, pancreatitis, or drugs such as amiodarone.) or low protein transudates from congestive heart failure (CHF), cirrhotic ascites, peritoneal dialysis, or nephrotic syndrome. *Symptoms* may be lacking or present as dyspnea and chest pain. Diagnosis is by clinical findings of ↓breath sounds and dullness on percussion, upright chest radiograph, ultrasound (especially useful for small pockets of fluid) CT scan, and thoracentesis if necessary, to diagnose condition or infections. *Treatment* includes:

- Therapy directed at underlying cause, such as diuretics for CHF.
- Needle/catheter thoracentesis to drain excessive fluid for large pleural effusions.
- Insertion of chest tube indicated for large amounts of fluid.
- Antibiotics as indicated for infection.

CYSTIC FIBROSIS

Cystic fibrosis (mucoviscidosis) is a progressive congenital disease that particularly affects the **pancreas and lungs** causing digestive and respiratory problems. It is caused by a genetic defect that affects sodium chloride movement in cells, including mucosal cells that line the lungs, causing the production of thick mucus that clogs the lungs and provides a rich medium for bacteria. While most patients with cystic fibrosis at one time died in childhood, the life expectancy is now about 30 years. Cystic fibrosis patients usually suffer from recurrent respiratory infections of the lower respiratory tract. The most common infective agents are Pseudomonas aeruginosa and Burkholderia cepacia complex. Patients with chronic infections serve as reservoirs for patient-to-patient transmission of infection, with proximity and duration of contact as precipitating factors. Cystic fibrosis patients should be maintained on universal and droplet precautions and, when hospitalized, placed in private rooms or cohorted with someone with the same pathogen.

SIDS AND ALTE

Infants with **apparent life-threatening event (ALTE)** are those who are lifeless and without respirations but are successfully resuscitated or begin breathing spontaneously. With **sudden infant death syndrome (SIDS)**, almost always related to respiratory arrest, the child cannot be resuscitated. There are numerous proposed causes for both ALTE and SIDS, so a careful history, including familial history of SIDS, and physical examination or post-mortem examination can provide important information, such as indications of child abuse or metabolic/infectious disorders. Diagnostic studies for ALTE include:

- CBC with serum electrolytes and chemical panel.
- ECG (12-lead).
- Blood, urine, and spinal fluid cultures.
- Stool culture and botulinum toxin testing.

Treatment includes continuing resuscitative efforts and stabilizing the patient. The child should be hospitalized for observation, further studies, and apnea monitoring as these children are at increased risk for SIDS. For SIDS patients, the FNP should provide support and information to the family. The protocol for reporting SIDS patients varies but usually involves notification of the coroner's office.

Cardiovascular

SKIN CHANGES AND ABNORMALITIES RELATED TO LEVD

Skin changes and abnormalities, in addition to edema, related to **lower-extremity venous disease (LEVD)** include:

- **Hemosiderin staining** occurs when hemosiderin, a brownish granular iron-containing pigment resulting from breakdown of hemoglobin, builds up in the interstitial fluid as a result of venous hypertension causing the erythrocytes to seep into the tissues. As the cells break down, the deposits along with melanin remain in the tissue. This causes a brownish, splotchy discoloration of the skin from the ankle to the anterior tibial area.
- **Lipodermatosclerosis** occurs in the lower leg area as the tissue becomes fibrotic from fibrin and protein (collagen) deposits, causing the skin to feel waxy and the tissue to harden with narrowing of the tissue around the ankle compared to proximal tissue above.
- **Venous (stasis) dermatitis** is inflammation of the epidermis and dermis resulting in scaly, erythematous, crusty, weepy, itchy skin, usually in the lower leg (ankle and tibia). It is progressive with redness and itching appearing before other symptoms. (Continued)
- **Malleolar flare** is caused by capillaries in a sunburst pattern inferior and distal to the medial malleolus.
- **Atrophie blanche lesions** are smooth white avascular sclerotic skin plaques that occur in about one-third of patients with LEVD. They are usually associated with torturous vessels and hemosiderin staining on the ankles or foot. They may appear similar to scarring from healed ulcers but actually have a high risk for deteriorating into ulcer formation.
- **Varicosities** (varicose veins) are veins where blood has pooled, causing them to become distended, twisted, and palpable, often appearing as blue rope-like vessels on back of the knee and calf or inside of the leg. They are the result of venous reflux and venous hypertension.
- **Ankle blowout syndrome** occurs when small vessels around the medial malleolus, creating a number of small very painful ulcers.

ASSESSMENT FOR LEND AND NEUROPATHIC/DIABETIC WOUNDS

The assessment for **lower extremity neuropathic disease (LEND)** and neuropathic/diabetic wounds includes:

- **History**: A history of general health and record of diabetes control and complications is critical. Risk factors should be identified and risks classified according to severity.
- **Physical examination**: The examination must identify any comorbid conditions, such as heart disease, arthritis, and peripheral arterial or venous insufficiency.
- **Lower extremity/foot examination**: A thorough examination of the lower extremity and foot should include screening for neuropathy and sensory loss, pain, musculoskeletal changes or abnormalities, and vascular status. The skin should be carefully assessed for corns, calluses, and pre-ulcerative lesions (such as blisters or cracks). Nails should be checked for fungus infections and thickening, which is common, and discolorations, such as red, black, or brown that may indicate trauma. Footwear should be examined for support and fit.
- **Evaluation and classification of the diabetic foot ulcer (DFU)**: Ulcers should be measured and classified according to standard classification systems, observing for signs of infection.

CHARACTERISTICS OF ARTERIAL AND VENOUS INSUFFICIENCY

	Arterial	Venous
Type of pain	Ranges from intermittent claudication to severe constant.	Aching and cramping.
Pulses	Weak or absent.	Present.
Skin of extremity	Rubor on dependency but pallor of foot on elevation. Skin pale, shiny, and cool with loss of hair on toes and foot. Nails thick and ridged.	Brownish discoloration around ankles and anterior tibial area.
Ulcers	Pain, deep, circular, often necrotic ulcers on toe tips, toe webs, heels, or other pressure areas.	Varying degrees of pain in superficial, irregular ulcers on medial or lateral malleolus and sometimes the anterior tibial area.
Extremity edema	Minimal.	Moderate to severe.

ARTERIAL, NEUROPATHIC, AND VENOUS ULCERS

There are distinct differences in arterial, neuropathic, and venous ulcers:

Characteristic	Arterial	Neuropathic	Venous
Location	End-of-toe pressure points, traumatic non-healing wounds	Plantar surface, metatarsal heads toes and sides of feet	Between knees and ankles, medial malleolus
Exudate	Slight amount, infection common	Moderate to large amount, infection common	Moderate to large amounts
Wound perimeters	Circular, well-defined	Circular, well-defined & often with callous formation	Irregular, poorly defined
Pain	Very painful	Often absent because of reduced sensation	Pain varies
Skin	Pale, friable, shiny, hairless with dependent rubor and elevational pallor	Ischemic signs (as in arterial) may be evident with comorbidity.	Brownish discoloration of ankles and shin, edema common

ASSESSMENT FOR DVT OF CALF

Deep vein thrombophlebitis (DVT) is usually related to poor circulation or damage to **vessels** and is more common in those over age 40. It can be induced by sitting for long periods without activity, as when flying long distances. Symptoms include pain or aching in the calf, especially on activity, and swelling. DVT should be differentiated from other injuries when athletes complain of calf pain. **Homan's sign** may be used to identify DVT:

- Person is lying in prone position with lower shin and foot extending over edge of the table.
- The examiner passively dorsiflexes the ankle while palpating the proximal calf.
- Positive findings are pain in the calf on dorsiflexion of the ankle or pain during the palpation.

ASSESSMENT OF PERFUSION OF LOWER EXTREMITIES

Assessment of perfusion can indicate venous or arterial abnormalities:

- **Venous refill time**: Begin with the patient lying supine for a few moments and then have the patient sit with the feet dependent. Observe the veins on the dorsum of the foot and count the seconds before normal filling. Venous occlusion is indicated with times >20 seconds.
- **Capillary refill**: Grasp the toenail bed between the thumb and index finger and apply pressure for several seconds to cause blanching. Release the nail and count the seconds until the nail regains normal color. Arterial occlusion is indicated with times >2-3 seconds. Check both feet and more than 1 nail bed.
- **Skin temperature**: Using the palm of the hand and fingers, gently palpate the skin, moving distally to proximally and comparing both legs. Arterial disease is indicated by decreased temperature (coolness) or a marked change from proximal to distal. Venous disease is indicated by increased temperature about the ankle.

ASSESSMENT OF PULSE AND BRUIT IN LOWER EXTREMITIES

Evaluation of the pulses of the lower extremities is an important part of assessment for peripheral arterial disease/trauma. Pulses should be first evaluated with the patient in supine position and then again with the legs dependent, checking bilaterally and proximally to distally to determine if intensity of pulse decreases distally. **Pedal pulses** should be examined at both the posterior tibialis and the dorsalis pedis. The pulse should be evaluated as to the rate, rhythm, and intensity, which is usually graded on a 0-4 scale:

> 0 = pulse absent
> 1 = weak, difficult to palpate
> 2 = normal as expected
> 3 = full
> 4 = strong and bounding

Pulses may be palpable or absent with **peripheral arterial disease**. Absence of pulse on both palpation and Doppler probe does indicate peripheral arterial disease. **Bruits** may be noted by auscultating over major arteries, such as femoral, popliteal, peroneal, and dorsalis pedis, indicating peripheral arterial disease.

EDEMA

Edema is usually checked by pressing the index finger into the tissue on top of each foot, behind the medial malleolus, and over the shin, starting distally and moving proximally to the highest level of edema, comparing both legs:

- Edema is rated on a 1-4-point **scale**:
  - 1+ slight pitting to about 2 mm (persists 10-15 seconds).
  - 2+ moderate pitting to about 4 mm (persists 10-15 seconds).
  - 3+ moderate-severe pitting to about 6 mm (persists >1 minute).
  - 4+ severe pitting to 8 mm or more (persists 2-5 minutes).

- **Venous edema**: edema from ankle to knee and may involve some limitation in ankle movement. Dependent pitting edema occurs, but may become non-pitting in chronic disease.

- **Lymphedema**: usually unilateral non-pitting hard edema from toes to groin. In advanced disease, elephantiasis with huge enlargement of extremity may occur.
- **Lipedema**: symmetrical bilateral soft rubbery tissue from ankle to groin and sometimes hips with pain on palpation and frequent bruising.

CORONARY ARTERY SYNDROMES

UNSTABLE AND VARIANT ANGINA

Unstable angina (also known as preinfarction or crescendo angina) is a progression of coronary artery disease and occurs when there is a change in the pattern of stable angina. The pain may increase, may not respond to a single nitroglycerin, and may persist for >5 minutes. Usually pain is more frequent, lasts longer, and may occur at rest. Unstable angina may indicate rupture of an atherosclerotic plaque and the beginning of thrombus formation so it should always be treated as a medical emergency as it may indicate a myocardial infarction.

Variant angina (also known as Prinzmetal's angina) results from spasms of the coronary arteries, either associated with or without atherosclerotic plaques, and is often related to smoking, alcohol, or illicit stimulants. Elevation of ST segments usually occurs with variant angina. Variant angina frequently occurs cyclically at the same time each day and often while the person is at rest. Nitroglycerin or calcium channel blockers are used for treatment.

STABLE ANGINA

Impairment of blood flow through the **coronary arteries** leads to ischemia of the cardiac muscle and angina pectoris, pain in the sternum, chest, neck, arms (especially the left) or back. The pain frequently occurs with crushing pain substernally, radiating down the left arm or both arms although this type of pain is more common in men than women, whose symptoms may appear less acute and include nausea, dyspnea, and fatigue. Elderly or diabetic patients may also have pain in arms, no pain at all (silent ischemia), or weakness and numbness in arms. **Stable angina** episodes usually last for <5 minutes and are caused by atherosclerotic lesions blocking >75% of the lumen of the effected coronary artery. Precipitating events include exercise, decrease in environmental temperature, heavy eating, strong emotions (such as fright or anger), or exertion, including coitus. Stable angina episodes usually resolve in less than 5 minutes by decreasing activity level and administering sublingual nitroglycerin. Angina decubitus occurs with the person lying supine because fluid redistribution increased cardiac workload.

CARDIOPULMONARY ARREST AND SCD

Over 60% of **sudden cardiac death (SCD)** from cardiovascular disease results from cardiopulmonary arrest, usually involving those with underlying cardiac disease, such as coronary atherosclerosis and/or enlarged heart. There are a number of causative events:

- **Ventricular tachyarrhythmias**, such as tachycardia or fibrillation, which may result from left ventricular hypertrophy.
  - *Treatment*: Prompt CPR and defibrillation.
- **Brady asystole** (cardiac rate <60 with periods of asystole) with failure of the electrical system of the heart, resulting from ischemia of the right coronary artery, ischemia of the AV node, systemic disease, hypoxia and hypercarbia, vagal stimulation, or sick sinus syndrome, a range of pacemaker disorders.
  - *Treatment*: Atropine, dopamine or epinephrine for sick sinus syndrome. Permanent ventricular or AV pacing is usually necessary.

- **Pulseless electrical activity** (PEA) is the present of organized rhythm without detectable pulse caused by marked decrease in cardiac output resulting from hypovolemia, shock, acidosis, hypothermia, electrolyte imbalances, cardiac dysfunction, or cardiotoxins (β-blockers, calcium channel blockers, and tricyclic antidepressants).
  - *Treatment*: Identify and treat underlying cause.

SHOCK

There are a number of different types of **shock**, but there are general characteristics that they have in common. In all types of shock, there is a marked decrease in tissue perfusion related to hypotension, so that there is insufficient oxygen delivered to the tissues and, in turn, inadequate removal of cellular waste products, causing injury to tissue:

- **Hypotension** (mean arterial pressure [MAP] below 65). This may be somewhat higher in those who are initially hypertensive.
- Tachycardia (>90).
- **Bradypnea** (<7) or **tachypnea** (>29). This varies depending upon the cause of shock.
- **Decreased urinary output** (<0.5 mL/kg/hr), especially marked in hypovolemic shock.
- Metabolic acidosis.
- **Hypoxemia** <90 mm Hg for children and adults, birth-50; < 80 mm Hg for those 51 to 70 and <70 for those over 70.
- Peripheral/cutaneous vasoconstriction/vasodilation.
- **Alterations in mental status** with dullness, agitation, anxiety, or lethargy.

Lymphatic

HODGKIN'S DISEASE

Hodgkin's disease is a malignancy of the **lymphatic system**. It originates in a single node and then spreads contiguously along the lymphatic system. Common symptoms are swollen lymph nodes, night sweats, weight loss, red bruising associated with decreased platelet count, low-grade fever, pruritus, hepatomegaly, and splenomegaly. It is staged according to spread, with substages (A and B) if specific symptoms (such as night sweats or weight loss) are present:

- **Stage I A/B**: Malignancy in 1 lymph node area (such as above the diaphragm on 1 side) or 1 area or organ (such as the stomach) outside of the lymph nodes.
- **Stage II A/B**: Malignancy in ≥2 lymph node areas on the same side of diaphragm OR malignancy is in only 1 area or organ outside of lymph nodes but the surrounding lymph nodes also have malignancy.
- **Stage III A/B**: Malignancy in lymph nodes on both sides of diaphragm and may spread to spleen or other organs near lymph nodes.
- **Stage IV**: Malignancy in organs outside of lymph nodes and may be in lymph nodes distant from organ involvement.

Treatment is chemotherapy and radiation or chemotherapy alone, depending on staging.

STAGES OF LYMPHEDEMA

Lymphedema is a dysfunction of the **lymphatic system**, resulting in a debilitating progressive disease. The healthy lymphatic system returns proteins, lipids, and fluids to the circulatory system from the interstitial spaces, but with lymphedema this accumulates, causing pronounced induration, edema, and fibrosis of tissues. As the fluid builds up, it causes distention, and the skin

69

becomes thick and fibrotic with orange discoloration (peau d'orange). Scaly keratotic debris collects, and the skin develops cracks and leakage of lymphatic fluid. Lymphedema may be **primary** (developmental abnormality) or **secondary**. It can occur after mastectomy and after radiation, infection, cancer or surgery, such as joint replacements and vascular procedures. Patients are at risk of infection, cellulitis and lymphangitis, as well as pain and limited mobility. Lymphedema has 3 stages:

- **Stage 1** is reversible pitting edema distally with no fibrosis.
- **Stage 2** is pitting or non-pitting edema with fibrosis and papillomatosis.
- **Stage 3** is elephantiasis with massive enlargement and distortion of limb, fibrosis and ulcerations.

Hepatic

HEPATIC CIRRHOSIS

Cirrhosis is a chronic hepatic disease in which normal liver tissue is replaced the fibrotic tissue that impairs liver function. There are 3 types:

- **Alcoholic** (from chronic alcoholism) is the most common type and results in fibrosis about the portal areas. The liver cells become necrotic, replaced by fibrotic tissue, with areas of normal tissue projecting in between, giving the liver a hobnail appearance.
- **Postnecrotic** with broad bands of fibrotic tissue is the result of acute viral hepatitis.
- **Biliary**, the least common type is caused by chronic biliary obstruction and cholangitis, with resulting fibrotic tissue about the bile ducts.

Cirrhosis may be either compensated or decompensated. **Compensated cirrhosis** usually involves non-specific symptoms, such as intermittent fever, epistaxis, ankle edema, indigestion, abdominal pain, and palmar erythema. Hepatomegaly and splenomegaly may also be present.

Decompensated cirrhosis occurs when the liver can no longer adequately synthesize proteins, clotting factors, and other substances so that portal hypertension occurs. Symptoms include:

- Hepatomegaly, portal obstruction resulting in jaundice and ascites.
- Chronic elevated temperature.
- Purpura resulting from thrombocytopenia, with bruising and epistaxis.
- Bacterial peritonitis may develop with ascites.
- Esophageal varices.
- Edema of extremities and presacral area resulting from reduced albumin in the plasma.
- Vitamin deficiency from interference with formation, use, and storage of vitamins, such as A, C, and K.
- Anemia from chronic gastritis and ↓dietary intake, anemia.
- Hepatic encephalopathy with alterations in mentation.
- Hypotension.
- Atrophy of gonads.

Treatment varies according to the symptoms and is supportive rather than curative as the fibrotic changes in the liver cannot be reversed: Dietary supplements and vitamins; diuretics (potassium sparing), such as Aldactone® and Dyrenium®, to decrease ascites; colchicine to reduce fibrotic changes; and liver transplant, the definitive treatment.

70

Gastrointestinal

PERITONITIS

Peritonitis (inflammation of the peritoneum) may be **primary** (from infection of blood or lymph) or, more commonly, **secondary**, related to perforation or trauma of the gastrointestinal tract. Common causes include perforated bowel, ruptured appendix, abdominal trauma, abdominal surgery, peritoneal dialysis or chemotherapy, or leakage of sterile fluids, such as blood, into the peritoneum. *Symptoms* of peritonitis are those of an acute abdomen:

- Diffuse abdominal pain with rebound tenderness (Blumberg's sign).
- Abdominal rigidity.
- Paralytic ileus.
- Fever (with infection).
- Nausea and vomiting.
- Sinus tachycardia.

Diagnosis is made according to clinical presentation, abdominal x-rays, which may show distention of the intestines or air in the peritoneum, and laboratory findings, such as leukocytosis. Blood cultures may indicate sepsis. *Treatment* includes:

- Intravenous fluids and electrolytes.
- Broad-spectrum antibiotics.
- Surgical consultation for laparoscopy as indicated to determine cause of peritonitis and effect repair.

APPENDICITIS

Appendicitis is inflammation of the **appendix** caused by luminal obstruction and pressure within the lumen as secretions build up and can eventually perforate the appendix. Appendicitis can occur in all ages, but infants <2 usually present with peritonitis or sepsis because of difficulty in early diagnosis. *Symptoms* include:

- Acute abdominal pain, which may be epigastric, periumbilical, right lower quadrant, or right flank with rebound tenderness.
- Anorexia.
- Nausea and vomiting.
- Positive psoas and obturator signs.
- Fever may develop after 24 hours.

Diagnosis is based on clinical presentation, complete blood count (although leukocytosis may not be present), urinalysis, and imaging studies (such as x-rays, ultrasound, and CT). *Treatment* includes: Antibiotics are usually begun on diagnosis, followed by surgical excision of the inflamed appendix. In rare cases of confined appendicitis (with mild symptoms), antibiotics alone may resolve the inflammation.

PEPTIC ULCER DISEASE

Peptic ulcer disease (PUD)/gastritis includes both ulcerations of the **duodenum** and **stomach**. They may be **primary** (usually duodenal) or **secondary** (usually gastric). Gastric ulcers are commonly associated with Helicobacter pylori infections (80%) but may be caused by aspirin and NSAIDs. H. pylori are spread in the fecal-oral route from person to person or contaminated water and causes a chronic inflammation and ulcerations of the gastric mucosa. PUD is 2-3 times more common in men and is associated with poor economic status resulting in a crowded unhygienic environment although it can occur in others. Usually others in the family have a history of ulcers as well. *Symptoms* include abdominal pain, nausea, vomiting and GI bleeding in children <6 with epigastric and post-prandial pain and indigestion in older children and adults. *Treatment* includes:

- **Antibiotics for H. pylori**: Amoxicillin, clarithromycin, metronidazole.
- **Proton pump inhibitors**: Lansoprazole or omeprazole.
- Sucralfate.
- **Histamine-receptor antagonists**: Cimetidine, ranitidine, famotidine.

> **Review Video: Peptic Ulcers and GERD**
> Visit mometrix.com/academy and enter code: 184332

ACUTE GASTROINTESTINAL HEMORRHAGE

Gastrointestinal (GI) hemorrhage (peptic ulcers) may occur in the upper or lower **gastrointestinal track**. The primary cause (50-70% of GI hemorrhage peptic ulcer disease [gastric and duodenal ulcers]), which results in deterioration of the gastro mucosal lining, compromising the glycoprotein mucous barrier and the gastroduodenal epithelial cells that provide protection from gastric secretions. The secretions literally digest the mucosal and submucosal layers, damaging blood vessels and causing hemorrhage. The primary causes are NSAIDs and infection with Helicobacter pylori. *Symptoms* include:

- Abdominal pain and distention.
- Hematemesis.
- Bloody or tarry stools.
- Hypotension with tachycardia.

Treatment includes:

- **Fluid replacement** with transfusions if necessary.
- **Antibiotic therapy** for Helicobacter pylori.
- **Endoscopic thermal therapy** to cauterize or injection therapy (hypertonic saline, epinephrine, ethanol) to cause vasoconstriction.
- **Arteriography** with intraarterial infusion of vasopressin and/or embolizing agents, such as stainless-steel coils, platinum microcoils, or Gelfoam pledgets.
- Vagotomy and pyloroplasty if bleeding persists.

CHOLECYSTITIS

Cholecystitis can result in obstruction of the **bile duct** related to calculi as well as pancreatitis from obstruction of the pancreatic duct. The disease is most common in overweight women 20-40 but can occur in pregnant women and people of all ages, especially those who are diabetic or elderly. Children may develop cholecystitis secondary to cystic fibrosis, obesity, or total parenteral nutrition. Symptoms range from asymptomatic to severe right upper quadrant or epigastric pain, persisting 2-6 hours per episode. Disease of the biliary tract may cause radiation of pain to the back and nausea and vomiting. Cholangitis may result in jaundice and altered mental status. Diagnosis is confirmed by ultrasound as laboratory findings may be within normal range. *Treatment* includes:

- **Antibiotics** for sepsis or ascending cholangitis.
- **Antispasmodic agents** (glycopyrrolate) for biliary colic and vomiting.
- **Analgesics** (meperidine for acute pain).

72

- **Antiemetics** (promethazine).
- **Surgical consultation** to determine if laparoscopic or open cholecystectomy is warranted.

DIVERTICULAR DISEASE

Diverticular disease (diverticulitis) is a condition in which diverticula (saclike pouchings of the bowel lining that extend through a defect in the muscle layer) occur anywhere within the **GI tract**. Diverticulitis occurs as diverticula become inflamed when food or bacteria are retained within diverticula. This may result in abscess, obstruction, perforation, bleeding, or fistula. *Symptoms* are similar to appendicitis and include:

- Steady pain in left lower quadrant.
- Change in bowel habits.
- Tenesmus.
- Dysuria from irritation.
- Toxic reactions: fever, severe pain, leukocytosis.
- Recurrent urinary infections from fistula.
- Paralytic ileus from peritonitis or intraabdominal irritation.

Diagnosis is per CT, as barium enema will show diverticula but not inflammation. *Treatment* includes:

- Rehydration and electrolytes per intravenous fluids
- Nothing by mouth initially
- Antibiotics, broad spectrum (IV if toxic reactions)
- NG suction if necessary, for obstruction
- Careful observation for signs of perforation or obstruction

GERD

Gastroesophageal reflux disease (GERD) is involuntary regurgitation of stomach contents into the **esophagus**, usually caused by decreased tone in the gastroesophageal valve and hiatal hernia, causing damage to the mucosal lining of the esophagus. Chronic esophagitis, strictures, Barrett's esophagus (abnormal changes in cells of distal esophagus), and esophageal cancer may develop. GERD symptoms include:

- Chronic cough, especially at night
- Dysphagia
- Earache
- Epigastric pain and "heartburn"
- Hoarseness
- Sinusitis

Treatment includes:

- Avoiding **large meals** or after dinner snacking and eating at least 3 hours before going to bed or lying down.
- Modifying **food intake** to avoid coffee, alcohol, fatty food, spicy foods, and cruciferous vegetables.
- Sleeping with head of the bed **elevated** and on **left side**.

73

- **Medications** include histamine-2 receptor blockers (famotidine and ranitidine), proton pump inhibitors, alginic acid (Gaviscon®), and antacids (without aluminum).
- **Surgical repair** (fundoplication) may be needed if medical treatment is not adequate.

CONTRIBUTING FACTORS TO BOWEL DYSFUNCTION

Contributing factors to **bowel dysfunction** range from those things that can be corrected and others that require compensation:

- **Dietary factors** include insufficient fiber and fluids as well as foods that cause diarrhea, constipation, and gas.
- **Clinical conditions** such as hemorrhoids may cause pain that delays defecation. Surgical treatment of hemorrhoids, fistulas, or the rectum may create trauma and injury to the sphincters. Chronic diseases, such as irritable bowel syndrome and multiple sclerosis, may be associated with bowel dysfunction. Dementia may result in the inability to manage toileting.
- **Delaying defecation**, often because of functional disability or dementia, is the leading cause of constipation, impaction, and fecal incontinence.
- **Pregnancy** can result in damage to anal sphincters, causing incontinence.
- **Medications** frequently cause constipation, but some, including antacids and antibiotics, may cause diarrhea. Laxative abuse causes laxative tolerance to develop.
- **Physical inactivity** decreases bowel motility and increases constipation.

ENCOPRESIS

Encopresis is the voluntary or involuntary passage of stool in places or manners that are inappropriate for a child, 80% of whom are male, 4 years or older. There are 2 types: retentive encopresis, which accounts for about 80% of those affected, and non-retentive, which accounts for the other 20%.

- **Retentive encopresis** is characterized by a history of long-term, painful constipation and the development of overflow diarrhea. The chronic constipation causes distention of the rectum and stretching of both the internal and external anal sphincters; as a result, the child may no longer feel the urge to defecate, so stool eventually leaks from the rectum, causing chronic fecal incontinence.
- **Non-retentive encopresis**, usually involving passage of normally formed stools on a daily basis, does not involve constipation or bowel abnormalities, except in a small subset that may have irritable bowel syndrome, but is generally a behavioral/psychological problem.

INFLAMMATORY BOWEL DISORDERS

CROHN'S DISEASE

Crohn's disease manifests with inflammation of the **GI system**. Inflammation is transmural (often leading to intestinal stenosis and fistulas), focal and discontinuous with aphthous ulcerations progressing to linear and irregular shaped ulcerations. Granulomas may be present. Common sites of inflammation are the terminal ileum and cecum. Condition is usually chronic, but an acute flare-up may mimic appendicitis. Children may have delayed development and stunted growth. There is a genetic component to the disease.

Symptoms:

- Perirectal abscess/fistula in advanced disease.
- **Diarrhea** is usually present with colonic disease. May have nocturnal bowel movements, watery stools, and rectal hemorrhage.
- **Anemia** may develop with chronic bleeding.
- **Abdominal pain** most common in lower right quadrant, usually indicating transmural inflammation; may include post-prandial pain and cramping,

Other symptoms include nausea and vomiting (usually related to strictures of small intestine), weight loss (with small intestine involvement), fever, and night sweats. *Treatment* includes:

- Corticosteroids and antibiotics for acute exacerbations.
- Immunomodulatory agents (cyclosporine, methotrexate).
- Antidiarrheals.

ULCERATIVE COLITIS

Ulcerative colitis is superficial inflammation of mucosa of **colon and rectum**, causing ulcerations in the areas where inflammation has destroyed cells. These ulcerations, ranging from pinpoint to extensive, may bleed and produce purulent material. The mucosa of the bowel becomes swollen, erythematous, and granular. Onset is usually between ages 15 and 30, and there is a genetic component. Ulcerative colitis may affect only the rectum (ulcerative proctitis), the entire colon (pancolitis), or only the left colon (limited or distal colitis).

Symptoms:

- **Abdominal pain** may be absent or mild unless severe disease.
- **Bloody diarrhea/rectal bleeding** in absence of infection may result in anemia and fluid and electrolyte depletion. Diarrhea more frequent as colonic involvement increases.
- Fecal urgency and tenesmus may occur.
- **Anorexia** resulting in weight loss, fatigue.
- **Systemic disorders** with eye inflammation, arthritis, liver disease, and osteoporosis as immune system triggers generalized inflammation.

Treatment:

- Aminosalicylates.
- Steroids.
- Immunomodulatory agents.
- Antispasmodics.

INTUSSUSCEPTION

Intussusception is a telescoping of 1 portion of the **intestine** into another, usually at the ileocecal valve, causing an obstruction. As the walls of the intestine come in contact, inflammation and edema cause decreased perfusion, which can result in infarction with peritonitis and death. Fecal material cannot move past the obstruction. It is most common between 3-12 months but can occur until 6 years and may relate to viral infections. *Symptoms* include:

- "Current jelly stool" composed of blood and mucous (occurs with 60%).
- Sudden acute episodes of severe abdominal pain during which child pulls knees to chest.
- Vomiting.

75

- Lethargy and weakness.
- Distended abdomen, painful to palpation.
- Sausage-shaped mass in RUQ of abdomen.
- Progressive fever and prostration if peritonitis occurs.

Treatment includes:

- **Barium or air enema** to diagnose and apply pressure that may resolve the intussusception.
- **Surgical repair** if there is shock, peritonitis, intestinal perforation, or failure to resolve with barium/air enema.

HYPERTROPHIC PYLORIC STENOSIS

Hypertrophic pyloric stenosis (PS) is obstruction of the pyloric sphincter between the gastric pylorus and small intestine, caused by hypertrophy and hyperplasia of the circular muscle of the pylorus so the enlarged tissue obstructs the sphincter. PS is more common in boys (especially firstborn) than girls and has a genetic predisposition (2-3 times more common in Caucasians). Onset of *symptoms* is usually >3 weeks:

- **Projectile vomiting** (1-4 feet) usually shortly after eating but may be delayed for a few hours. Emesis may be blood-tinged but non-bilious.
- Child is hungry and eats readily, but shows **weight loss** and signs of **dehydration**.
- **Upper abdominal distention** with palpable mass in epigastrium (to right of umbilicus).
- Visible left to right **peristaltic waves**.

Diagnosis is based on ultrasound. Decreased sodium and potassium levels may not be evident with dehydration.

Treatment:

- **Intravenous fluids** to restore hydration and electrolyte balance.
- **Surgical pyloromyotomy**: longitudinal incisions through the circular muscle fibers down to the submucosa to release the restriction and allow the muscle to expand.

BOWEL OBSTRUCTION/INFARCTION

Bowel obstruction occurs when there is a mechanical obstruction of the **passage of intestinal contents** because of constriction of the lumen, occlusion of the lumen, or lack of muscular contractions (paralytic ileus). Obstruction may be caused by congenital or acquired abnormalities/disorders. Symptoms include:

- Abdominal pain and distention.
- Abdominal rigidity.
- Vomiting and dehydration.
- Diminished or no bowel sounds.
- Severe constipation (obstipation).
- Respiratory distress from diaphragm pushing against pleural cavity.
- Shock as plasma volume diminishes and electrolytes enter intestines from bloodstream.
- Sepsis as bacteria proliferates in bowel and invades bloodstream.

Bowel infarction is ischemia of the intestines related to severely restricted blood supply. It can be the result of a number of different conditions, such as strangulated bowel or occlusion of arteries of the mesentery, and may follow untreated bowel obstruction. People present with acute abdomen and shock, and mortality rates are very high even with resection of infarcted bowel.

CONSTIPATION AND IMPACTION

Constipation is a condition with bowel movements less frequent than normal for a person, or hard, small stool that is evacuated fewer than 3 times weekly. Food moves through the gastrointestinal from the small intestine to the colon in semi-liquid form. Constipation results from the colon, where fluid is absorbed. If too much fluid is absorbed, the stool can become too dry. People may have abdominal distention and cramps and need to strain for defecation.

Fecal impaction occurs when the hard stool moves into the rectum and becomes a large, dense, immovable mass that cannot be evacuated even with straining, usually as a result of chronic constipation. In addition to abdominal cramps and distention, the person may feel intense rectal pressure and pain accompanied by a sense of urgency to defecate. Nausea and vomiting may also occur. Hemorrhoids will often become engorged. Fecal incontinence, with liquid stool leaking about the impaction is common.

DIAGNOSTIC PROCEDURES FOR CONSTIPATION

Medical procedures to evaluate causes of **constipation** should be preceded by a careful history as this may help to define the type of diarrhea and guide the choice of diagnostic procedures. Most tests are necessary only for severe constipation that does not respond to treatment. Medical diagnostic procedures may include the following:

- **Physical exam** should include rectal exam and abdominal palpation to assess for obvious hard stool or impaction.
- **Blood tests** can identify hypothyroidism and excess parathyroid hormone.
- **Abdominal x-ray** may show large amounts of stool in the colon.
- **Barium enema** can indicate tumors or strictures causing obstruction.
- **Colonic transit studies** can show defects of the neuromuscular system.
- **Defecography** shows defecation process and abnormalities of anatomy.
- **Anorectal manometry studies** show malfunction of anorectal muscles.
- **Colonic motility studies** measure the pattern of colonic pressure.
- **Colonoscope** allows direct visualization of the lumen of the rectum and colon.

INTESTINAL PERFORATION

Intestinal perforation is a complete rupture or penetration of the **intestinal wall**. There are a number of causes:

- Traumatic injuries, such as gunshot or knife wounds.
- NSAIDs and/or aspirin, especially in elderly with diverticulitis.
- Acute appendicitis.
- Peptic ulcer disease.
- Iatrogenic causes: laparoscopy, endoscopy, colonoscopy, radiotherapy.
- Bacterial infections.
- Inflammatory bowel diseases, such as Crohn's disease or ulcerative colitis.
- Ingestion of toxic substances (acids) or foreign bodies (toothpicks).

The danger posed by infection after perforation varies depending upon the site. The stomach and proximal portions of the small intestine have little bacteria, but the distal portion of the small intestine contains aerobic bacteria, such as E. coli, as well as anaerobic bacteria. *Symptoms* include abdominal pain and distention and rigidity, fever, guarding and rebound tenderness, tachycardia and paralytic ileus with nausea and vomiting. *Treatment* is as for peritonitis, with antibiotics and surgical repair.

BRISTOL STOOL FORM

The **Bristol Stool Form** is named for Bristol University in England, where it was designed as a general description of stool constancy or form. The form is often given to people when they do a bowel diary so that they can more clearly identify for healthcare providers what types of stools they are passing.

The scale has descriptions and pictures to help people identify the correct type of stool:

- **Type 1**: Separate small hard lumps of stool that are difficult to pass.
- **Type 2**: Sausage-shaped lumpy stool.
- **Type 3**: Sausage-shaped and lumpy but with cracks on the surface.
- **Type 4**: Long, smooth, soft, snake-like stool.
- **Type 5**: Soft blobs of stool that are easily passed and have clear-cut edges.
- **Type 6**: Mushy, fluffy pieces of stool with uneven ragged edges.
- **Type 7**: Watery stool that is entirely liquid with no solid pieces.

Reproductive

VAGINAL BLEEDING/ABORTION

Vaginal bleeding during the first trimester of pregnancy may indicate spontaneous abortion, ectopic pregnancy, gestational trophoblastic disease, or infection. All women of childbearing age with an intact uterus presenting with abdominal pain or vaginal bleeding should be assessed for pregnancy. Abortion classifications:

- **Threatened**: Vaginal bleeding during first half of pregnancy without cervical dilatation.
- **Inevitable**: Vaginal bleeding with cervical dilatation.
- **Incomplete**: Incomplete loss of products of conception, usually between 6-14 weeks.
- **Complete**: Complete loss of products of conception, before 20 weeks.
- **Missed**: Death of fetus before 20 weeks without loss of products of conception within 4 weeks.
- **Septic**: Infection with abortion.

Diagnostic tests include:

- Pelvic examination.
- CBC, Rh factor, antibody screen, urinalysis, quantitative serum β-hCG level.
- Ultrasound to rule out ectopic pregnancy.

Treatment includes:

- Suctioning of vaginal vault with Yankauer suction tip with pathologic examination of tissue.
- Evacuation of uterus for incomplete abortion.
- RhoGAM (50-150µg) for bleeding in unsensitized Rh-negative women.

Nausea and Vomiting and Hyperemesis Gravidarum Related to Pregnancy

About 60-80% of pregnant woman suffer from nausea and vomiting (NV), especially during the first trimester, but only about 2% suffer severe (sometimes intractable) nausea and vomiting, known as **hyperemesis gravidarum (HG),** associated with weight loss, dehydration, hypokalemia, or ketonemia. Nausea and vomiting may be associated with numerous disorders, including cholelithiasis, pancreatitis, hepatitis, and ectopic pregnancy; it is especially accompanied by abdominal pain. *Diagnosis* includes:

- Physical examination to rule out other disorders.
- CBC with serum electrolytes, BUN, creatinine, and urinalysis.

Ketonuria is an indication of inadequate nutrition. *Treatment* includes:

- Intravenous fluids with 5% glucose in normal saline or Ringer's lactate.
- Oral fluids after nausea and vomiting controlled.
- Antiemetic drugs.

Hypertensive Disorders of Pregnancy During the Second Half of Pregnancy

Hypertensive disorders of pregnancy comprise a continuum ranging from mild to severe:

- **Hypertension**: BP ↑140/90 or 20-mm Hg ↑ in systolic or 10-mm diastolic. May be chronic or transient without signs of preeclampsia or eclampsia.
- **Preeclampsia**: Hypertension associated with proteinuria (300 mg/24 h) and edema (peripheral or generalized) or ↑ of ≥5 pounds of weight in 1 week after 20th week of gestation. Severe preeclampsia is BP ≥160/110. Symptoms include headache, abdominal pain, and visual disturbances.
- **Eclampsia**: Preeclampsia with seizures occurring at 20th week of gestation to 1 month after delivery.
- **HELLP syndrome** (hemolysis, elevated liver enzymes (AST and ALT), and low platelets (<100,000). Usually accompanied by epigastric or right upper quadrant pain.

Treatments include:

- **Chronic hypertension**: Methyldopa beginning with 250 mg every 6 hours.
- Preeclampsia, eclampsia, HELLP:
  o Delivery of fetus (may be delayed with mild pre-eclampsia if < 37 weeks gestation)
  o Magnesium sulfate IV 4-6 g over 15 minutes initially and then 1-2 g per hour.
  o Antihypertensive drugs.

Abruptio Placentae and Placenta Previa

An **abruptio placenta** occurs when the placenta separates prematurely from the wall of the uterus. *Symptoms* include:

- Vaginal bleeding.
- Tender uterus with ↑resting tone.
- Uterine contractions (hypertonic or hyperactive.
- Nausea and vomiting (in some patients).
- Dizziness.

Complications include fetal distress, hypotension and DIC, as well as fetal and/or maternal death. Fetal death is common with ≥50% separation.

Diagnosis includes:

- Ultrasound.
- CBC and type and cross match.
- Coagulation studies (50% have coagulopathy).

Treatment includes:

- Gynecological consultation.
- Crystalloids to increase blood volume.
- Fresh frozen plasma for coagulopathy.

Placenta previa occurs when the placenta implants over the cervical opening. Implantation may be complete (covering the entire opening), partial, or marginal (to the edge of the cervical opening). Symptoms include painless bleeding after 20th week of gestation. Diagnosis is per ultrasound. Vaginal examination with digit or speculum should be avoided.

PRETERM LABOR AND PROM

Preterm or premature labor occurs within weeks 20-37. **Premature rupture of membrane (PROM)** occurs when the membranes rupture before the onset of labor, and may lead to premature labor. There are numerous causes for PROM, including infections and digital pelvic exams. When a woman presents in labor, the estimated date of delivery (EDD) should be obtained by questioning the date of the last menstrual period (LMP) and using a gestation calculator wheel or estimating with Nägele's rule:

First day of LMP minus 3 months plus 7 days = EDD

Fetal viability is very low before 23 weeks of gestation but by 25 weeks, delaying delivery for 2 days can increase survival rates by 10%. Tocolytic drugs, which have many negative side effects, may be used to delay delivery in order to administer glucocorticoids, such as betamethasone or dexamethasone, to improve fetal lung maturity between weeks 24-36. **Tocolytics** include:

- β-Adrenergics
- Magnesium sulfates
- Calcium channel blockers
- Prostaglandin synthetase inhibitors

ECTOPIC PREGNANCY

Ectopic pregnancy occurs when the fertilized ovum implants **outside the uterus** in an ovary, fallopian tube (the most common site), peritoneal cavity, or cervix. Early symptoms may include:

- Indications of pregnancy: amenorrhea, breast tenderness, nausea and vomiting.
- Positive Chadwick's sign (blue discoloration of cervix).
- Positive Hegar's sign (softening of isthmus).
- Bleeding may be the first indication as hormones fluctuate.
- Hormone hCG present in blood and urine.

Symptoms of **rupture** include:

- One-sided or generalized abdominal pain.
- ↓ Hemoglobin and hematocrit.
- Hypotension with hemorrhage.
- Right shoulder pain because of irritation of the subdiaphragmatic phrenic nerve.

Diagnostic studies include: vaginal exam, pregnancy test, transvaginal sonography (TVS) to rule out intrauterine pregnancy, hCG titers (increase more slowly with ectopic pregnancy), and progesterone level >22 to rule out ectopic pregnancy. Treatments include: Methotrexate IM or IV if unruptured and <3.5 cm in size to inhibit growth and allow body to expel and laparoscopic linear salpingostomy or salpingectomy.

OVARIAN CYSTS

Ovarian cysts can grow within or on the **ovaries**:

- **Functional**: follicular cyst usually resolves in 1-3 months; corpus luteum usually resolve in a few weeks but cyst may grow to 4 inches, causing torsion and pain.
- **Cystadenoma forma** on exterior of ovary and may enlarge and cause pain.
- **Endometrioma** attaches to ovaries and cause pain during menses and sexual activity.
- **Dermoid cyst** may enlarge and cause pain.
- **Polycystic ovaries** may have multiple cysts.
- Ovarian cysts may cause problems if they rupture or hemorrhage and if they twist or become infected. Presenting *symptoms* include:
  - Hypotension and hypovolemia if hemorrhage occurs, pain (often acute) and tenderness in lower abdomen on affected side and/or lower back pain, dysuria, and weight gain.

Diagnostic studies include:

- Pregnancy test to rule out ectopic pregnancy, ultrasound with Doppler flow.

Treatment depends upon the type of cyst and complications:

- Emergency surgery for torsion.
- **Antibiotics** for infection.
- **Hormone therapy** may be useful for endometrioma.

PELVIC ORGAN PROLAPSE

Pelvic organ prolapse occurs when pelvic floor muscles weaken with age or trauma and cannot support the pelvic organs. The uterus is the only organ that can fall into the vagina. Other organs can push against and cause a protrusion in the wall of the vagina.

- **Cystocele** is the bladder falling toward the vagina, causing an anterior vaginal wall protrusion.
- **Urethrocele** is the urethra pushing against the anterior vaginal wall, near the vaginal orifice, often occurring with a cystocele and called a cystourethrocele.
- **Enterocele** is part of the small intestine falling into the space between the rectum and posterior vaginal wall.
- **Rectocele** is the rectum protruding into the posterior vaginal wall while a rectal prolapse is the rectum falling through the anus.

- **Uterine prolapse** is the uterus falling into the vagina.
- **Vaginal vault prolapse** is the top of the vagina falling in on itself after hysterectomy.

Vulvovaginitis

Vulvovaginitis is inflammation of **vulvar and vaginal tissues**:

- **Bacterial vaginosis** (Gardnerella or other bacteria).
- **Fungal infections** (usually Candida albicans).
- **Parasitic infections** (Trichomonas vaginalis.).
- **Allergic contact vaginitis** (from soaps or other irritants).
- **Atrophic vaginitis** (post-menopause).

Symptoms include vaginal odor, swelling, vaginal discharge or bleeding, pain and discomfort, severe itching (common with Candida albicans). *Diagnostic studies* include:

- Physical exam and culture of discharge, pH testing with Nitrazine paper:
  - **>4.5** is typical of bacterial and Trichomonas infections.
  - **<4.5** is typical of fungal infections.

Treatment includes:

- **Bacterial** infections:
  - Metronidazole 500 mg orally BID 7 days.
  - Metronidazole gel 0.75% intravaginally BID 5 days.
  - Clindamycin cream 2% intravaginally at bedtime 7 days.
- **Fungal** infections:
  - Diflucan® 150 mg tablet in 1 dose.
  - Vaginal creams, tablets, or suppositories, such as Femstat® 2% cream 3 days or Vagistat 6.5% ointment for 1 dose.
- **Parasitic** (Trichomonas)
  - Metronidazole 2 g orally in 1 dose.

Bartholin Cyst

The **Bartholin glands** are small glands located on both sides of the vagina in the lips of the labia minora. The glands help to lubricate the vulvar area. A Bartholin **cyst** occurs when a duct to 1 gland becomes obstructed, usually because of infection or trauma, resulting in swelling and formation of a cyst (usually 1-3 cm but may be much larger with infection). Bartholin cyst is most common in women in their 20s. Blockage may result from tumors as well, but usually in women over 40. *Symptoms* of a Bartholin cyst include:

- Palpable mass on 1 side of the vagina (usually painless).
- Pain and tenderness and increasing size of lesion if infection and abscess occurs.

Treatment includes:

- Warm moist compresses or sitz baths.
- Antibiotics for infection.
- Surgical incision and drainage may be necessary in some cases.

PID

Pelvic inflammatory disease (PID) comprises infections of the **upper reproductive system**, often ascending from vagina and cervix, and includes salpingitis, endometritis, tubo-ovarian abscess, peritonitis, and perihepatitis. Neisseria gonorrhoeae and Chlamydia trachomatis are implicated in most cases but some infections are polymicrobial. Complications include increase in ectopic pregnancy and tubal factor infertility. *Symptoms* include lower abdominal pain, vaginal pain, discharge, or bleeding, dyspareunia, dysuria, fever, and nausea and vomiting. *Diagnostic studies* include:

- Pregnancy test. Vaginal secretion testing, endocervical culture.
- Complete blood count (CBC). Syphilis, HIV, and hepatitis testing.
- Transvaginal pelvic ultrasound.
- Endometrial biopsy.
- Laparoscopy for definitive diagnosis.

Treatments include:

- Broad spectrum **antibiotics**:
  - (In-patient) Cefotetan 2 g IV every 12 hours or every 6 hours with doxycycline 100 mg every 12 hours.
  - (Out-patient) Ofloxacin 400 mg twice daily for 1 week with or without Metronidazole 500 mg twice daily for 2 weeks.
- **Laparoscopy** to drain abscesses if symptoms do not improve <72 hours.
- **Treatment** specific to associated disorders (such as human immunodeficiency virus [HIV] or hepatitis).

PHIMOSIS AND PARAPHIMOSIS

Phimosis and paraphimosis are both restrictive disorders of the **penis** that occur in males who are uncircumcised or incorrectly circumcised. **Phimosis** is the inability to retract the foreskin proximal to the glans penis, sometimes resulting in urinary retention or hematuria. *Treatments* include:

- Dilating the foreskin with a hemostat (temporary solution).
- Circumcision.
- Application of topical steroids (triamcinolone 0.025% twice daily) from end of foreskin to glans corona for 4-6 weeks.

Paraphimosis occurs when the foreskin tightens above the glans penis and can't be extended to normal positioning; resulting in edema of the foreskin and circulatory impairment of the glans penis, sometimes progressing to gangrene so immediate treatment is critical. *Symptoms* include pain, swelling, and inability to urinate. *Treatments* include:

- **Compression** of the glans to reduce edema (wrapping tightly with 2-inch elastic bandage for 5 minutes).
- Reducing edema by making several **puncture wounds** with 22-25-gauge needle.
- Local **anesthetic** and dorsal **incision** to relieve pressure.

PROSTATITIS AND BENIGN PROSTATIC HYPERTROPHY

Prostatitis is an acute infection of the prostate gland, commonly caused by Escherichia coli, Pseudomonas, Staphylococcus, or other bacteria. *Symptoms* include:

- Fever and chills
- Lower back pain
- Urinary frequency
- Dysuria
- Painful ejaculation
- Perineal discomfort

Diagnosis is based on clinical findings of perineal tenderness and spasm of rectal sphincter.

Treatment includes:

- **Ciprofloxacin** 500 mg orally twice daily for 1 month (treatment of choice).
- **Trimethoprim/sulfamethoxazole** (TMP/SMX) DS twice daily for 1 month.
- **Urethral culture** to check for sexually transmitted diseases (STDs).

Benign prostatic hypertrophy/hyperplasia usually develops after age 40. The prostate may slowly enlarge, but the surrounding tissue restrains outward growth, so the gland compresses the urethra. The bladder wall also goes through changes, becoming thicker and irritated, so that it begins to spasm, causing frequent urinations. The bladder muscle eventually weakens and the bladder fails to empty completely. *Symptoms* include urgency, dribbling, frequency, nocturia, incontinence, retention, and bladder distention. *Diagnosis* may include intravenous pyelogram (IVP), cystogram, and prostate-specific antigen (PSA).

Treatment includes:

- Catheterization for urinary retention/bladder distention.
- Surgical excision.

EPIDIDYMITIS AND ORCHITIS

Epididymitis, infection of the epididymis, is often associated with infection in a **testis** (epididymo-orchitis). In children, infection may be related to congenital anomalies that allow reflux of urine. In sexually active males under 35, it is usually related to sexually transmitted diseases (STDs). In males >40, it is usually related to urinary infections or benign prostatic hyperplasia (BPH) with urethral obstruction. Symptoms include progressive pain in lower abdomen, scrotum and/or testicle. Late symptoms include large tender scrotal mass. Diagnosis includes:

- Clinical examination
- Pyuria
- Sonography
- Urethral culture for sexually transmitted diseases (STDs)

Orchitis alone is rare but occurs with mumps, other viral infections, and epididymitis. Ultrasound may be needed to rule out testicular torsion.

Treatment for both conditions depends upon the cause, but epididymitis usually resolves with **antibiotics**:

- <35-40 associated with STDs: Ceftriaxone 250 mg IM and doxycycline 100 mg orally twice daily for 10 days.
- >35-40 associated with other bacteria:
  - Ciprofloxacin 500 mg twice daily for 10-14 days.
  - Levofloxacin 250 mg daily for 10-14 days.
  - Trimethoprim/sulfamethoxazole (TMP/SMX) DS twice daily for 10-14 days.

Renal/GU

RENAL AND URETERAL CALCULI

Renal and urinary calculi occur frequently, more commonly in male patients, and can relate to diseases (hyperparathyroidism, renal tubular acidosis, gout) and lifestyle factors, such as sedentary work. Additionally, some medications can precipitate calculi. Calculi can form at any age, most composed of **calcium**, and can range in size from very tiny to >6 mm. Those <4 mm can usually pass in the urine easily. *Symptoms* occur with obstruction and are usually of sudden onset and acute:

- Severe flank pain radiating to abdomen and ipsilateral testicle or labium majus, abdominal, or pelvic pain (young children).
- Nausea and vomiting.
- Diaphoresis.
- Hematuria.

Diagnostic studies include:

- Clinical findings.
- Urinalysis.
- Pregnancy test to rule out ectopic pregnancy.
- Blood urea nitrogen (BUN) and creatinine if indicated.
- Helical computed tomography (CT [non-contrast]) is diagnostic, ultrasound (for pregnant women and children), IV urography.

Treatments include:

- Analgesia: opiates and nonsteroidal inflammatory drugs (NSAIDs).
- Instructions and equipment for straining urine.
- Antibiotics if concurrent infection.
- Referral to urologist for large calculi.

URINARY TRACT INFECTIONS

CYSTITIS

Urinary infections, cystitis, are common and often-chronic low-grade **kidney infections** develop over time, so observing for symptoms of urinary infections and treating promptly are very important:

- Changes in **character** of urine:
  - *Appearance*: The urine may become cloudy from mucus or purulent material. Hematuria may be present.
  - *Color*: Urine usually becomes concentrated and may be dark yellow/orange or brownish in color.
  - *Odor*: Urine may have a very strong or foul odor.
  - *Output*: Urinary output may decrease markedly.
- **Pain**: There may be lower back or flank pain from inflammation of the kidneys.
- **Systemic**: Fever, chills, headache, and general malaise often accompany urine infections. Some people suffer lack of appetite as well as nausea and vomiting. Fever usually indicates that the infection has affected the kidneys. Children may develop incontinence or loose stools and cry excessively.

Treatment includes:

- Increased fluid intake.
- Antibiotics.

PYELONEPHRITIS

Pyelonephritis is a potentially organ-damaging bacterial infection of the parenchyma of the kidney. Pyelonephritis can result in abscess formation, sepsis, and kidney failure. Pyelonephritis is especially dangerous for those who are immunocompromised, pregnant, or diabetic. Most infections are caused by *Escherichia coli. Diagnostic studies* include urinalysis, blood and urine cultures. Patients may require hospitalization or careful follow-up.

Symptoms vary widely but can include:

- Dysuria and frequency, hematuria, flank and/or low back pain.
- Fever and chills.
- Costovertebral angle tenderness.
- Change in feeding habits (infants).
- Change in mental status (geriatric)

Young women often exhibit symptoms more associated with lower urinary infection, so the condition may be overlooked.

Treatment includes:

- Analgesia.
- Antipyretics.
- Intravenous fluids

86

- Antibiotics: started but may be changed based on cultures.
    - IV ceftriaxone with fluoroquinolone orally for 14 days.
    - Monitor BUN. Normal 7-8 mg/dL (8-20 mg/dL >age 60). Increase indicates impaired renal function, as urea is end product of protein metabolism.

Ophthalmic

GLAUCOMA

Glaucoma comprises a group of eye conditions characterized by damage to the optic nerve and vision impairment. Risk factors include:

- >40 years.
- Family history.
- Cardiovascular disease.
- Myopia.
- Migraine syndromes.
- Corticosteroid use.
- Diabetes.
- African American.

With glaucoma, **intraocular pressure** (normally 10-21 mm Hg) increases as aqueous fluid is inhibited from flowing because of impairment of the drainage system and a decreased angle (<45°) between the iris and cornea. There are a number of different types of glaucoma, but symptoms are similar: blurred vision, halos about lights, lack of focus, eye discomfort, headache, and difficulty seeing in low light. Referral should be made to an ophthalmologist for evaluation. Treatment may include topical β-blockers, miotics, adrenergic agonists, carbonic anhydrase inhibitors, and prostaglandins. Surgical management includes laser trabeculoplasty, laser iridotomy, filtering procedures, trabeculectomy, and drainage implants/shunts.

> **Review Video: Glaucoma and Cataracts**
> Visit mometrix.com/academy and enter code: 279024

ACUTE ANGLE-CLOSURE GLAUCOMA

Acute angle-closure glaucoma is a medical emergency that involves increased intraocular pressure and impairment of vision in those without previous history of glaucoma because of occlusion of drainage, which forces the iris forward. This condition is most common in the elderly. *Symptoms* include:

- 2 of these: eye pain (periorbital) associated with headache, nausea and vomiting, ↓visual acuity with halos AND
- 3 of these: intraocular pressure >21 mm Hg (may be as high as 50), conjunctival injection, edema of epithelium of cornea, pupil non-reactive and mid-dilated, and shallower anterior chamber.

Treatment aims to reduce pressure in the eye by reducing production of aqueous humor:

- Topic β-blocker (Timoptic® 0.5%) one drop.
- Topical a-agonist (Iopidine® 0.1%) one drop.

- Topical steroid (Pred Forte® 1%) one drop every 15 minutes for 1 hour and then every hour.
- Acetazolamide (Diamox®) 500 mg IV or by mouth.
- Mannitol 1-2 g/kg IV.
- Pilocarpine 1-2% after pressure reduced.
- Continued monitoring of intraocular pressure every hour.

CORNEAL ABRASIONS

Corneal abrasion results from direct scratching or scraping trauma to the eye, often involving contact lenses, causing a defect in the epithelium of the cornea. Infection with corneal ulceration can occur with abrasions. *Symptoms* include:

- Pain.
- Intense photophobia.
- Tearing.

Determining the cause and source of the abrasion is important for treatment as organic sources pose the danger of fungal infection and soft contact lenses pose the danger of Pseudomonas infection. *Diagnosis* includes:

- **Topical anesthetic** prior to testing for visual acuity.
- **Fluorescent staining** and examination with cobalt blue light.
- **Eversion of eyelid** to check for foreign body.
- Examine **cornea** and assess anterior chamber with slit lamp.

Treatments include:

- **Cycloplegic agent** to relieve spasm and pain: cyclopentolate 1%.
- **Erythromycin ophthalmic ointment** 4 times daily with or without eye patch if not related to contact lens AND without eye patch if related to organic source.
- **Tobramycin ophthalmic ointment** 4 times daily without eye patch if related to contact lens.

CHEMICAL EYE BURNS

Chemical burns are caused by splashing of chemicals (solid, liquid, or fumes) into any part of the eye, often related to facial burns. Chemical burns may damage the **cornea and conjunctiva** although other layers of the eye may also be damaged, depending upon the chemical and degree of saturation. Many injuries are work-related and involve alkali (> 7 pH), acid (< 7 pH) (muriatic acid or sulfuric acid), or other irritants (neutral pH) such as pepper spray. Alkali chemicals (such as ammonia, lime, and lye) usually cause the most serious injuries. Symptoms include pain, blurring of vision, tearing, and eyelid edema.

Diagnosis includes:

- History of event.
- Eye exam showing corneal irritation.

Treatment includes:

- Irrigate eye and other areas of contact with copious amounts of water or normal saline.
- Litmus paper exam of eye to determine residual pH and continue irrigation until pH returns to neutral.
- Cycloplegic agent to relieve spasm and pain: Cyclopentolate 1%.
- Antibiotic ointment to prevent infection.

CATARACTS

A **cataract** is opacity of the **lens** that can occur at any age but is most common in the elderly. Cataracts can occur in 1 eye or bilaterally and usually progress slowly. There are 3 primary types of age-related cataracts:

- **Nuclear**: Associated with myopia and tends to worsen myopia and blur vision.
- **Cortical**: Involves the anterior, posterior or equatorial lens cortex, with vision worse in bright light.
- **Posterior subcapsular**: Anterior to the posterior capsule, tends to develop in younger people or those on chronic corticosteroids. Eye becomes increasingly photophobic and near vision diminishes.

Patients most commonly complain of blurring of vision without pain. Other *symptoms* may be astigmatism, diplopia, color shift, and reduction in light transmission. There is no medical *treatment*. Patients should be referred to ophthalmologists for evaluation. Surgical repair is done when decreased vision interferes with activities.

INFECTIOUS CONJUNCTIVITIS

Infectious conjunctivitis (pink eye) is inflammation of the conjunctiva of the eye from bacteria or viruses. If it occurs <30 days of birth, it is referred to as ophthalmia neonatorum and is commonly acquired during delivery:

- **Pathogenic agents** include Chlamydia trachomatis, Neisseria gonorrhea, and herpesvirus.
- **Antibiotic drops** are applied to the newborns eyes to prevent conjunctivitis. Intravenous acyclovir is given to infants exposed to herpesvirus.

Infectious conjunctivitis in older children (or adults) is usually caused by Staphylococci, Streptococci, Pneumococci, or viruses and is extremely contagious, so good hand hygiene is essential. It is difficult to differentiate between bacterial and viral infections without cultures. The child should be kept from school and other children for 24 hours after starting treatment or until *symptoms* subside:

- Red, swollen, itchy conjunctiva.
- Eye pain.
- Purulent discharge.
- Scratchy feeling under eyelids.
- Mild photophobia.

Treatment is usually antibiotic drops or ointment and cool compresses although many cases are caused by viruses and the condition often disappears without treatment in 3-5 days.

KERATITIS

Keratitis is inflammation of the **cornea**, and it may be superficial or deep, which usually results in scarring. There are multiple causes for keratitis, including bacterial, fungal, viral, and parasitic infections as well as allergic response to antigens and photokeratitis from exposure to ultraviolet rays. It can also arise from wearing contact lenses. Any corneal ulceration can allow pathogens to enter the eye and cause infection. *Symptoms* include:

- Pain and tearing.
- Photophobia.
- ↓Visual acuity.
- Discharge.

Diagnosis includes:

- Careful examination with slit lamp.
- Culture of discharge.

Treatment includes:

- Antifungal or antibacterial drops as indicated.
- Trifluridine (Viroptic®) every 2-3 hours during awake hours to maximum of 9 drops daily for herpes simplex until healing and then 4 x daily for about 1 week.
- Artificial tears.
- Analgesia.

ULTRAVIOLET KERATITIS

Ultraviolet (UV) keratitis results from injury to the **corneal epithelium** from exposure to UV rays from the sun (as in snow blindness where the snow reflects UV rays into the eyes) or from artificial light sources, such as tanning beds, halogen lights, or welding torches (flash burn). *Symptoms* usually occur 6-12 hours after exposure and include pain, tearing, photophobia, ↓visual acuity, spasm of eyelids, and exam shows punctate irregularities of corneal surface and corneal haze. An accurate history that details exposure to UV rays should be done. *Diagnostic studies* include:

- Examination of eye and lids.
- Slit lamp exam with fluorescein staining.

Treatment includes:

- **Cycloplegic agent** to relieve spasm and pain: cyclopentolate 1%.
- Antibiotic ophthalmic ointment, such as Erythromycin.
- **Analgesia**: opiate (oxycodone) and nonsteroidal anti-inflammatory drugs (NSAIDs; e.g., ibuprofen 600 mg 4 times daily).
- **Topical NSAIDs** are sometimes used.
- Healing should be evident within 24-48 hours.

Neurological/Neurovascular

ALS

Amyotrophic lateral sclerosis (ALS) is a progressive degenerative disease of the **upper and lower motor neurons**, resulting in progressively severe symptoms, such as spasticity,

90

hyperreflexia and muscle weakness and paralysis that can cause dysphagia, cramping, muscular atrophy, and respiratory dysfunction. ALS may be sporadic or familial (rare). Speech may become monotone; however, cognitive functioning usually remains intact. Eventually, patients become immobile and cannot breathe independently. *Diagnosis* is based on history, electromyography, nerve conduction studies, and magnetic resonance imaging (MRI). Treatment includes riluzole to delay progression of the disease. Patients may develop an acute complication, such as acute respiratory failure, aspiration pneumonia, or other trauma. *Treatment* includes:

- **Nebulizer treatments** with bronchodilators and steroids.
- **Antibiotics** for infection.
- Mechanical **ventilation**.

If ventilatory assistance is needed, it's important to determine if the patient has a living will expressing the wish to be ventilated or not or has assigned power of attorney for health matters to someone to make this decision.

> **Review Video: Amyotrophic Lateral Sclerosis (ALS)**
> Visit mometrix.com/academy and enter code: 178603

MULTIPLE SCLEROSIS

Multiple sclerosis is an autoimmune disorder of the central nervous system in which the **myelin sheath** around the nerves is damaged and replaced by scar tissue that prevents conduction of nerve impulses. Symptoms vary widely and can include problems with balance and coordination, tremors, slurring of speech, cognitive impairment, vision impairment and nystagmus, pain, and bladder and bowel dysfunction. *Symptoms* may be relapsing-remitting or progressive or a combination. Onset is usually 20-30, with incidence higher in females. Patient may initially present with problems walking or falling or optic neuritis (30%) causing loss of central vision. Males may complain of sexual dysfunction as an early symptom. Others have dysuria with urinary retention. *Diagnosis* is based on clinical and neurological examination and magnetic resonance imaging (MRI). *Treatment* is symptomatic and includes treatment to shorten duration of episodes and slow progress.

- **Glucocorticoids**: methylprednisolone.
- **Immunomodulator**: Interferon-β, glatiramer acetate, natalizumab.
- Immunosuppressant: Mitoxantrone.
- **Hormone**: Estriol (for females).

MYASTHENIA GRAVIS

Myasthenia gravis (MG) is an autoimmune disorder of the **neuromuscular system** in which acetylcholine receptors are damaged at neural synapses, preventing transmission of impulses to contract muscles. The thymus gland develops abnormalities and sometimes thymoma. *Symptoms* of MG are muscle weakness, which decreases with rest. Eye muscles are often affected first, resulting in ptosis and visual disturbances such as diplopia. General weakness in extremities, neck, and face as well as dysphagia and slurred speech occur. Acute respiratory failure can occur as part of myasthenic crisis before diagnosis or related to fever, infection, or drug therapy. *Diagnosis* of MG is from history, neurological exam, antibody testing, edrophonium chloride testing to differentiate exacerbation of disease from cholinergic crisis, electromyogram, and pulmonary function tests. *Treatments*:

- **Crisis**: mechanical ventilation and treatment of underlying cause.
- **Thymectomy**: relieves symptoms in 70%.
- **Immunosuppressants**: azathioprine, cyclosporine, and prednisone.
- Acetyl-cholinesterase inhibitors: pyridostigmine.

Many drugs can trigger respiratory failure, so drug lists should be checked and ventilatory equipment available when treating MG patients.

> **Review Video: Myasthenia Gravis**
> Visit mometrix.com/academy and enter code: 162510

BELL'S PALSY

Bell's palsy is caused by inflammation of cranial nerve VII, usually from a herpes simplex I or II infection, and generally affects only 1 side of the paired nerves. Onset is generally sudden, and symptoms peak by 48 hours with a wide range of presentation. *Symptoms* usually subside within 2-6 months but may persist for 1 year:

- Mild weakness on 1 side of face to complete paralysis with distortion of features.
- Drooping of eyelid and mouth.
- Tearing in affected eye.
- Taste impairment.

Diagnosis includes:

- Neurological, eye, parotid gland, and ear exam to rule out other cranial nerve involvement or conditions.

Treatment includes:

- **Artificial tears** during daytime with lubricating ophthalmic ointment and patch at night to protect eye.
- **Optional treatments** (not completely supported by data): Prednisone 60 mg daily for 5 days with tapering over 5 days AND
- **Acyclovir** 400 mg 5 times daily for 10 days.

PARKINSON'S DISEASE

Parkinson's disease (PD) is an **extrapyramidal movement motor system disorder** caused by loss of brain cells that produce dopamine. Typical symptoms include tremor of face and extremities, rigidity, bradykinesia, akinesia, poor posture, and lack of balance and coordination, causing increasing problems with mobility, talking, and swallowing. Some may suffer depression and mood changes. Tremors usually present unilaterally in an upper extremity. Diagnosis includes:

- Cogwheel rigidity test: extremity put through passive range of motion causes ↑muscle tone and ratchet-like movements.
- Physical and neurological exam.
- Complete history to rule out drug-induced Parkinson's akinesia.

92

Treatment includes:

- Symptomatic support.
- **Dopaminergic therapy**: Levodopa, amantadine, and carbidopa.
- **Anticholinergics**: trihexyphenidyl, benztropine.
- Drug-induced Parkinson's: terminate drugs.

Drug therapy tends to decrease in efficiency over time, and patients may present with marked ↑ in symptoms. Discontinuing the drugs for 1 week may exacerbate symptoms initially, but functioning may improve when drugs are reintroduced.

> **Review Video: <u>Parkinson's Disease</u>**
> Visit mometrix.com/academy and enter code: 110876

ALZHEIMER'S DISEASE

Alzheimer's disease is the most common cause of dementia. Alzheimer's disease causes the **cerebral cortex** to shrink, particularly about the hippocampus, where memories are stored, and the ventricles to enlarge. Damage occurs within the network of neurons, disrupting electrical charges and neurotransmitters. Sticky β-amyloid protein plaques form between neurons, and tangles form from the tau protein as the neurons begin to collapse and die. There are 2 types of Alzheimer's disease, but the *symptoms* are the same:

- **Late-onset** Alzheimer's occurs >65 years and affects 5 million Americans.
- **Early-onset** <65 years usually begins in the 50s but may occur earlier. This is an inherited form of Alzheimer's with a defective gene on chromosome 1, 4, or 21.

Diagnosis is based on history, physical exam to rule out other causes of dementia, and assessment of cognition with Mini-mental state exam (MMSE) or Mini-cog. *Treatment* to slow progression of the disease is with anti-cholinesterase drugs, such as Aricept® (donepezil) and Exelon® (rivastigmine) and/or Namenda® (memantine).

ASSESSMENT OF COGNITION/DEMENTIA

Patients with evidence of dementia or short-term memory loss, often associated with **Alzheimer's disease**, should have cognition assessed. The Mini-mental state exam (MMSE) or the Mini-cog test is commonly used. Both require the patient to carry out specified tasks:

- MMSE:
  - Remembering and later repeating the names of 3 common objects.
  - Counting backward from 100 by 7s or spelling "world" backward.
  - Naming items as the examiner points to them.
  - Providing the location of the examiner's office, including city, state, and street address.
  - Repeating common phrases.
  - Copying a picture of interlocking shapes.
  - Following simple 3-part instructions, such a picking up a piece of paper, folding it in half, and placing it on the floor.
- Mini-cog:
  - Remembering and later repeating the names of 3 common objects.
  - Drawing the face of a clock with all 12 numbers and the hands indicating the time specified by the examiner.

There are a number of methods for **staging Alzheimer's disease**. Staging is done by a combination of physical exam, history (often provided by family or caregivers), and mental assessment, as there is no definitive test for Alzheimer's. The 7-stage classification system (developed by Barry Reisberg, MD) is used by the Alzheimer's Association:

- **Stage 1**: Preclinical with no evident impairment although slight changes may be occurring within the brain.
- **Stage 2**: Very mild cognitive decline with some misplacing of items and forgetting things or words, but impairment is not usually noticeable to others or found on medical examination.
- **Stage 3**: Mild, early-stage cognitive decline with short term memory loss, problems with reading retention, remembering names, handling money, planning, and organizing. May misplace items of value.
- **Stage 4**: Moderate cognitive decline with decreased knowledge of current affairs or family history, difficulty doing complex tasks, and social withdrawal. This stage is more easily recognized on exam and may persist for 2-10 years, during which the patients may be able to manage most activities of daily living and hygiene.
- **Stage 5**: Moderately-severe cognitive decline as the cerebral cortex and hippocampus shrink and the ventricles enlarge. Patients are obviously confused and disoriented to date, time, and place. Patients may have difficulty using/understanding speech and managing activities of daily living. They may forget address and telephone number. They may dress inappropriately, forget to eat and lose weight, or eat a poor diet. They may be unable to do simple math, such as counting backward by 2s.
- **Stage 6**: Moderately severe cognitive decline as the brain continues to shrink and neurons die. Patients are profoundly confused and unable to care for themselves and may undergo profound personality changes. They may confuse fiction and reality. They may fail to recognize family members, experience difficulty toileting, and begin to pace obsessively or wander away. Sundowner's syndrome, in which the person has disruption of waking/sleeping cycles and tends to get restless and wander about at night, is common. Patients may develop obsessive behaviors, such as tearing items, pulling at the hair, or wringing hands. This stage (with stage 7) may be prolonged, lasting 1-5 years.
- **Stage 7**: Very severe cognitive decline during which most patients are wheelchair bound or bedbound and lose most ability to speak beyond a few words. They are incontinent of urine and feces and may be unable to sit unsupported or hold head up. They choke easily and have increased weakness and rigidity of muscles.

EPIDURAL HEMATOMA

Epidural hematoma occurs with bleeding between the **skull and the dura mater**. Epidural hematomas usually result from blunt trauma and usually are associated with skull fractures. *Symptoms* can include loss of consciousness after trauma with a lucent period and then a relapse into unconsciousness although some never lose consciousness and others never regain consciousness. *Diagnosis* is by computed tomography (CT) scan. Epidural hematomas are usually arterial but may be venous (20%) and are always medical emergencies and require craniotomy with evacuation before compression damage to the brain occurs. Prognosis is good if corrected early because underlying brain damage is rarely severe. *Treatment*: Evacuation of hematomas can be done in a number of different ways, including burr holes; needle aspiration, direct surgical craniotomy, or endoscope. If no neurosurgical care is available, bilateral burr holes may need to be done in an emergency department to prevent herniation from arterial bleeding.

SUBDURAL HEMORRHAGE

Subdural hemorrhage is bleeding between the **dura and the cerebrum**, usually from tears in the cortical veins of the subdural space. It tends to develop more slowly than epidural hemorrhage and can result in a subdural hematoma. If the bleeding is acute and develops within minutes or hours of injury, the prognosis is poor. Subacute hematomas that develop more slowly cause varying degrees of injury. Subdural hemorrhage is a common injury related to trauma but it can result from coagulopathy or aneurysms. *Symptoms* of acute injury may occur within 24-48 hours, but subacute bleeding may not be evident for up to 2 weeks after injury. Chronic hemorrhage occurs primarily in the elderly. Symptoms vary and may include bradycardia, tachycardia, hypertension, and alterations in consciousness. *Treatment*: Older children and adults usually require surgical evacuation of the hematoma.

ACUTE BRAIN INJURY IN INFANTS AND SMALL CHILDREN

Infants and small children often exhibit symptoms of **acute brain injury** that are non-specific or different than the typical symptoms of adults. There may be associated injuries, such as laceration or bruising evident:

- **Mild injuries**: Children may be irritable and restless or somnolent and listless. They may lose consciousness or have periods of confusion. Pallor and vomiting are common.
- **Progressive injuries**: As the condition worsens, alterations of consciousness appear, and children may be difficult to rouse. There may be agitation and marked fluctuations in vital signs, as well as focal neurological deficits (paralysis, spasticity, paresis, or lack of sensation in 1 part of the body).
- **Severe injuries**: Children may show signs of increased intracranial pressure, retinal hemorrhage, hemiparesis/hemiplegia or quadriparesis/quadriplegia, thermal deregulation with elevated temperature. Older children may exhibit uncoordinated gait and papilledema.

SHAKEN BABY/SHAKEN IMPACT SYNDROME

Shaken baby syndrome is believed to be the result of vigorous shaking of an infant, causing **acute subdural hematoma** with subarachnoid, and retinal hemorrhages. It is believed that the shaking of the brain causes both coup and contrecoup damage as well as damaging vessels and nerves with resultant cerebral edema. Some authorities, however, believe that the extent of injuries typically seen with these infants precludes just shaking and that they must also suffer blunt impact, as the injuries are more compatible with the head striking against a solid surface with great force, so the newer terminology is shaken impact syndrome, which includes shaking AND impact. *Symptoms* include:

- Mortality rate of about 50%.
- Severe residual problems that may include vision and hearing defects, seizures, intellectual disability or impaired cognition, paralysis, or coma.

Sometimes children may not exhibit obvious neurological symptoms immediately after trauma but have learning disabilities and behavioral disorders that appear in school. *Treatment* includes:

- Stabilizing patient.
- Neurosurgical consult.

GUILLAIN-BARRÉ SYNDROME

Guillain-Barré syndrome (GBS) is an autoimmune disorder of the **myelinated motor peripheral nervous system**, often triggered by a viral gastroenteritis or Campylobacter jejuni infection.

Symptoms include: numbness and tingling with increasing weakness of lower extremities that may become generalized, sometimes resulting in complete paralysis and inability to breathe without ventilatory support. Deep tendon reflexes are typically absent, and some people experience facial weakness and ophthalmoplegia (paralysis of muscles controlling movement of eyes). *Diagnosis* is by history, clinical symptoms, and lumbar puncture, which often shows ↑ protein with normal glucose and cell count although protein may not ↑ for a week or more. *Treatment* is supportive. Patients should be hospitalized for observation and placed on ventilator support if forced vital capacity is <2 L. While there is no definitive treatment, plasma exchange or IV immunoglobulin shorten the duration of symptoms.

> **Review Video: Guillain-Barre Syndrome**
> Visit mometrix.com/academy and enter code: 742900

SEIZURE DISORDERS

Seizures are sudden involuntary abnormal **electrical disturbances in the brain** that can manifest as alterations of consciousness, spastic tonic and clonic movements, convulsions, and loss of consciousness. Seizures may be partial, affecting part of the brain or generalized, affecting the whole brain. Seizures are a symptom of underlying pathology. Many seizures are transient. Some seizures may result from pathology, such as meningitis, cerebral edema, brain trauma, or brain tumors. Others are idiopathic, predisposing the person to recurrent seizures, usually of the same type. Seizures are characterized as focal (localized), focal with rapid generalization (spreading) and generalized (widespread). Seizure disorders with onset in childhood <4 usually cause more neurological damage than those that have a later onset. *Diagnosis* may include:

- Serum glucose, pregnancy test, serum electrolytes, blood urea nitrogen (BUN), toxicology screening.
- Computed tomography (CT) or magnetic resonance imaging (MRI) to rule out lesions.
- Electroencephalogram (EEG).

Treatment includes protecting patient from injury during active seizures:

- Anticonvulsants: Phenytoin, carbamazepine, phenobarbital, primidone, valproic acid.
- Referral to neurologist for new onset.

PARTIAL SEIZURES

Partial seizures are caused by an electrical discharge to a localized area of the **cerebral cortex**, such as the frontals, temporal, or parietal lobes with seizure characteristics related to area of involvement. They may begin in a focal area and become generalized, often preceded by an aura.

- **Simple partial**: unilateral motor symptoms including somatosensory, psychic, and autonomic.
  - o *Aversive*: eyes and head turned away from focal side
  - o *Sylvan* (usually during sleep): tonic-clonic movements of the face, salivation, and arrested speech.
- **Special sensory**: various sensations (numbness, tingling, prickling, or pain) spreading from 1 area. May include visual sensations, posturing or hypertonia. Rare <8 years.

- **Complex** (Psychomotor): No loss of consciousness, but altered consciousness and non-responsive with amnesia. May involve complex sensorium with bad tastes, auditory or visual hallucinations, feeling of déjà vu, strong fear. May carry out repetitive activities, such as walking, running, smacking lips, chewing, or drawling. Rarely aggressive. Seizure usually followed by prolonged drowsiness and confusion, and occurs 3 through adolescence.

GENERALIZED SEIZURES

Generalized seizures lack a focal onset and appear to involve **both hemispheres**, usually presenting with loss of consciousness and no preceding aura.

- **Tonic-clonic** (Grand Mal): Occurs without warning.
  - *Tonic period* (10-30 seconds): Eyes roll upward with loss of consciousness, arms flexed, stiffen in symmetric tonic contraction of body, apneic with cyanosis and salivating.
  - *Clonic period* (10 seconds to 30 minutes, but usually 30 seconds). Violent rhythmic jerking with contraction and relaxation. May be incontinent of urine and feces. Contractions slow and then stop.
  - Following seizures, there may be confusion, disorientation, impairment of motor activity, speech and vision for several hours. May involve headache, nausea, and vomiting. Person often falls asleep and awakens conscious.
- **Absence** (Petit Mal): Onset between ages 4 and 12 and usually ends in puberty. Onset is abrupt with brief loss of consciousness for 5-10 seconds and slight loss of muscle tone but often appears to be daydreaming. May include lip smacking or eye twitching.

STATUS EPILEPTICUS

Status epilepticus (SE) is usually **generalized tonic-clonic seizures** that are characterized by a series of seizures with intervening time too short for regaining of consciousness. The constant assault and periods of apnea can lead to exhaustion, respiratory failure with hypoxemia and hypercapnia, cardiac failure, and death. There are a number of causes of SE:

- Uncontrolled epilepsy or non-compliance with anticonvulsants. Infections, such as encephalitis.
- Encephalopathy or brain attack, brain trauma, neoplasms.
- Drug toxicity (isoniazid).
- Metabolic disorders.

Treatment includes:

- **Anticonvulsants**, usually beginning with fast-acting benzodiazepine (Ativan®), often in steps, with administration of medication every 5 minutes until seizures subside.
- If cause is undetermined, **acyclovir and ceftriaxone** may be administered.
- If there is no response to the first 2 doses of anticonvulsants (refractory SE), **rapid sequence intubation** (RSI), which involves sedation and paralytic anesthesia may be done while therapy continues. Combining phenobarbital and benzodiazepine can cause apnea, so intubation may be necessary.
- Phenytoin and phenobarbital are added.

97

BRAIN ATTACKS/STROKES
ISCHEMIC

Brain attacks (strokes, cerebrovascular accidents) result when there is interruption of the blood flow to an area of the brain. The 2 basic types are ischemic and hemorrhagic. About 80% are **ischemic**, resulting from **blockage of an artery** supplying the brain:

- **Thrombosis** in large artery, usually resulting from atherosclerosis, may block circulation to a large area of the brain. It is most common in the elderly and may occur suddenly or after episodes of transient ischemic attacks.
- **Lacunar infarct** (penetrating thrombosis in small artery) is most common in those with diabetes mellitus and/or hypertension.
- **Embolism** travels through the arterial system and lodges in the brain, most commonly in the left middle cerebral artery. An embolism may be cardiogenic, resulting from cardiac arrhythmia or surgery. An embolism usually occurs rapidly with no warning signs.
- **Cryptogenic** has no identifiable cause.

HEMORRHAGIC

Hemorrhagic brain attacks account for about 20% and result from a **ruptured cerebral artery**, causing not only lack of oxygen and nutrients but also edema that causes widespread pressure and damage:

- **Intracerebral** is bleeding into the substance of the brain from an artery in the central lobes, basal ganglia, pons, or cerebellum. Intracerebral hemorrhage usually results from atherosclerotic degenerative changes, hypertension, brain tumors, anticoagulation therapy, or some illicit drugs, such as crack and cocaine. Onset is often sudden and may cause death.
- **Intracranial aneurysm** occurs with ballooning cerebral artery ruptures, most commonly at the Circle of Willis.
- **Arteriovenous malformation** (AVM) is a tangle of dilated arteries and veins without a capillary bed. This is a congenital abnormality. Rupture of AVMs is a cause of brain attack in young adults.
- **Subarachnoid hemorrhage** is bleeding in the space between the meninges and brain, resulting from aneurysm, AVM, or trauma. This type of hemorrhage compresses brain tissue.

RIGHT HEMISPHERE

Brain attacks most commonly occur in the **right or left hemisphere**, but the exact location and the extent of brain damage affects the type of presenting symptoms. If the frontal area of either side is involved, there tends to be memory and learning deficits. Some symptoms are common to specific areas and help to identify the area involved:

- **Right hemisphere**: This results in left paralysis or paresis and a left visual field deficit that may cause spatial and perceptual disturbances so that people may have difficulty judging distance. Fine motor skills may be impacted, resulting in trouble dressing or handling tools. People may become impulsive and exhibit poor judgment, often denying impairment. Left-sided neglect (lack of perception of things on the left side) may occur. Depression is common as well as short-term memory loss and difficulty following directions. Language skills usually remain intact.

LEFT HEMISPHERE, BRAIN STEM, AND CEREBELLUM

Symptoms of **brain attacks** vary according to the area of the brain affected:

- **Left hemisphere**: This results in right paralysis or paresis and a right visual field defect. Depression is common and people often exhibit slow, cautious behavior, requiring repeated instruction and reinforcement for simple tasks. Short-term memory loss and difficulty learning new material or understanding generalizations is common. Difficulty with mathematics, reading, writing, and reasoning may occur. Aphasia (expressive, receptive, or global) is common.
- **Brain stem**: Because the brain stem controls respiration and cardiac function, a brain attack frequently causes death, but those who survive may have a number of problems, including respiratory and cardiac abnormalities. Strokes may involve motor or sensory impairment or both.
- **Cerebellum**: This area controls balance and coordination. Brain attacks in the cerebellum are rare but may result in ataxia, nausea and vomiting, and headaches and dizziness or vertigo.

AMERICAN STROKE ASSOCIATION CLASSIFICATION SYSTEM

The American Stroke Association developed a brain attack outcome classification system to standardize descriptions of **stroke injuries**:

- Number of **impaired domains** (motor, sensory, vision, language, cognition, and affect):
  o Level 0: none.
  o Level 1: one impaired.
  o Level 2: two impaired.
  o Level 3: >2 impaired.
- **Degree** of impairment:
  o A (minimal).
  o B (moderate) 1 or more domains involved.
  o C (severe) 1 or more domains involved.
- Assessment of **function** determines the ability to live independently. Level III requires much assistance and Levels IV and V cannot live independently.
  o I—Independent in basic activities of daily living (BADL), such as bathing, eating, toileting, and walking; and instrumental activities of daily living (IADL) such as telephoning, shopping, maintaining a household, socializing, and using transportation.
  o II—Independent in BADL but partially dependent in IADL.
  o III—Partially dependent in BADL (<3 areas) and IADL.
  o IV—Partially dependent in BADL (3 or more areas).
  o V—Completely dependent in BADL (5 or more areas) and IADL.

RUPTURED CEREBRAL ANEURYSMS

Cerebral aneurysms, weakening and dilation of a **cerebral artery**, are usually congenital (90%). Aneurysms usually range from 2-7 mm and commonly occur in the Circle of Willis at the base of the brain. A rupturing aneurysm may decrease perfusion as well as increasing pressure on surrounding brain tissue. With dissecting aneurysm, the vessel wall is torn apart and blood enters layers, sometimes occurring during angiography or secondary to trauma or disease. *Symptoms* of ruptured aneurysm may include severe headache, nausea and vomiting, buccal rigidity, visual disturbances, or loss of consciousness.

99

Diagnosis:

- Computed tomography (CT) scan shows subarachnoid hemorrhage.
- Cerebral angiography to isolate bleeding.

Treatment: Surgical clipping of a ruptured aneurysm is usually necessary because of the danger of rebleeding, 4% in the first 24 hours and 1-2% each day for the next month. Embolization, including endovascular coiling, may be done as an alternative to clipping in some cases.

ARTERIOVENOUS MALFORMATION

Arteriovenous malformation (AVM) is a congenital abnormality with a tangle of **dilated arteries and veins without a capillary bed**. AVMs can occur anywhere in the brain and may cause no significant problems. Usually the AVM is "fed" by 1 or more cerebral arteries, which enlarge over time, shunting more blood through the AVM. The veins also enlarge in response to increased arterial blood flow because of the lack of a capillary bridge between the two. Because vein walls are thinner and lack the muscle layer of an artery, the veins tend to rupture as the AVM becomes larger, causing a subarachnoid hemorrhage. Chronic ischemia that may be related to the AVM can result in cerebral atrophy. Sometimes small leaks, usually accompanied by headache and nausea and vomiting, may occur before rupture. AVMs may cause a wide range of neurological *symptoms*, including changes in mentation, dizziness, sensory abnormalities, confusion, and dementia. *Treatment* includes:

- Supportive management of symptoms.
- Surgical repair or focused irradiation (definitive treatments).

HEADACHES

Headaches may be primary or secondary. **Primary headaches** include migraines, cluster and tension headaches, usually with low rates of morbidity; however, secondary headaches, such as those caused by brain tumors, meningitis, sinusitis, severe hypertension, dental abscesses, and other disorders may result in severe morbidity and death. Symptoms of **secondary headache** include sudden onset and severe pain, and may be associated with fever, nausea and vomiting, and altered mental status. It may occur after head trauma. Diagnosis includes: complete history and physical, including neurological examination. A complete description of the headache should be included: location, quality, frequency, precipitating factors, aggravating factors, time of day, and associated symptoms. Allergy and family history may provide clues to the cause as well. If there are abnormalities on the neurological exam or severe onset of symptoms, computed tomography (CT), angiography, or magnetic resonance imaging (MRI) may be indicated as well as complete blood count (CBC), erythrocyte sedimentation rate (ESR), and chemical panels. *Treatments*:

- Nonsteroidal inflammatory drugs (NSAIDs).
- Triptans and ergotamines for migraines).
- Corticosteroids (cerebral arteritis).
- Neurological consult as needed.

AUTONOMIC DYSREFLEXIA

Autonomic dysreflexia (hyperreflexia) is a complication of **central cord lesions** at or above T6. This may be precipitated by urinary infection, bladder distention, or kidney stones or fecal impaction, but numerous other stresses, such as ingrown toenail, pressure ulcers, sunburns, sexual intercourse, or tight clothing can cause the disorder. *Symptoms* include: hypertension with ↑ 20-40 mm Hg systolic blood pressure, vasoconstriction, pallor, piloerection below lesion, severe pounding headache, nasal congestion, restlessness and apprehension. *Diagnosis* is based on clinical findings and hypertension. *Treatment* includes:

- **Antihypertensives**: Nitroprusside, nitrates.
- Placement of **urinary catheter** if necessary (using lidocaine jelly to decrease stimulation) or checking catheter for obstruction.
- Check for **fecal impaction** after blood pressure (BP) stabilizes, placing lidocaine jelly into the rectum 5 minutes before disimpaction.
- If there are no bladder or bowel problems, a **complete examination** needs to be done to identify other causes.
- Patient should be **monitored** for 2 hours after hypertension and symptoms subside.

THORACIC OUTLET SYNDROME

Thoracic outlet syndrome comprises a number of disorders affecting the nerves of the brachial plexus as well as nerves and vessels that travel from the neck to the axilla. Traumatic thoracic outlet syndrome most commonly affects those who participate in sports and relates to **repetitive hyperextension of the arm**. Muscle weakness causes narrowing of the thoracic outlet, which is between the clavicle and the first rib, resulting in pressure on both the nerves and vessels. *Symptoms* include lack of sensation, tingling, burning, pain in neck, shoulder, and arm and decreased circulation to arms and hands. The collateral circulation of the hand may also be impaired from other types of injuries or occlusion of arteries from thrombophlebitis. The Allen test and Adson test may be done to evaluate thoracic outlet syndrome and circulation in the radial and ulnar arteries.

ALLEN TEST AND ADSON TEST

The **Allen test** is done to evaluate circulation of the **radial and ulnar arteries** at the wrist:

- The person is sitting with the shoulder abducted (90°) and externally rotated (90°) and elbow flexed (90°).
- The person makes a tight fist and maintains it for at least 20 seconds before testing.
- The examiner grasps the hand, applying pressure against both the radial and ulnar arteries at the wrist.
- The person opens the hand, which should blanche.
- The ulnar artery is released first and if circulation is normal, color will rebound within 5-7 seconds. If ulnar blockage, color remains blanched until the radial artery is released.
- The test is repeated, releasing the radial artery first.

The **Adson test**: The person takes a deep breath, hyperextends the neck, and turns the head to the right while examiner palpates the left radial pulse. A positive finding is a reduction of pulse strength. The test is repeated on the opposite side.

GLASGOW COMA SCALE

The **Glasgow coma scale (GCS)** measures the depth and duration of coma or impaired consciousness. The GCS measures 3 parameters: Best eye response, best verbal response, and best motor response, with a total possible score that ranges from 3-15:

- Eye opening
  - 4: Spontaneous.
  - 3: To verbal stimuli.

- o 2: To pain (not of face).
- o 1: No response.
- Verbal
  - o 5: Oriented.
  - o 4: Conversation confused, but can answer questions.
  - o 3: Uses inappropriate words.
  - o 2: Speech incomprehensible.
  - o 1: No response.
- Motor
  - o 6: Moves on command.
  - o 5: Moves purposefully respond pain.
  - o 4: Withdraws in response to pain.
  - o 3: Decorticate posturing (flexion) in response to pain.
  - o 2: Decerebrate posturing (extension) in response to pain.
  - o 1: No response.

Injuries are **classified** according to the total score: 3-8 Coma; < 8 Severe head injury; 9-12 Mod. head injury; 13-15 Mild head injury.

NEUROLOGICAL MOTOR TESTING AND TESTING FOR NUCHAL RIGIDITY

Neurological motor testing requires careful observation for involuntary or spastic movements and examination of muscles for lack of symmetry or atrophy with observation of gait. **Muscle tone** is examined by flexing and extending the upper and lower extremities, observing for flaccid or spastic changes. **Muscle strength** is examined by having the patient press fingers, wrists, elbows, hips, knees, ankles, and plantar area against resistance, graded 0 (no movement) to 5 (normal).

Pronator drift is an indication of disease of the **upper motor neurons**. The patient stands with eyes closes and both arms extended horizontally in front with the palms facing upwards (supination). The patient should be told to hold the arms still and not move them while the examiner taps downward on the arm. If motor neuron disease is present, the patient's arms will drift downward and hands will drift toward pronation.

Nuchal rigidity is tested by placing the hands behind the patient's head and flexing the neck gently to determine if there is increased resistance.

CRANIAL NERVE ASSESSMENT

The FNP should be familiar with **cranial nerve assessment** as part of evaluation for suspected head injury or neurological disorders:

1. **Olfactory** (smell): The person is asked to smell and identify a substance, such as coffee or soap, with 1 nostril held closed, and the other.
2. **Optic** (vision): Test visual acuity and the ability to recognize color. Test each eye separately. Red desaturation is tested by having the person look at a red object with first 1 eye and then the next to determine if the color looks the same with both eyes or is dull with 1 eye.
3. **Oculomotor** (eye muscles and pupil response): Using a penlight, the examiner checks eyes for size, shape, reaction to light and accommodation. Eyes are checked for rotation and conjugate movements. The lids should be examined for ptosis.
4. **Trochlear** (eye muscles—upward movement): Eye movement is checked by having the person follow a moving finger with the eyes on the vertical plane.

5. **Trigeminal** (chewing muscles, sensory): The person closes eyes for the sensory examination and is instructed to indicate when part of the face is stroked (light stroke with cotton). The forehead, cheek, and jaw are stroked. The same areas are then examined for sharp or dull. The eye should be observed for blinking and tearing, but touching the cornea with cotton or other items should be avoided as it can cause abrasion. The jaw muscles are assessed by having the person hold the mouth open as well as palpating the muscles on each side to determine if they are equal in size and strength.

6. **Abducens** (eye muscles—lateral movement): The person is also asked to follow the finger from the 1 o'clock position clockwise to the 11 o'clock position. At the horizontal and vertical axis, the eyes should be checked for deviation or nystagmus, which may occur normally only in the extreme lateral position.

7. **Facial nerve** (facial expression, tears, taste, and saliva): Usually, only the motor portion is evaluated for nerve VII, and taste is examined with testing of cranial nerve IX, but one can test the ability to discriminate between salt and sugar. Motor functions are assessed by asking the person to frown, smile, puff out the cheeks, and wrinkle the forehead. The muscles are observed for symmetry. The person is asked to hold the eyes tightly closed while the examiner attempts to open the lids with the thumb on the lower lid and the index finger on the upper lid, using care not to apply pressure to the eye.

8. **Vestibulocochlear** (balance and hearing): Balance is checked with tandem gait and Romberg's test. Hearing is checked (with the person's eyes closed) by rubbing fingers together or holding ticking watch next to 1 ear and then the other. Weber's test may be done to evaluate lateralization and Rinne's test for bone and air conduction.

   a. **Weber's test:** A vibrating tuning fork is touched to the top of the head or the forehead and person asked if sound is equal in both ears. Hearing deficit in 1 ear suggests sensorineural hearing loss.

   b. **Rinne's test:** A vibrating tuning fork is held on the mastoid bone and the time measured until sound ceases. Then the vibrating tuning fork is held at the external ear. Sound is normally heard twice as long through air as through bone. If there is conductive hearing loss, the sound is heard longer through the bone. If there is sensorineural hearing loss, the sound is heard longer through the air.

9. **Glossopharyngeal** (taste, mouth sensation): This test is not usually performed unless the person complains of lack of taste or abnormalities of taste. The mouth must be moist for accurate assessment, so the person should drink water if possible before the test and the testing substance should be in solution. The person is tested for recognition of sweet, sour, bitter, and salt.

10. **Vagus** (swallowing, gag reflex): The examiner has the person open the mouth and say "aw." The uvula and palate should elevate equally on both sides. The gag reflex is usually tested if the person reports difficulty swallowing or changes in speech. Gag reflex is tested by lightly touching the tongue blade to the soft palate. Some people are hyper-responsive, so accurate testing of the gag reflex may be difficult.

11. **Spinal accessory** (muscle movement—sternocleidomastoid, trapezius): These muscular movements are tested by the examiner placing the hands along the side of the face and asking the person to turn the face first 1 side and then the other against resistance to determine if strength is normal and equal. Then, the examiner places hands on the person's shoulders and asks the person to shrug the shoulders, elevating them upward, against resistance to determine if the strength is normal and equal.

103

12. **Hypoglossal** (tongue): The examiner asks the person to stick out the tongue to determine if it deviates to 1 side, indicating a lesion on that side of the brain. To determine if there is equal strength on both sides of the tongue, a tongue blade is held against the side of the tongue and the person asked to push against it with the tongue. Both sides are checked to determine if strength is normal and equal.

PERIPHERAL NERVE ASSESSMENT

PERONEAL AND RADIAL

- **Peroneal**: The peroneal nerve branches from the sciatic nerve, which arises from the L4, L4 and S1, S2, and S3 dorsal nerves and travels down the leg. The peroneal nerve enervates the lower leg, foot, and toes. Sensation is evaluated by pricking the webbed area between the great and second toe. Movement is evaluated by having the person dorsiflex and extend the foot.
- **Radial**: The radial nerve branches from the brachial plexus and enervates the dorsal surface of the arm and hand, including the thumb and fingers 2, 3, and 4. Sensation is evaluated by pricking in skin in the webbed area between the thumb and the index finger. Movement is evaluated by having the person extend the thumb, the wrist, and fingers at the metacarpal joint.

MEDIAN, TIBIAL, AND ULNAR

A musculoskeletal evaluation should include **peripheral nerve assessment** to determine if injury has impaired nerve function. Nerve function should be assessed for both sensation and movement. Assessment of sensation is done with a sharp or pointed instrument, using care not to prick the skin. The person should feel a slight prick if the sensory function is intact:

- **Median**: The median nerve branches from the brachial plexus, which arises from C5, C6, C7, C8, and T1. The median nerve travels down the arm and forearm, through the carpal tunnel. Sensation is evaluated by pricking the top or distal surface of the index finger. Movement is evaluated by having the person touch the ends of the thumb and little finger together and having the person flex the wrist.
- **Tibial**: The tibial nerve branches from the sciatic nerve. The tibial nerve travels down the back of the leg, through the popliteal fossa at the back of the knee and terminates at the planter side of the foot. Sensation is evaluated by pricking the medial and lateral aspects of the plantar surface of the foot. Movement is evaluated by having the person plantar flex the toes and then the ankle.
- **Ulnar**: The ulnar nerve branches from the brachial plexus and travels down the arm from the shoulder, traveling along the anterior forearm beside the ulna, to the palm of the hand. Sensation is evaluated by pricking the distal fat pad at the end of the small finger. Movement is evaluated by having the person extend and spread all fingers.

Emergency Situations

MEDICAL EMERGENCIES

RETINAL DETACHMENT

Retinal detachment occurs when the **retinal pigment epithelial (RPE) layer** separates from the **underlying sensory layer**. There are 4 types of detachment:

- **Rhegmatogenous**: a tear occurs in the sensory retina and liquid vitreous seeps through, detaching the RPE.
- **Traction**: bands of scar tissue provide traction that pulls on retina, usually related to diabetes, vitreous hemorrhage, or retinopathy of prematurity.
- **Exudative**: the choroid produces serous fluid under the retina, usually related to uveitis or macular degeneration.
- **Combination** of other types.

Symptoms include:

- Painless visual changes, such as floaters, "cobwebs," photopsia (flashes of light), shadow over vision, or loss of central vision.
- *Diagnosis* includes:
  - Checking visual acuity.
  - Dilated fundus exam with indirect ophthalmoscope and Goldman 3-mirror to create a detailed retinal diagram.

Treatment consists of immediate referral to retinal surgeon for surgical repair.

INGESTION OR EXPOSURE TO INSECTICIDES

Insecticides, organophosphorus compounds and carbamates can cause severe **central nervous system (CNS) toxicity**, usually within 8-24 hours of exposure by ingestion, inhalation, or contact. *Symptoms* may include:

- Salivation, lacrimation
- Urinary and fecal incontinence
- GI irritation with nausea and vomiting.
- Bradycardia, heart block, ventricular dysrhythmias.
- Bronchorrhea and bronchospasm.
- Hydrocarbon or garlic odor.
- 1-4 days after ingestion: paralysis of neck flexor, proximal limb and respiratory muscles may occur.
- 1-3 weeks after ingestion: Irreversible neurological and neurobehavioral abnormalities and paralysis may occur.

Diagnosis: history, clinical exam, cholinesterase assays, and tests for specific compounds. Staff must use protective measures caring for patients with external contamination. *Treatment* includes:

- Supportive treatment.
- Gastric decontamination (if ingested orally).
- Decontamination (varies according to type of insecticide).

- Oxygen (100%), oximetry, and cardiac monitoring.
- Antidotes: Atropine 1 mg (adult) or 0.01-0.04 mg/kg (children) IV initially and may be repeated and Pralidoxime 1-2 g (adults) or 20-40 mg/kg (children) in NS over 10 minutes or IM to resolve paralysis.

REYE'S SYNDROME

Reye's syndrome is a serious, sometimes fatal, **systemic disorder** that follows a viral infection, such as chicken pox, upper respiratory infections, and influenza, usually in children. The primary problems include fatty accumulation in the liver and other organs and encephalopathy. Early diagnosis is critical for prevention of permanent brain damage or death. There is an association with the use of salicylates (aspirin, aspirin compounds) for viral infections, so children under 19 should not receive salicylates. *Symptoms* usually appear as a viral infection recedes:

- **Infants**: diarrhea with or without vomiting, hyperventilation or periods of apnea, seizures.
- **Others**: Sudden onset of vomiting, usually without diarrhea, alterations in mental status with lethargy, agitation, stupor, extensor spasms, decerebrate rigidity, and coma. Symptoms common to salicylate poisoning may occur.

Diagnosis is based on ↑serum glutamic oxaloacetic transaminase (SGOT)-serum glutamic pyruvic transaminase (SGPT) ≥200 units but no jaundice, ↑ blood NH_3. Hypoglycemia is common in infants. *Treatment* includes:

- IV 10% hypertonic glucose.
- Supplemental oxygen and ventilation as necessary.
- Supportive care to reduce cerebral edema and as indicated.

ANAPHYLAXIS SYNDROME

Anaphylaxis syndrome is a sudden acute systemic immunoglobulin E (IgE) or non-immunoglobulin E (non-IgE) inflammatory response affecting the cardiopulmonary and other systems.

- **IgE-mediated response** (anaphylactic shock) is an antibody-antigen reaction against an allergen, such as milk, peanuts, latex, insect bites, drugs, or fish. This is the most common type.
- **Non-IgE-mediated response** (anaphylactoid reaction) is a systemic reaction to infection, exercise, radio contrast material or other triggers. While the response is almost identical to the other type, it does not involve IgE.
- Typically, with IgE-mediated response, an **antigen** triggers release of substances, such as histamine and prostaglandins, which affect the skin, cardiopulmonary, and gastrointestinal systems. Histamine causes initial erythema and edema by inducing vasodilation. Each time the person has contact with the antigen, more antibodies form in response, and allergic reactions worsen. Anaphylactic shock related to anesthesia is rare, although anaphylactoid reactions may occur with opioids, hypnotics, and muscle relaxants. Antibiotics (penicillin, sulfonamides, and cephalosporins) and latex allergy cause most medication/treatment-related anaphylaxis.

Anaphylaxis syndrome may present with a few symptoms or a wide range that encompasses cardiopulmonary, dermatological, and gastrointestinal responses. *Symptoms* may recur after the initial treatment (biphasic anaphylaxis) so careful monitoring is essential:

- Sudden onset of weakness, dizziness, confusion.
- Severe generalized edema and angioedema. Lips and tongue may swell. Urticaria.
- Increased permeability of vascular system and loss of vascular tone.
- Severe hypotension leading to shock.
- Laryngospasm/bronchospasm with obstruction of airway causing dyspnea and wheezing.
- Nausea, vomiting, and diarrhea.
- Seizures, coma and death.

Treatment includes:

- Establish patent **airway** and intubate if necessary, for ventilation.
- Provide **oxygen** at 100% high flow.
- Monitor **VS**.
- Administer **epinephrine** (Epi-pen® or 1:1000 solution t 0.1 mg/kg/wt).
- 2.5 mg **albuterol** per nebulizer for bronchospasm.
- **Intravenous fluids** to provide bolus of fluids for hypotension.
- **Diphenhydramine** 1.0 mg/kg/wt (to 25 mg) if shock persists.
- **Methylprednisolone** 2.0 mg/kg/wt if no response to other drugs.

RAPE AND SEXUAL ABUSE

Rape and sexual abuse victims (both male and female) should be treated sensitively and questioned privately. Examination should include:

- **Assault history** that includes what happened, when, where, and by whom. Questioning should determine if there is a possibility of drug-induced amnesia or activities, such as douching or showering, which might have destroyed evidence.
- **Medical history** to determine if there is a risk of pregnancy and when and if the last consensual sex occurred that might interfere with laboratory findings.
- **Physical examination** should include examination of the genitals, rectum, and mouth. The body should be examined for bruising or other injuries. Toluidine dye should be applied to the perineum before insertion of a speculum into the vagina to detect small vulvar lacerations.

Forensic evidence must be collected within 72 hours and requires informed consent and the use of a rape kit. Forensic evidence includes:

- Victim samples for control.
- Assailant-identifying samples.
- Evidence of sexual activity.
- Evidence of force or coercion.

FEBRILE SEIZURE

Febrile seizure is a generalized seizure associated with fever (usually >38.8°C, 101.8° F) from any type of infection (e.g., upper respiratory, urinary) but without intracranial infection or other cause, occurring between 6 months and 5 years of age. Careful clinical examination must be conducted to

107

rule out more serious disorders. Laboratory tests are conducted in relation to symptoms. Lumbar puncture is not usually indicated unless intracranial infection is suspected. Seizures usually last <15 minutes and are without subsequent neurological deficit. *Treatment* includes:

- **Fever control**: Acetaminophen 10-15 mg/kg every 4 hours OR ibuprofen 10 mg/kg every 6-8 hours.
- Tepid water bath (NOT alcohol).
- Repeat seizures or history of febrile seizures: **Phenobarbital** 15 mg/kg IV and 4-6 mg/kg each day until improvement.
- **Anti-epileptic drugs** (AEDs) are usually not advised unless seizures are complex, child is <6 months, or there is a pre-existing neurological disorder: Diazepam 0.2-0.5 mg/kg every 8 hours during fever. (May cause lethargy.)

ANIMAL BITES

There is no one typical therapy for **traumatic wounds** because they vary so widely in the type and degree of injury. A cat scratch on the knee is treated very differently from a shark attack that involves massive tissue injury or tissue loss. Animal bites, including human, are frequent causes of traumatic injury. Treatment includes:

- **Cleanse** wound by flushing with 10-35 cc syringe with 18-gauge Angiocath to remove debris and bacteria using normal saline or dilute Betadine® solution.
- Hand, puncture, and infected wounds or those more than 12 hours old may be closed by **secondary intention**.
- **Moisture-retentive dressings** as indicated by the size and extent of injury of wound left open. **Dry dressings** may be applied to injuries with closure by primary intention.
- **Topical antibiotics** may be indicated although systemic antibiotics are commonly prescribed for animal bites.
- **Tetanus toxoid** or **immune globulin** is routinely administered.

TICK BITES

Ticks, blood-feeding parasites, are the primary vector of infectious diseases in the United States. Ticks transmit a wide variety of **pathogens**, including bacteria such as Rickettsiae, protozoan parasites, and viruses. **Lyme disease** is the most common tick-borne disease, but there are increasing reports of other diseases, such as babesiosis, human anaplasmosis, and ehrlichiosis. Many tick-borne diseases present with similar non-specific flu-like symptoms and can easily be misdiagnosed. Ticks should be carefully removed if still feeding:

- Using fine-tipped **tweezers**, tick is grasped close to the skin and pulled upward with even and steady pressure, avoiding jerks or twists that may break mouthparts.
- The tick must not be handled with **bare hands**.
- **Disinfect** skin site.
- Tick should be saved for **identification**: place tick in a plastic bag, date, and place in freezer in case illness occurs in 2 to 3 weeks.

People should be cautioned to immediately seek medical attention for **flu-like or neurological symptoms** or **erythema migrans** (bullseye rash) typical of Lyme disease.

BEE STINGS

Bees and wasps sting by puncturing the skin with a hollow stinger and injecting **venom**. Wasps and bumblebees can sting more than once but honeybees have barbs on their stingers, and the barbs keep the stinger hooked into the skin. Local reactions to bee sting:

- Raised white **weal** with central red spot of about 10 mm appearing within a few minutes and lasting 20 minutes (honeybees)
- **Edema and erythema**, which may last several days (Vespid wasps).
- Pain, swelling, and redness confined to **sting site**.
- Swelling may extend **beyond the sting site** and may, for example involve swelling of an entire limb.

Some people may develop an **anaphylactic reaction**, including a biphasic reaction, in which the symptoms recede and then return 2-3 hours later. About 50% of deaths occur within 30 minutes of the sting, and 75% within 4 hours. Symptoms of an allergic reaction/anaphylaxis may become increasingly severe with generalized urticaria, edema, hypotension, and respiratory distress.

TREATMENT

Treatment of **bee stings** initially includes:

- **Wash** the site with soap and water.
- **Remove** stinger using a 4x4-inch gauze wiped over the area or by scraping a sharp instrument over the area.
- NEVER **squeeze** the stinger or use tweezers, as this will cause more venom to go into the skin.
- Apply **ice** to reduce the swelling (10-20 minutes on/10-20 minutes off for 24 hours).
- **Antihistamines** may be prescribed.
- A paste of **baking soda and water** or meat tenderizer and water may reduce itching.
- **Topical corticosteroids** may relieve itching.
- Tetanus toxoid or tetanus immune globulin as needed.

Allergic responses/anaphylaxis require **immediate aggressive medical intervention**: Epinephrine, antihistamines, corticosteroids, oxygen and other supportive treatment, and IV fluids as needed. People with extensive local or anaphylactic reactions should be advised to carry an EpiPen® for emergency use if stung.

SPIDER BITES

Spider bites are frequently a misdiagnosis of a Staphylococcus aureus or methicillin-resistant Staphylococcus aureus (MRSA) infection, so unless the spider was observed, the wound should be cultured and antibiotics started. If the wound responds to the antibiotic, then it probably wasn't a spider bite. There are 2 main types of venomous spider bites:

- Producing **neurological symptoms** (Black widow).
- Producing **local necrosis** (brown recluse, yellow sac, and hobo spiders).

Treatment includes:

- Cleanse wound and apply cool compress and elevate body part if possible.
- Black widow bites:
    - Narcotic analgesics.

109

- o Nitroprusside to relieve hypertension.
- o Calcium gluconate 10% solution IV for abdominal cramps.
- o Latrodectus antivenin for those with severe reaction.
- Necrotic/ulcerated bites (brown recluse, etc.).
  - o There is no consensus on the best treatment as ulceration caused by the venom may be extensive and surgical repair with grafts may be needed.
  - o Treatment as for other necrotic ulcers, with moisture retentive dressings as indicated.
  - o Hyperbaric oxygen therapy (HBOT) used in some cases.

SNAKE BITES

About 45,000 **snake bites** occur in the United States each year, with about 8000 poisonous. In the United States, about 25 species of snakes are venomous. There are 2 types of snakes that can cause serious injury, classified according to the type of fangs and venom.

CORAL SNAKES

Coral snakes have short fixed permanent fangs in the upper jaw and venom that is primarily neurotoxic, but may also have hemotoxic and cardiotoxic properties:

- Wounds show no fang marks but there may be scratches or semi-circular markings from teeth.
- There may be little local reaction, but neurological symptoms may range from mild to acute respiratory and cardiovascular failure.

Treatment includes:

- Cleansing wound thoroughly of dirt and debris and leave open or cover with dry dressing.
- Antibiotics not usually needed.
- Administering antivenin immediately even without symptoms, which may be delayed.
- Tetanus toxoid or immune globulin.

PIT VIPERS

A second type that can cause serious injury are the **pit vipers. Rattlesnakes, copperheads, and cottonmouths** have erectile fangs that fold until they are aroused, and venom is primarily hemotoxic and cytotoxic but may have neurotoxic properties.

- Wounds usually show 1-2 fang marks.
- Edema may begin immediately or may be delayed up to 6 hours.
- Pain may be severe.
- There may be a wide range of symptoms, including hypotension and coagulopathy with defibrination that can lead to excessive blood loss, depending upon the type and amount of venom.
- There may be local infection and necrosis.

Treatment includes:

- Cleansing wound thoroughly and dressings as indicated.
- Tetanus toxoid or immune globulin.
- Analgesics, such as morphine sulphate
- Avoiding NSAIDs and aspirin because of anticoagulation properties.
- Marking edema every 15 minutes.
- Antivenin therapy if indicated (observation for serum sickness if horse serum used).
- Prophylactic antibiotics for severe tissue necrosis.
- Platelets, plasma, or packed RBCs for coagulopathy.

Musculoskeletal

DEVELOPMENTAL HIP DYSPLASIA

Developmental **hip dysplasia** is hip instability resulting from **misalignment of the femoral head and acetabulum**. Hip instability may present as dislocation, subluxation, or acetabular dysplasia (abnormal structural development of the joint). Symptoms may not be evident until after the neonatal period and involvement of the left hip is more common than the right. There appears to be a genetic tendency and an association with breech birth. Signs include:

- **<3 months**: Positive Barlow's test (pressing on the knees to apply pressure to the head of the femur when hips are flexed causes posterior subluxation). Positive Ortolani test (hips rotated through range of motion and click heard at abduction as femoral head slips).
- **>3 months**: Limp, decreased abduction, thigh fold asymmetry, and disparity in length of legs. Allis's sign is positive (one knee higher than the other when knees flexed).

Referral to orthopedist is indicated for application of Pavlik harness for infants (<3 months) or skin traction, surgery and spica cast, bracing for older children.

RESTLESS LEG SYNDROME

Restless leg syndrome (RLS) is characterized by **pain and paresthesia in the legs at rest**, especially in the evening and at night. Some people also have periodic jerking of limbs. The discomfort in the legs is relieved by moving the legs, but this often results in difficulty sleeping and resultant exhaustion during the daytime. Neurological examination is typically normal, but family history of RLS is common. In some cases, the symptoms may relate to iron deficiency anemia, so hemoglobin and hematocrit should be checked. Treatment includes:

- **Ropinirole** (Requip®) and **pramipexole** (Mirapex®) have been approved by the FDA specifically for RLS.
- **Levodopa/carbidopa** (Sinemet®) 25/100 mg SR ½ tab at HS.
- **Opioids**: Propoxyphene, tramadol
- Cyclobenzaprine 10 mg HS
- **Anticonvulsants**: Gabapentin 100 mg/HS.
- Iron replacement therapy if indicated.

Some people have relief of symptoms if they reduce caffeine, alcohol, and tobacco use.

MARFAN SYNDROME

Marfan syndrome is a genetic disorder of the **connective tissue** that may put people at risk. Connective tissue, such as tendons, ligaments, heart valves, and blood vessels are often defective

111

and weak. Depending upon the severity of the disorder, people diagnosed with this disorder may be restricted from strenuous activities, such as team sports, especially contact sports that may result in chest trauma, or isometric exercises, such as weight lifting. The patient with symptoms of Marfan syndrome should be referred to a specialist for assessment of aortic abnormalities. *Traits* can include:

- Tall, thin stature with loose joints, with the long bones disproportionately long.
- Scoliosis.
- Flat feet.
- Pectus carinatum (pigeon chest) or pectus excavatum (funnel chest).
- Long, narrow face with high arched roof of mouth and crowding of teeth.
- Dislocation of lenses of eyes and sometimes retinal detachment, myopia.
- Aortic dilatation (with risk of dissection)
- Cardiac valve disorders with heart murmur.
- Stretch marks.
- Sleep apnea (rare).

HERNIAS

Hernias are protrusions into or through the **abdominal wall** and may occur in children and adults. Hernias may contain fat, tissue, or bowel. There are a number of types:

- **Direct inguinal hernias** occur primarily in adults and rarely incarcerate.
- **Indirect inguinal hernias** related to congenital defect are most common on the right in males and can incarcerate, especially during the first year and in females.
- **Femoral hernias** occur primarily in women and may incarcerate.
- **Umbilical hernias** occur in children, especially African-American and rarely incarcerate. They may also occur in adults, primarily women, and may incarcerate.
- **Incisional hernias** are usually related to obesity or wound infections and may incarcerate.

Hernias are evident on clinical examination. *Symptoms* of incarceration include severe pain, nausea and vomiting, soft mass at hernia site, tachycardia, and ↑ temperature. *Treatment* for hernias includes reduction if incarceration is very recent with patient in Trendelenburg position and gentle compression or surgical excision and fixation and broad-spectrum antibiotics.

BURSITIS AND TENDINITIS

Bursitis is inflammation of the **bursa**, fluid-filled spaces or sacs that form in tissues to reduce friction, causing thickening of the lining of the bursal walls. This can be the result of infection, trauma, crystal deposits, or chronic friction from trauma. **Tendinitis** is inflammation of the long, tubular **tendons and tendon sheaths**, adjacent to the bursa. Causes of tendinitis are similar to bursitis, but tendinitis may also be caused by quinolone antibiotics. Frequently, both bursa and tendons are inflamed. Common types of bursitis include shoulder, olecranon (elbow), trochanteric (hip) and prepatellar (front of knee).

Common types of tendinitis include wrist, Achilles, patellar, and rotator cuff. *Symptoms* include pain with movement, edema, dysfunction, and decreased range of motion. *Diagnosis* is by clinical examination although x-rays may rule out fractures. *Treatment* for bursitis and tendinitis includes:

- Rest and immobilization.
- Nonsteroidal inflammatory drugs (NSAIDs).

- Application of cold packs to affected area.
- Steroid injections.

GOUT

Gout (metabolic arthritis) is a group of conditions associated with a defect of **purine metabolism** that results in hyperuricemia with oversecretion of uric acid, decreased excretion of uric acid, or a combination. The increased uric acid levels can cause monosodium urate crystal depositions in the joints, resulting in severe articular and periarticular inflammation. With chronic gout, sodium urate crystals, called tophi, accumulate in peripheral body areas, such as the great toe (75%), hands, and ears although other joints may be affected as well. *Symptoms* include abrupt onset of pain with erythema and edema lasting 3-10 days. Attacks become more frequent over time and some may develop kidney stones. *Diagnosis* is based on clinical examination, history, and uric acid level >7 mg/dL. *Treatment* includes:

- Restriction of high purine foods (organ meats) and alcohol.
- Weight control methods.
- Acute medications:
    o Nonsteroidal inflammatory drugs (NSAIDs).
    o Colchicine.
- Prophylactic medications for chronic episodes:
    o Probenecid (to prevent tophi formation).
    o Allopurinol (to prevent formation of uric acid).

LUMBOSACRAL PAIN

Lumbosacral (low back) pain may be related to strain, muscular weakness, osteoarthritis, spinal stenosis, herniated disks, vertebral fractures, bony metastasis, infection, or other musculoskeletal disorders. Disk herniation or other joint changes put pressure on nerves leaving the spinal cord, causing pain to radiate along the nerve. Pain may be acute or chronic (>3 months). *Symptoms* include: local or pain radiating down the leg (radiculopathy), impaired gait and reflexes, difference in leg lengths, decreased motor strength, and alteration of sensation, including numbness. *Diagnosis* is by careful clinical examination and history as well as x-ray (fractures, scoliosis, dislocations), computed tomography (CT; identifies underlying problems), magnetic resonance imaging (MRI; spinal pathology), and/or electromyography (EMG) and nerve conduction studies. Diagnostic studies may be deferred in many cases for 4-6 weeks as symptoms may resolve over time. *Treatments* for non-specific back pain include:

- **Analgesia**: acetaminophen, nonsteroidal anti-inflammatory drugs (NSAIDs), opiates.
- Encourage **activity** to tolerance but not bed rest.
- **Muscle relaxants**: diazepam 5-10 mg every 6-8 hours.
- Cold compresses and/or heat compresses.

STRAINS AND SPRAINS

A **strain** is an overstretching of a part of the musculature ("pulled muscle") that causes microscopic **tears in the muscle**, usually resulting from excess stress or overuse of the muscle. Onset of pain is usually sudden with local tenderness on use of the muscle. A **sprain** is damage to a **joint**, with a partial rupture of the supporting ligaments, usually caused by wrenching or twisting that may occur with a fall. The rupture can damage blood vessels, resulting in edema, tenderness at the joint, and pain on movement with pain increasing over 2-3 hours after injury. An avulsion fracture (bone fragment pulled away by a ligament) may occur with strain, so x-rays may be indicated to rule out

113

fractures. Current best practice guidelines call for using the Ottawa rules to decide if x-ray of the knee, foot, or ankle are indicated. Treatment for both strains and strains include:

- **RICE protocol**: rest, ice, compression, and elevation.
- **Ice compresses** (wet or dry) should be applied 20-30 minutes intermittently for 48 hours and then intermittent heat 15-20 minutes 3-4 times daily.
- **Monitor** neurovascular status (especially for sprain).
- **Immobilization** as indicated for sprains for 1-3 weeks.

OSTEOARTHRITIS AND RHEUMATOID ARTHRITIS

There are many different types of arthritis, but the 2 most common are osteoarthritis and rheumatoid arthritis. There are distinctive differences:

- Osteoarthritis:
  - *Cause*: Idiopathic or previous injury.
  - *Onset*: Slowly progressive with symptoms >60 years.
  - *Destruction*: Cartilage deterioration
  - Symptoms:
    - ❖ Pain increases with use/weight-bearing
    - ❖ Stiffness develops
    - ❖ Involvement: Local and unilateral
  - *Treatment*: Nonsteroidal anti-inflammatory drugs (NSAIDs), heat, weight reduction, joint rest, orthotic devices, postural exercises, osteotomy, arthroplasty (with joint replacement)
- Rheumatoid arthritis:
  - *Cause*: Systemic autoimmune inflammatory disorder (etiology unknown).
  - *Onset*: Acute onset beginning in hands, wrists, feet at 25-50 years.
  - *Destruction*: Joint inflammation and deformity
  - Symptoms:
    - ❖ Pain, stiffness, swelling, erythema, nodules, and lack of function in affected joints
    - ❖ Generalized weakness, fatigue, weight loss, and fever
    - ❖ Involvement: Systemic and bilateral and symmetric.
  - *Treatment*: Light exercise to prevent contractures.
  - *Medications*: Salicylates (acetylsalicylic acid [ASA]), NSAIDs, Cox-2 inhibitors (Celebrex® [celecoxib]), disease-modifying antirheumatic drugs (gold-containing compounds, methotrexate, azathioprine, adalimumab), immunomodulators (abatacept), Interleukin 1 receptor inhibitors (anakinra), and glucocorticoids (prednisone) and topical analgesics.

FIBROMYALGIA

Fibromyalgia is a complex syndrome of disorders that include fatigue, chronic generalized muscle pain, and focal areas of tenderness persisting for at least 3 months. The cause of fibromyalgia is not clear and has only recently been recognized as a distinct disorder. *Symptoms* vary widely but can include:

- Pain and stiffness unresponsive to treatment, persisting for months.
- Sleep disorders.
- Irritable bowel syndrome.

- Stiffness in neck and shoulders associated with headache and pain in face.
- Sensitivity to odor, noises, and lights.
- Mood disorders, such as depression and anxiety.
- Dysmenorrhea.
- Paresthesia in hands and feet.

Diagnosis is by clinical exam and ruling out other disorders. *Treatment* includes:

- **Analgesia**: Acetaminophen, tramadol, or nonsteroidal anti-inflammatory drugs (NSAIDs).
- **Antidepressants**, such as amitriptyline, nortriptyline, or fluoxetine (Prozac®). Cymbalta® (duloxetine) and Effexor® (venlafaxine) have been shown to reduce pain.
- **Pregabalin** (Lyrica®) is the first FDA-approved treatment for the pain of fibromyalgia.
- Referral for physical therapy and/or cognitive therapy.

CARPEL TUNNEL SYNDROME

Carpel tunnel syndrome occurs when the **median nerve** is compressed within the carpel tunnel, formed from ligaments and bones, between the forearm and the hand. The carpal tunnel also contains tendons. Initial symptoms include numbness, tingling, or burning in the hand, especially the palm, thumb, index, and middle fingers with eventual weakening and inability to grip. Compression increases when the wrist is flexed, so the symptoms may worsen during sleep. Positive tests include:

- **Tinel's sign**: Percussion or pressure directly over the carpal tunnel elicits thumb and first 3 fingers, but this test is not always reliable.
- **Phalen's test**: Placing the dorsum (backs) of the hands together and flexing the wrist to the full extent, holding light pressure for 1 minute elicits symptoms.
- **Oriental prayer test**: Palms of hands are placed together with fingers and thumb fully abducted, and thumbs don't touch.

Treatment includes steroid injection, splint, modification of activities, and decompression surgery with loss of sensation.

TENNIS ELBOW

Tennis elbow is inflammation of the **lateral epicondyle**, affecting the tendon of the extensor carpi brevis muscle. This injury occurs in sports and activities that involve repetitive wrist extension against resistance, such as badminton and squash, and often relates to poor technique or incorrect grip size. It is more common in those over 30. Symptoms include lateral elbow pain, stiffness, and forearm pain.

Tests include the **Tennis elbow test**:

- The person is in sitting position.
- The elbow on the affected arm is extended (with severe pain, flexed to 90°), wrist flexed and hand in a fist.
- The examiner supports the elbow with 1 hand.
- The forearm is pronated, and the wrist is extended and deviated radially against resistance.
- A positive finding is pain at the lateral epicondyle on the outside of the elbow.

TENDINITIS SCREENING

Tendinitis (or tendonitis) is inflammation of the **long, tubular tendons and tendon sheaths**, adjacent to bursa. Causes of tendinitis are similar to bursitis. Frequently, both bursa and tendons are inflamed. Injury to athletes often occurs in the tendons of the upper extremities of those participating in water sports, baseball, football, and other throwing sports. Poor conditioning may contribute to tendinitis. Common types of tendinitis include wrist and rotator cuff in the arm and Achilles and patellar in the leg. Biceps tendinitis (bicipital tenosynovitis) occurs from repetitive throwing motions from playing tennis or pitching.

Speed's test is commonly used to assess biceps tendonitis although studies show it's only about 50% effective in diagnosis:

- The person stands and holds the arm out at a 60° angle and attempts to flex the arm while the examiner applies isometric resistance.
- Pain at the bicipital groove is positive, indicating there may be inflammation.

ROTATOR CUFF ASSESSMENT

The **rotator cuff** comprises the muscles and ligaments of the **shoulder joint**. The bones in the joint include the scapula and the humerus. Muscles (subscapularis, supraspinatus, infraspinatus, spines minor) and tendons anchor to the head of the humerus so that the arm can move in all directions, and ligaments connect the bones. Part of the rotator cuff is under the scapula. The bursa is between the rotator cuff and shoulder joint, providing protection. Injury may result from trauma, such as a fall, forced external rotation (football) or repetitive stress, such as from pitching a baseball. Tears may occur in the ligaments and muscles as well as tendonitis or bursitis. *Symptoms* include pain in shoulder, weakness, and limited range of movement. Bone spurs may cause inflammation and pain. Most injuries respond to physical therapy for strengthening and range of motion exercises although in some cases nonsteroidal inflammatory drugs (NSAIDs), corticosteroid injections, or surgical repair may be indicated.

ROTATOR CUFF/SUPRASPINATUS TENDON ASSESSMENT

The most common injury to the rotator cuff is a tear in the **supraspinatus tendon**, so that the tendon is separated from its attachment. Typically, the athlete complains of pain in the lateral shoulder, increasing at night and with movement, such as lifting the arm. There may be weakness both in lifting the arm and externally rotating it. Tests include (sitting or standing):

- Drop arm test:
  - Arm is abducted (90°) and slowly lowered.
  - Positive findings for tear/pathology are if arm drops or lowering is jerky.
  - If trainer lightly taps on abducted arm, arm may drop suddenly.
- "Empty can" or supraspinatus strength test:
  - The arms are held in scaption (30° horizontal adduction with the shoulder abducted to 90°) so the arms are out straight in front.
  - The trainer applies downward pressure to the arms while the person tries to hold the arms stable, resisting pressure.
  - If the person cannot resist the pressure and the affected arm falls, this positive result indicates supraspinatus damage.

- Painful arc:
  - Person stands with arm resting at the side of the body.
  - Arm is passively and/or actively abducted (raised from the side to straight overhead in a half-circle arc).
  - Positive for supraspinatus pathology: Pain between 120-170°. Note: external rotation during abduction may relieve pain by decreasing pressure, so close observation is necessary.
  - Positive for AC joint pathology: Pain between 140-180°.
- Apley's scratch test:
  - Person sits for testing.
  - Person reaches with injured arm behind head and tries to touch the outer rim of the superior medial scapula.
  - Pathology of the rotator cuff (usually the supraspinatus) is indicated by pain or failure to reach target area.
- Ludington sign:
  - Person sits for test.
  - Person is directed to place both hands behind the neck.
  - A tear in the rotator cuff is indicated by failure to carry out action with the affected arm or the need for compensatory movement to carry out action.

POSTERIOR CRUCIATE LIGAMENT ASSESSMENT

The **posterior cruciate ligament** (back of the knee joint) is 1 of the 4 ligaments supporting the knee. It provides support to the knee, preventing hyperextension, side to side, and rotational movement. The injury may result from blunt trauma to the knee while the knee is flexed, forcing the tibia posteriorly and stretching or tearing the ligament. There is usually less swelling than with an anterior cruciate tear, but the knee may be stiff and somewhat unstable. The **posterior drawer test** is the most sensitive test for evaluation:

- Note: The person's position is similar to that of the anterior drawer test, supine with hip flexed at 45°, knee at 80° and foot in neutral position.
- The examiner anchors the person's foot and palpates the hamstrings to ensure they are relaxed.
- The examiner places both hands immediately below the knee and applies pressure posteriorly to the tibial head.
- Subluxation of the tibia posterior to the femur is positive for posterior cruciate defect.

ANTERIOR CRUCIATE LIGAMENT ASSESSMENT

The **anterior cruciate ligament** is 1 of the 4 ligaments that support the knee. It provides stability, prevents the tibia from moving anterior to the femur, and limits rotation. A tear or partial tear can result from marked twisting of the joint or blunt trauma. Symptoms usually include pain and swelling of the joint as well as instability of the knee, depending upon the degree of damage. The **anterior drawer test** is used to evaluate stability of the knee:

- The person lies supine on an examining table with the foot on the affected side at the side of the table, the hip flexed to 45° and the knee at 90°.
- An assistant stabilizes the foot or (alternately) the examiner sits on the foot, using the buttocks to stabilize the foot.
- The test is performed with the foot in 3 positions: neutral, externally rotated 15° and 30°.

117

- The examiner places both hands on the upper calf at the head of the tibia and pulls anteriorly with even pressure.
- A positive sign of damage to the anterior cruciate ligament is palpable anterior tibial displacement.

This technique should be used with care in acute or multiple knee injuries as it can cause further damage. In acute injuries, the muscles may contract reflexively to protect the joint, and this may result in false positive results because the knee may appear stable. Additionally, pain may restrict flexion.

SUPINE LACHMAN TEST

In acute injuries, the supine Lachman test may be used:

- The person lies in supine position with the hip flexed to 45° and the knee to 20-30°.
- The examiner uses 1 hand to grasp and stabilize the distal thigh above the knee and the other hand to grasp the upper calf at the head of the tibia, which is then pulled anteriorly to evaluate for displacement.

ACHILLES TENDON AND THOMPSON'S TEST

A ruptured **Achilles tendon** can occur from blunt trauma to the tendon, excessive forced dorsiflexion of the ankle, or injury to a taut tendon. The injury occurs about 2-3 cm above the area where the tendon attaches the gastrocnemius (calf muscle) to the calcaneus (heel bone). The area of injury is usually tender to palpation, edematous, and bruised with a palpable gap where the tendon ruptured. **Thompson's test** is used to evaluate the injury:

- Place the person in prone position (face down) with the knee of the uninjured leg flexed to 90° and the foot relaxed.
- Squeeze the gastrocnemius muscle of the uninjured leg, causing it to contract and the foot to flex, noting the degree of response for comparison.
- Repeat test for the injured leg.
- If the Achilles tendon is partially or completely intact, plantar flexion of the foot occurs (negative finding).
- If plantar flexion is absent (positive finding), then this is indicative of a ruptured tendon.

TIBIAL STRESS FRACTURE AND THE TALAR BUMP/HEEL PERCUSSION TEST

One of the most common sports injuries is the **tibial stress fracture**, which may result from overtraining or training beyond level of strength and endurance. Symptoms may be non-specific but may involve point tenderness or increasing pain during activity. Stress fractures may not be evident on X-ray and may need a bone scan. Stress fractures may be difficult to differentiate from other injuries. The **Talar bump test** (Heel percussion test) may be done to differentiate the tibial stress fracture (talus or calcaneus) from the medial tibial stress syndrome:

- The person is in supine position with the knee and proximal calf on the table and the rest of the leg extending over the edge.
- The examiner holds the foot in neutral position with 1 hand.
- With the other open palm, the examiner applies percussive force (slapping) against the plantar surface of the foot.
- A positive sign of fracture is pain at the point of injury during percussion.

118

Allergic Reactions

ALLERGIC CONTACT DERMATITIS

Contact dermatitis is a localized response to contact with an **allergen**, resulting in a rash that may blister and itch. Common allergens include poison oak, poison ivy, latex, benzocaine, nickel, and preservatives, but there is a wide range of items preparations and products to which people may react.

Treatment includes:

- Identifying the **causative agent** through evaluating the area of the body affected, careful history, or skin patch testing to determine allergic responses.
- **Corticosteroids** to control inflammation and itching.
- Soothing oatmeal baths.
- **Caladryl®** (pramoxine) lotion to relieve itching.
- **Antihistamines** to reduce allergic response.
- **Lesions** should be gently cleansed and observed for signs of secondary infection.
- **Antibiotics** are used only for secondary infections as indicated.
- **Rash** is usually left open to dry.
- **Avoidance** of allergen will prevent recurrence.

ACUTE LATEX SENSITIVITY

Latex sensitivity is increasing in frequency, especially among those who are exposed to latex regularly through work, such as rubber industry workers, or have repeated contact with the healthcare system. Children with myelomeningocele have a high incidence of latex sensitivity. Latex sensitivity may manifest as 3 different types of reactions:

- **Irritant** (non-immune): Erythematous irritation from contact
- **Contact dermatitis** (type 4): Dry erythema beyond area of contact with pruritus, weeping, and blistering and results from chemicals (thiuram and thiazoles) used in production of latex
- **IgE** (type I) (immune reaction): Response to proteins in latex with urticaria, rhinitis, angioedema, asthma, laryngeal edema, anaphylactic shock, and death

Treatment for type I reaction includes:

- Establish patent **airway** and intubate if necessary, for ventilation.
- High flow **oxygen** (100%).
- Monitor **vital signs** (VS).
- Administer **epinephrine** (Epi-pen® or solution).
- **Albuterol** per nebulizer for bronchospasm.
- **Intravenous fluids** to provide bolus of fluids for hypotension.
- **Diphenhydramine** if shock persists.
- **Methylprednisolone** if no response to other drugs.

Integumentary

SKIN STRIPPING AND LACERATIONS

Mechanical trauma may result in stripping of the epidermis and sometimes the dermis of the skin or lacerations. Mechanical trauma may occur from tape removal or blunt trauma, such as colliding with furniture. Skin tears are categorized with the Payne-Martin Classification System:

1. Skin tear leaves avulsed skin adequate to cover wound. Tears may be linear or flap-type.
2. Skin tear with loss of partial thickness, involving either scant (<25% of epidermal flap over tear is lost) to moderate-large (> 25% of dermis in tear is lost).
3. Skin tear with complete loss of tissue, involving a partial-thickness wound with no epidermal flap.

Treatment includes:

- Recognizing fragile skin and treating carefully.
- Applying emollients, skin sealants, and skin barriers as indicated.
- Applying and removing tape appropriately.
- Avoiding adhesives when possible.
- Using hydrocolloids, Steri-strips®, and transparent dressings to stabilize flaps.

ACNE

Acne is acute or chronic **inflammation of the sebaceous hair follicles** on the face and trunk (chest and upper back), believed to be caused by increased sebum and androgen. The sebum blocks the follicular canals, which become inflamed and infected with anaerobic Propionibacterium. About 85% of teenagers 12-15 suffer from some degree of acne, which can cause severe emotional distress and low self-esteem. Acne must be differentiated from recent outbreaks of folliculitis caused by Staphylococcus aureus and community-acquired methicillin-resistant Staphylococcus aureus (MRSA). Acne is categorized and treated by grades:

- **Grade I**: Comedonal acne, treated with Retin-A® daily and salicylic acid/
- **Grade II**: Papulopustular acne, treated with 2.5% benzoyl peroxide and Retin-A® twice daily; topical clindamycin, erythromycin, or tetracycline twice daily.
- **Grade III**: Cystic acne, treated with Retin-A® and benzoyl peroxide twice daily and oral antibiotics, such as tetracycline.
- **Grade IV**: Severe pustulocystic nodular, treated with Accutane®.

FOLLICULITIS AND IMPETIGO

Folliculitis is bacterial infection of the **hair follicles**, often on the face, resulting in pustules, erythema, and crusts that are painful and itchy. Recently, there has been an increase in cases of community-acquired methicillin-resistant Staphylococcus aureus folliculitis infections. Folliculitis may occur as a primary or secondary infection and may result from chronic nasal colonization of methicillin-resistant Staphylococcus aureus (MRSA).

Treatment includes:

- Antibacterial soaps.
- Topical (Bactroban®) and oral antibiotics.

Impetigo is a contagious itchy bacterial infection of the skin, commonly on the face or hands, causing clusters of blisters or sores, especially in children. Group A Streptococcus usually causes small blisters that crust over. Staphylococcus aureus usually causes larger blisters that may be bullous and cause lesions 2-8 cm in size that persists for months. *Treatment* includes:

- Avoid scratching itches.
- Gently cleanse area with soap and water.
- Topical Bactroban® 3 times daily until healed.

CANDIDIASIS

Candidiasis, infection of the epidermis with Candida spp. (commonly referred to as "yeast" or "thrush"), causes a pustular erythematous papular rash that is commonly scaly, crusty, and macerated with a white cheese-like exudate. It may burn and is usually extremely pruritic and grows in warm moist areas of the skin, such the perineal area, aggravated by the use of disposable diapers. Candidiasis must be differentiated from bacterial infections because antibiotic treatment will worsen the condition. *Treatment* includes:

- Preventing humid moist conditions of skin.
- Controlling **hyperglycemia**.
- Careful **cleansing** and exposing area to air as much as possible.
- **Topical antifungal creams** (nystatin) with each diaper change or 4 times daily.
- **Zinc chloride ointment** over antifungal to provide barrier protection.
- Topical antifungal powders for mild cases.
- **Oral antifungal** (Diflucan®) for severe cases.

TATTOOS AND PIERCING

Tattoos and piercing have both been implicated in methicillin-resistant Staphylococcus aureus (MRSA) infections. **Tattooing** uses needles that inject dye, sometimes resulting in local infection with erythema, edema, and purulent discharge. **Body piercing** for insertion of jewelry carries similar risks. Piercings of concern include the upper ear cartilage, nipples, navel, tongue, lip, penis, and nose. Some people who do piercings use reusable piercing equipment that is difficult to adequately clean and sterilize. Infections resulting from piercing in cartilage are often resistant to antibiotics because of lack of blood supply. *Treatment* includes:

- **Cleansing wounds**. Jewelry may need to be removed in some cases.
- **Antibiotics**: Culture should be obtained, but medications for community-acquired-MRSA should be started immediately:
  - Mupirocin (Bactroban®) may be used topically 3 times daily for 7-10 days with or without systemic antimicrobials.
  - Trimethoprim-sulfamethoxazole 1-2 DS tablets (160 mg TMP/800 mg SMX) twice daily. Children, dose based on TMP: 8-12 mg TMP per kg/day in 2 doses.

121

Infectious Disease

LYME DISEASE

Lyme disease, first identified in 1975, is contracted through the bite of a tick infected with the bacterium **Borrelia burgdorferi**. There is a wide range of *symptoms*:

- **Early localized**: Erythema migrans (EM) bullseye rash occurs 3-30 days after bite in 70-80%, flu-like symptoms.
- **Early disseminated**: Migratory pain in joints, additional EMs, flu-like symptoms, fever, fatigue, headache, stiff neck, vision changes.
- **Late** (weeks, months): Arthritis of 1-2 large joints, neurological problems (confusion, memory loss, disorientation, peripheral numbness), cardiovascular disorders.

Diagnosis requires 2 steps: Enzyme-linked immunosorbent assay (ELISA) of indirect fluorescent antibody (IFA) with positive results confirmed by Western blot test. *Treatment*:

- **Oral antibiotics**: Doxycycline or Amoxicillin, 21-28 days although some studies show 10 days is sufficient.
- **IV antibiotics** (for more serious symptoms): Ceftriaxone (Rocephin) or Penicillin G 4-6 weeks.
- **NO vaccine** is currently available as it was withdrawn from the market.
- **Prophylaxis** after tick bite in highly endemic area where an engorged tick is found and removed: Doxycycline, single 200-mg dose.

> **Review Video: Lyme Disease**
> Visit mometrix.com/academy and enter code: 505529

BACTERIAL GASTROENTERITIS

A wide range of bacterial and viral pathogens can cause mild to severe life-threatening diarrhea:

- *Campylobacter jejuni* transmitted from pets to children younger than 7 years through contaminated food and water, usually in the summer. Diarrhea with fever, vomiting, and abdominal pain persists 7 to 12 days. *Treatment:* (in complicated cases) levofloxacin 500 mg orally for 3 days or until symptoms improve.
- *Clostridium difficile* occurs secondary to antibiotic use as normal flora of the gut is killed and c. difficile colonizes the GI tract. Some people are asymptomatic carriers, but severe illness is life-threatening with bloody diarrhea and abdominal pain leading to megacolon. *Treatment:* stop inciting antibiotic, contact precautions with soap and water instead of hand sanitizer to remove spores. Metronidazole (moderate) or vancomycin for 10-14 days (severe).
- *Yersinia enterocolitica* found in uncooked pork or unpasteurized milk causes secretory diarrhea with fever, foul, green, bloody stool, and pain in RLQ of abdomen. Usually resolves in 3-4 days.
- *Shigella* is transmitted fecal-oral route from contaminated food and water and occurs primarily in children from 6 to 36 months of age. Characterized by bloody diarrhea, abdominal pain, and fever. *Treatment:* Tailored to cultures but use fluoroquinolones once daily x 3 days while waiting for culture results or Trimethoprim-sulfamethoxazole (TMP-SMZ): TMP 8 mg/kg and SMZ 40 mg/kg per day given orally in 2 divided doses every 12 hours for 5 days.

Salmonella Gastroenteritis

Salmonella causes up to 4 million infections in the United States, resulting in 500 deaths, primarily of young children. There are two main types of salmonella, with nontyphoidal salmonella being the most common in the United States. **Nontyphoidal *Salmonella*** is spread by the fecal-oral route through ingestion of contaminated food or water, including all meats, milk, eggs, and vegetables. Raw or undercooked meat, unpasteurized milk, and unwashed produce are high risk. *Salmonella* may be found in the feces of pets, particularly reptiles such as snakes and turtles. *Symptoms* appear 12 to 72 hours after infection and include bloody diarrhea with abdominal pain, fever, and vomiting. Most cases resolve within 7 to 10 days, and are often indistinguishable from any other gastroenteritis. The mainstay of treatment is keeping the patient from becoming hypovolemic and keeping electrolytes balanced. In some cases, life-threatening sepsis may occur, requiring *treatment* with antibiotics, and fluoroquinolones are the antibiotics of choice. Antibiotic prophylaxis is usually contraindicated except in children younger than 1 year of age who are at risk for bacteremia or those who are immunocompromised. Patients who handle food as an occupation and those who are healthcare workers should not return to work until symptoms abate.

Escherichia Coli Gastroenteritis

E. coli strains are part of the normal flora of the intestines and serves to inhibit other bacteria, but some serotypes can cause intestinal disease and severe diarrhea. Onset of symptoms is generally about 4 days after being exposed. Some strains of *E. coli* are more common in developing countries and may occur in people who are traveling in areas where feces have contaminated food supplies and water. Severe outbreaks of *E. coli* infection have occurred in the United States with a toxic strain, O157:H7, known as an **enterohemorrhagic *E. coli***. This strain produces a toxin that can cause damage to the intestinal lining, including blood vessels, resulting in hemorrhage and watery diarrhea that becomes bloody, especially in children and elderly persons. This hemorrhagic colitis usually clears with supportive treatment after 10 days. However, about 15% of children develop sepsis and hemolytic uremic syndrome with kidney failure, hemolytic anemia, and thrombocytopenia. Death rates are 3% to 5%, but residual renal and neurological damage may result. *Treatment* is supportive with IV therapy, blood transfusions, and kidney dialysis. Antibiotics and antidiarrheals are contraindicated because they may worsen *E. coli* infections.

Giardia Lamblia Gastroenteritis

Giardia lamblia is a protozoan that infects water supplies and spreads through the fecal-oral route. It is the most common cause of nonbacterial diarrhea in the United States, causing about 20,000 cases of infection each year in all ages. Children often become infected swallowing recreational waters (pools, lakes) or putting contaminated items into the mouth. *Giardia* lives and multiplies within the small intestine where cysts develop. *Symptoms* occur 7 to 14 days after ingestion of 1 or more cysts and include: diarrhea with greasy floating stools (rarely bloody), stomach cramps, nausea, and flatulence, lasting 2 to 6 weeks. Chronic infection may develop. *Diagnosis* is based on 3 stool specimens, ELISA, or PCR for DNA. *Treatment* includes correcting fluid and electrolyte issues and antibiotics for symptomatic patients or patients who are food handlers, immunocompromised, or children who attend day care type settings:

- Metronidazole 250 mg 3 times daily for 5 days (drug of choice).
- Pediatric dosage: 15 mg/kg/day in 3 doses for 5 days.

123

OR

- Nitazoxanide 500 mg twice daily for 3 days.
- Pediatric dosage: 1 to 3 years, 100 mg every 12 hours for 3 days; 4 to 11 years, 200 mg every 12 hours for 3 days.
- Foods that contain lactose should be avoided for one month after treatment.

RUBEOLA

Rubeola (measles) is a viral disease characterized by fever and rash but can cause serious morbidity and death. It is highly infectious by droplets 4 days before and 4 days after onset of rash and has an incubation period of 7 to 18 days.

Symptoms include:

- Flu-like symptoms: cough, fever, running nose.
- Red maculopapular rash.
- Koplik spots on mucous membranes.
- Complications include: pneumonia, seizures, severe neurological damage from encephalitis.

Vaccination (MMR) or previous infection provides immunity. The vaccine may be used as a prophylaxis for 72 hours after exposure while immunoglobulin may provide protection if given within 6 days.

Treatment for measles is supportive because nothing eradicates the virus:

- Acetaminophen or ibuprofen.
- Vitamin A (small children).
- Standard barrier precautions.

MUMPS

Mumps is a viral disease that causes fever and swollen parotid glands but can cause deafness, meningitis, and swelling of the testicles. Mumps is spread through contact with saliva or aerosolized droplets from someone infected. The incubation period is 2 to 3 weeks. Incidence has decreased since vaccinations have become routine.

Diagnosis is by clinical exam and virus culture if necessary. *Symptoms* include:

- Painful swelling of glands on one or both sides of the face.
- Fever.
- Weakness, fatigue.
- Complications (rare) include orchitis, encephalitis, meningitis, ovarian inflammation, pancreatitis, and permanent hearing loss.

Treatment is supportive. There is no effective prophylaxis after exposure, although vaccination is not harmful and may protect against future infections if exposure does not cause disease. There is no effective treatment for mumps except for **supportive care**:

- Acetaminophen or ibuprofen.
- Standard barrier precautions.

RUBELLA

Rubella, also known as German measles, is a viral disease that can cause rash, fever, and arthritis, but the big danger is that it can cause a woman who is pregnant to miscarry or deliver a child with serious birth defects. Transmission is through airborne droplets. The incubation period is 2 to 3 weeks after exposure.

Symptoms persist 2 to 3 days and include:

- Fever 102°F or lower.
- Rhinitis.
- Conjunctivitis.
- Poor appetite, nausea.
- Rash, red or pink and sometimes itchy, starts on the face and moves down the body with the face clearing of rash as it progresses.
- Inflamed lymph nodes behind ears and at back of neck.

Children born with congenital rubella may shed the virus in stool and urine, which can infect caregivers. There is no effective prophylaxis after exposure.

Treatment is supportive:

- Acetaminophen or ibuprofen.
- Referral to obstetrician/gynecologist (pregnant women).
- Barrier precautions.

CHAGAS DISEASE

Chagas disease, caused by the protozoan parasite Trypanosoma cruzi, is endemic to much of Mexico, Central, and South America, and is transmitted when a **triatomine insect** bites the skin and deposits contaminated feces in the wound. The parasite invades organs and is transmitted through blood and organ donations. Chagas is an emerging disease in the United States where a large Latin American immigrant population has brought between 100,000 to 625,000 cases. Chagas has 3 stages: **acute** with either no or flu-like symptoms for most people, an **intermediate** stage that is asymptomatic, and a **chronic** stage that occurs about 30 years after infection, presenting with severe cardiomyopathy and digestive problems. People are often unaware that they are infected but pose a danger to the blood supply. Treatment is often ineffective after the acute stage. Centers for Disease Control (CDC) recommends treatment for those with acute disease and those who are immunocompromised or have congenital infection.

TREATMENT

Only 2 medications are available to treat **Chagas disease** and both are available from the Centers for Disease Control (CDC) only as investigational drugs:

- Benznidazole:
    - <12 yrs.: 10 mg/kg/day in 2 doses x 30-90 days
    - >12 yrs.: 5-7 mg/kg/day in 2 divided doses x 30-90 days
- Nifurtimox:
    - 1-10 yrs.: 15-20 mg/kg/day in 4 doses for 90 days
    - 11-16 yrs.: 12.5-15 mg/kg/day in 4 doses for 90 days
    - >16: 8-10 mg/kg/day in 3-4 doses for 90-120 days

Side effects are frequent and include gastrointestinal disturbance, anorexia, subsequent weight loss, epigastric pain, nausea and vomiting, headache, and/or vertigo. In rare cases, central nervous system (CNS) toxicity may occur with resultant confusion, nystagmus, psychosis, ataxia, tremors, and seizures. Studies have indicated that treatment of non-acute Chagas with medications in the early stages, prior to cardiac abnormalities, may have better outcomes. Magnetic resonance imaging (MRI) may be used to monitor heart function during the chronic stage of the disease.

AIDS

Acquired immunodeficiency syndrome (AIDS) is a progression of infection with **human immunodeficiency virus (HIV)**. AIDS is diagnosed when the following criteria are met:

- HIV infection.
- CD4 count less than 200 cells/mm^3.
- AIDS defining condition, such as opportunistic infections (cytomegalovirus, tuberculosis), wasting syndrome, neoplasms (Kaposi sarcoma), or AIDS dementia complex.

Because there is such a wide range of AIDS defining conditions, the patient may present with many types of *symptoms*, depending upon the diagnosis, but more than half of AIDS patients exhibit:

- Fever.
- Lymphadenopathy.
- Pharyngitis.
- Rash.
- Myalgia/Arthralgia.

It is important to review the following:

- CD4 counts, to determine immune status.
- WBC and differential for signs of infection.
- Cultures to help identify any infective agents.
- CBC to evaluate for signs of bleeding or thrombocytopenia.

Treatment aims to cure or manage opportunistic conditions and control underlying HIV infection through highly active anti-retroviral therapy (HAART), 3 or more drugs used concurrently.

WEST NILE VIRUS

West Nile virus (WNV), an RNA virus, is spread by infected mosquitoes. Infection has been traced to donor organs, blood transfusions, and breast milk although the blood supply has been monitored since 2003. While WNV is more common in adults, especially the elderly, it can affect infants and children. Infected children show symptoms more readily than adults. The incubation period ranges from 2-14 days. There are 3 types of infection:

- **Viremia**: 80%, infection but no symptoms.
- **Mild**: 20% (West Nile fever), characterized by fever, malaise, lymphadenopathy, headache, rash, nausea, and vomiting. The acute stage is usually is self-limiting within a few days, but symptoms can persist for weeks, including muscular weakness, fatigue, concentration problems, fever, and headache. About 30% require hospitalization.
- **Severe**: <1%, severe neurological symptoms, with meningitis and associated symptoms being the most common in children and young adults.

Treatment is supportive during illness and preventive (insect repellant).

The FDA has approved a human globulin (Omr-IgG-am) for treatment of WNV, primarily for those with neurological involvement.

BACTERIAL MENINGITIS

Bacterial meningitis may be caused by a wide range of pathogenic organisms, with the predominant agents in patients varying with age:

- **1 month or younger**: E.coli, group B streptococci, Listeria monocytogenes, and Neisseria meningitidis.
- **1 to 2 months**: group B streptococci.
- **Older than 2 months**: Streptococcus pneumoniae, N. meningitidis.
- **Unvaccinated** (Hib vaccine) children are at risk for *Haemophilus influenzae.* These are most common in adults.

Bacterial infections usually arise from spread distant infections, although they can enter the CNS from surgical wounds, invasive devices, nasal colonization, or penetrating trauma. The infective process includes inflammation, exudates, white blood cell accumulation, and tissue damage with the brain showing evidence of hyperemia and edema. Purulent exudate covers the brain and invades and blocks the ventricles, obstructing CSF and leading to increased intracranial pressure. Since antibodies specific to bacteria do not cross the blood/brain barrier, the body's ability to fight the infection is very poor. *Diagnosis* is usually based on lumbar puncture examination of cerebrospinal fluid and symptoms.

AGE-RELATED SYMPTOMS

Bacterial meningitis may manifest differently, depending upon age:

- **Neonates**: Signs may be very nonspecific, such as weight loss, hypo- or hyperthermia, jaundice, irritability, lethargy, irregular respirations with periods of apnea. More specific signs may include increasing signs of illness, difficulty feeding with loss of suck reflex, hypotonia, weak cry, seizures, and bulging fontanels (may be a late sign). Nuchal rigidity does not usually occur with neonates.
- **Infants and young children**: Classic symptoms usually do not appear until at least 2 years. Signs may include fever, poor feeding, vomiting, irritability, and bulging fontanel. Nuchal rigidity in some children.
- **Older children and adolescents/adults**: Abrupt onset, including fever, chills, headache, and alterations of consciousness with seizures, agitation, and irritability. May have photophobia, hallucinations, aggressive or stuporous behavior, and lapsing into coma. Nuchal rigidity progressing to opisthotonos. Reflexes are variable but positive Kernig and Brudzinski signs. Signs may relate to particular bacteria, such as rashes, sore joints, or draining ear.

MONONUCLEOSIS

Mononucleosis is an infectious disorder caused by the **Epstein-Barr virus**. It is spread through saliva and airborne droplets and occurs most common in teenagers and young adults. Incubation period is 4 to 6 weeks. *Symptoms* are usually similar to an upper respiratory tract infection or flu, with adults affected more than children, and may persist for weeks:

- Weakness.
- Headaches.
- Fever.

- Persistent sore throat.
- Enlarged lymph nodes in neck and axillae.
- Enlarged tonsils.
- Generalized red macular rash.
- Enlarged spleen, rupture may occur in rare cases.

Diagnosis may include clinical examination, antibody tests (such as Monospot), and CBC.

Treatment is primarily supportive as there is no treatment for the virus:

- Rest and restricted activity to avoid spleen rupture.
- Acetaminophen or ibuprofen.
- Adequate fluid intake.

MYCOBACTERIUM TUBERCULOSIS

Mycobacterium tuberculosis is a nonmotile obligate aerobic bacillus that forms chains, which are associated with a toxic surface component called cord factor. *M. tuberculosis* is neither gram-negative nor positive. As an extracellular agent, it needs oxygen, so it is attracted to the upper respiratory tract. It is also a facultative intracellular invader, allowing it to evade the immune system. Humans serve as the reservoir for this pathogen. The virulence is increased because of a unique cell wall composed of peptidoglycan, as well as complex lipids that provide antibiotic resistance and include acids that protect the cell, cord factor that is toxic to host cells, and Wax-D, which protects the cell envelope. The host immune system attempts to control the spread of *M. tuberculosis* by walling it off with macrophages, causing a positive skin reaction (cell-mediated immune response) but no infection. Resistant strains are an increasing cause of concern. Nosocomial outbreaks have occurred, often related to failure to identify an infected source.

DIAGNOSTICS AND PRECAUTIOUS

TB, caused by *Mycobacterium tuberculosis,* is not a new disease, but an increase in resistant strains has brought control and prevention of tuberculosis to the forefront of infectious disease control. TB is a particular danger to those who are immunocompromised, with 8% to 10% of those with HIV developing TB. Patients with TB may develop weight loss, general debility, night sweats, and fever. With pulmonary involvement, a progressive cough resulting in dyspnea and bloody sputum is common.

Diagnosis is based on skin and sputum testing as well as x-ray. Transmission is from airborne particles small enough to suspend in the air, so anyone in contact to someone with active TB is at risk of inhaling particles.

Precautions:

- Prompt diagnosis and anti-tuberculosis drugs per protocol.
- Airborne infection isolation.
- Skin testing/x-rays of those in contact.
- Preventive isoniazid therapy for those with latent infection or newly converted to positive on TB testing.

PNEUMONIA

Pneumonia is inflammation of the **lung parenchyma**, filling the alveoli with exudate. It is common throughout childhood and adulthood. Pneumonia may be a primary disease or may occur secondary to another infection or disease, such as lung cancer. Pneumonia may be caused by

128

bacteria, viruses, parasites, or fungi. Common causes for community-acquired pneumonia (CAP) include:

- Streptococcus pneumoniae.
- Legionella species.
- Haemophilus influenzae.
- Staphylococcus aureus.
- Mycoplasma pneumoniae.
- Viruses.

Pneumonia may also be caused by chemical damage. Pneumonia is characterized by location:

- **Lobar** involves one or more lobes of the lungs. If lobes in both lungs are affected, it is referred to as "bilateral" or "double" pneumonia.
- **Bronchial/lobular** involves the terminal bronchioles and exudate can involve the adjacent lobules. Usually the pneumonia occurs in scattered patches throughout the lungs.
- **Interstitial** involves primarily the interstitium and alveoli where white blood cells and plasma fill the alveoli, generating inflammation and creating fibrotic tissue as the alveoli are destroyed.

VIRAL PNEUMONIA

Viral pneumonia is more common in adults than children. However, the **respiratory syncytial virus** (RSV), which causes upper respiratory tract infections and bronchiolitis, can progress to pneumonia and is most commonly found in children younger than 5. A number of other viruses, such as adenoviruses, parainfluenza, cytomegalovirus, and coronavirus, may be implicated. The viruses invade the cells that line the airways and alveoli, causing death of the cells.

Symptoms related to viral pneumonia are similar to those of bacterial pneumonia, although the onset is often slow with pneumonia preceded by a respiratory infection that progressively worsens, with increasing cough, fever, dyspnea, cyanosis, and respiratory distress. There are few effective treatments for viral pneumonia, and one danger is that a viral pneumonia increases susceptibility to bacterial infection of the lungs.

Treatment may include:

- Rest and adequate fluids and nutrition.
- Antipyretics, such as acetaminophen.
- Oxygen therapy with intubation and mechanical ventilation may be required in the presence of severe disease and respiratory compromise.
- Ribavirin aerosol is used for severe RSV disease and pneumonia.

STREPTOCOCCUS PNEUMONIAE

S. pneumoniae (a gram-positive coccus) is part of the normal flora of the upper respiratory tract and is the most frequent cause of **bacterial pneumonia**, often secondary to an upper respiratory tract infection. The overall incidence has dropped since the heptavalent pneumococcal conjugate vaccine (PCV-7) was introduced in 2000, with the most significant effect on those younger than 2 years of age (78% drop in cases). However, a vaccinated infant that is febrile with toxic symptoms and a leukocyte count of at least 15,000 cells/mL is at risk for pneumonia. The bacteria induce an acute inflammatory response causing the alveoli and interstitium to fill with protein-rich fluid. The infection spreads quickly, often to multiple lobes, causing consolidation, pleural effusions, super infections, and bacteremia (15% to 25%). Pericarditis may occur. *Symptoms* include an abrupt onset with high fever (at least 105°F), chills, diaphoresis, cyanosis, chest pain, tachypnea, tachycardia, altered consciousness, and cough productive of rusty or green-tinged mucus. Although + sputum cultures and consolidations on chest x-ray indicate pneumonia, diagnosis is differentiated by blood culture or urinary antigen.

Treatment may include:

- Antipyretics and analgesics.
- Respiratory support.
- Antibiotics: penicillins or others.

COMMUNITY-ACQUIRED PNEUMONIA

MRSA

Community-acquired methicillin-resistant *Staphylococcus aureus (MRSA)* has emerged as a documented cause of **pneumonia** since 1997, although, pneumococcus remains the most predominant pathogen for community acquired pneumonia. CA-MRSA tends to be more susceptible to antibiotics than hospital acquired, but it is often more destructive with higher mortality, often causing a necrotizing pneumonia. CA-MRSA is suspected when a patient who is already known to be colonized with CA-MRSA (often those living in crowded places, prisoners, those who play contact sports) develops pneumonia. CA-MRSA pneumonia also often follows influenza in patients that are elderly or very young, and should be suspected, especially if pulmonary necrosis is present on imaging.

Symptoms are the same for other types of pneumonia.

Diagnosis: Blood cultures, Chest x-ray, assessment, history, and sputum cultures (will show gram-positive cocci in clusters).

Treatment includes:

- **Linezolid** (treatment of choice) 600 mg IV every 12 hours for 7-21 days.
- **Vancomycin** 45-60 mg/kg/day divided every 8 hours for 7-21 days, and keeping target trough levels between 15-20 mcg/mL.

MYCOPLASMA PNEUMONIAE

Mycoplasma pneumoniae is caused by pleomorphic (variously shaped) microorganisms that interfere with the function of the **cilia** and produce hydrogen peroxide, which disrupts **cell functions**. They also activate an inflammatory response. Only about 3% of those infected develop pneumonia, affecting primarily children and young adults between the ages of 4 and 20. Mycoplasma pneumoniae occurs seasonally in the fall in a regular 4- to 8-year cycle of epidemics. The onset is usually gradual, and children tend to be less obviously ill than with other types of pneumonia.

Symptoms may include a paroxysmal cough, low-grade fever, myalgia, diarrhea, erythematous rash, and pharyngitis. The pneumonia presents as interstitial infiltrates on x-ray. While complications, such as myocarditis, endocarditis, and aseptic meningitis and encephalitis, may occur, most infections clear without sequelae. *Treatment* includes:

- **Antibiotic therapy**: erythromycin, tetracycline, macrolide, or fluoroquinolone.
- **Symptomatic support**: antidiarrheals, antipyretics, and analgesics.

INTESTINAL PARASITES
ASCARIS LUMBRICOIDES/ROUNDWORMS

Worldwide, there are numerous **helminths (worms)** that can cause intestinal infections. Studies estimate that 50 million children in the United States are infected with worms.

Risk factors include:

- Young age.
- Going barefoot.
- Poor sanitation of food and water.
- Poor hygiene.
- Living in or traveling to an endemic area.
- Immigrant status, especially from Mexico.

Roundworms (Ascaris lumbricoides) can grow 6 to 13 inches in length, and a child may have up to 100 worms. After ingestion of eggs from contaminated raw foods or vegetables, the worms migrate to the intestines but can migrate to other organs, such as the lungs, and cause serious damage. They may also multiply in clumps and cause intestinal obstruction or may penetrate the intestinal wall causing peritonitis.

Symptoms include malnutrition, abdominal discomfort, and passing worms in stool or emesis.

Treatment includes albendazole 400 mg orally once OR mebendazole 100 mg times 3 days OR pyrantel pamoate 11 mg/kg in 1 dose. Piperazine citrate 75 mg/kg/day for 2 days for intestinal obstruction.

ENTEROBIUS VERMICULARIS/PINWORMS

Enterobius vermicularis (pinworms) are tiny (3 to 13 mm) worms that hatch in the small intestine after ingestion of eggs. The mature worms crawl through the rectum to lay eggs in the perianal folds, causing intense itching, often resulting in repeat self-infection; the person scratches and touches the hand to the mouth or contaminates food. Infection may result from contact with contaminated surfaces as well. The larvae hatch in the small intestines, but the adults live in the colon. Pinworms are the most common helminthic infection in the United States, affecting about 40 million people, especially children. Many are asymptomatic except for intense perianal itching, although some may have abdominal discomfort and anorexia or develop secondary infections from scratching. Girls may develop vulvovaginitis from invasion of the genital tract.

Diagnosis is made by the "scotch tape" test or anal swabs.

Treatment includes albendazole 400 mg for 1 dose repeated in 2 weeks or mebendazole 100 mg for 1 dose repeated in 2 weeks or pyrantel pamoate 11 mg/kg for 1 dose repeated in 2 weeks.

NECATOR AMERICANUS/HOOKWORMS

Necator americanus is the most common species of hookworm found in the southeastern United States. Hookworm larvae may be swallowed directly or penetrate the skin, often the feet of children going barefoot, and migrate to the lungs, where they are coughed up and swallowed, and then carried to the small intestines, where they attach themselves to the walls to suck blood and multiply. Severe infection can result in hypochromic, microcytic anemia along with hypoproteinemia and malnutrition. Infection with hookworms can result in dyspnea, cardiomegaly, and arrhythmias, and can be fatal in infants. Infected children may have restricted growth and mental development, which may be irreversible.

Diagnosis is with serial stool specimens.

Symptoms include itching and rash at the site of infection, followed by abdominal pain, diarrhea, anorexia, weight loss, and anemia.

Treatment includes albendazole 400 mg once OR mebendazole 100 mg times 3 days. Iron supplements may be necessary. Stools must be rechecked 1 week after treatment so that repeat treatment can be done if needed.

TINEA CAPITIS AND TINEA CORPORIS

Tinea capitis is a fungal infection of the scalp, usually affecting children between 1 and 10. It is spread through the sharing of combs, brushes, or caps.

Symptoms include circumscribed areas of hair loss with fine scaling and superficial pustules with mild itching.

Treatment includes:

- **Griseofulvin** orally 8 to 12 weeks.
- **Selenium sulfide shampoo** 2 to 3 times weekly, leaving shampoo on scalp for 10 minutes before rinsing.

Tinea corporis is a fungal infection of the skin of the trunk, although it can occur on the face or other parts of the body. It is spread by direct contact.

Symptoms include one or multiple circular patches that may be scaly and erythematous with slightly raised borders.

Treatment includes:

- **Selenium sulfide shampoo** wash of area before applying medication.
- **Topical antifungal** (clotrimazole, miconazole, tolnaftate, naftifine, terbinafine) 2 times daily for 4 weeks.
- **Systemic agents**: terbinafine, fluconazole, and itraconazole.

TINEA CRURIS AND TINEA PEDIS

Tinea cruris (jock itch) is a fungal infection of the perineal area, penis, inner thighs, and inguinal creases, but may also occur under breasts in women and beneath abdominal folds where skin is warm and moist. It rarely occurs before adolescence.

Symptoms include scaly, itching, erythematous rash that may contain papules or vesicle and is usually bilateral and symmetrical.

Treatment includes:

- **Selenium sulfide shampoo** wash of area before applying medication.
- **Topical antifungal** (clotrimazole, miconazole, tolnaftate, naftifine, terbinafine) 2 times daily for 4 weeks.

Tinea pedis (athlete's foot) is a fungal infection of the feet and toes. It is rare before adolescence and is more common in males. *Symptoms* include:

- Severe itching with vesicles or erosion of instep and with peeling maceration and fissures between toes.
- Dry, scaly, mildly erythematous patches on plantar and lateral foot surfaces.

Treatment includes:

- Same as tinea cruris.
- Keep feet dry with absorbent talc.
- Allow feet to air dry and use 100% cotton socks, changed twice daily.

TAPEWORMS

Cestodes, or **tapeworms**, are parasitic worms that live in the intestinal tracts of some animals/fish. There are several different species that can infect humans who eat raw or undercooked meat or fish that contains the immature form of the tapeworm. The worms mature and lay eggs that usually undergo maturation in the small bowel (autoinfection) or pass through the host feces. Many infections are asymptomatic, but heavy infections can cause nausea, vomiting, weight loss, diarrhea, and epigastric and abdominal pain. Pork tapeworms may invade the subcutaneous tissue and CNS, causing epilepsy and neurological compromise. Fish tapeworm may cause pernicious anemia.

Diagnosis: stool ova and parasites.

Treatment includes:

- **Praziquantel** 5 to 10 mg/kg one-time (drug of choice for all types)
- **Nitazoxanide** 500 mg for 3 days (dwarf tapeworm)
  - 1 to 3 years, 100 mg twice daily for 3 days
  - 4 to 11 years, 200 mg twice daily for 3 days
- **Niclosamide** 1 g one time (beef, pork, fish, and double-pored dog tapeworm)
  - 50 mg/kg one-time pediatric dose.

PEDICULOSIS

Pediculosis is infestation with **lice**, transmitted by direct contact with someone who is infested:

- Head lice (most common in children).
- Body lice (most common in transient populations). They feed on the body but live in clothing or bedding and are spread by sharing bedding, clothes, or towels.
- Pubic lice spread by sexual contact or (rare) sharing clothes or bedding, and may infest the genital area, eyebrows, eyelids, lower abdomen, and beard.

Symptoms include persistent itch (usually worse at night), irritation, excoriation, and sometimes secondary infection.

Diagnosis is by clinical exam and finding of lice or nits.

Treatment includes:

Permethrin 1% (treatment of choice): This is a cream rinse applied after body or hair is shampooed with a nonconditioning shampoo and then towel dried. It is left on for 10 minutes and then rinsed off, leaving residue designed to kill nymphs emerging from eggs not killed with the first application. Treatment is often repeated in 7 to 10 days. Nits should be manually removed.

SCABIES

Scabies is caused by a microscopic mite, *Sarcoptes scabiei hominis,* which tunnels under the outer layer of skin, raising small lines a few millimeters long. Mites prefer warm areas, such as between the fingers and in skin folds, but can infest any area of the body. As the mites burrow, they cause intense itching and subsequent scratching can result in excoriation and secondary infections. Some develop a generalized red rash. Scabies is spread very easily through person-to-person contact and has become a problem in nursing homes and extended-care facilities where staff spread the infection. Incubation time is 6 to 8 weeks and itching usually begins in about 30 days, so people may be unaware they are transmitting scabies. Most infestations involve only about a dozen mites, but a severe form of scabies infection, Norwegian or crusted scabies, can occur in elderly patients or those who are immunocompromised, and usually causes less itching. However, lesions can contain thousands of mites, making this type highly contagious.

DIAGNOSIS AND TREATMENT

Diagnosis of **scabies** is through skin scrapings, but because so few adult females usually infest a person, a negative finding does not mean that the person does not have scabies. When examining a patient with suspected scabies, it is helpful when searching for burrows to use a magnifying glass and a small flashlight held at an oblique angle.

Treatment for scabies includes:

- Scabicide:
  - **Permethrin** 5% cream (drug of choice) applied from chin to toes and left on for 12 hours and then showered off with a repeat treatment in 1 week.
  - **Sulfur** in petrolatum 10% concentration applied to entire body below the head on 3 successive nights and then bathe 24 hours after each application (safe for small children and pregnant women).
- Oral medication:
  - **Ivermectin oral medication** in 2 doses, 1 week apart, especially effective for crusted form.
- Itching: Antihistamines.
- Secondary infections: **Antibiotics**.

SYPHILIS

Syphilis is caused by the spirochete *Treponema pallidum* and has increased in incidence over the last 10 years; it is associated with risk-taking behavior such as drug use. The disease has 3 phases, with an incubation period of about 3 weeks:

- **Primary**: chancre (painless) in areas of sexual contact, persisting 3 to 6 weeks.
- **Secondary**: General flu-like symptoms (sore throat, fever, headaches) and red papular rash on trunk, flexor surfaces, palms, and soles, and lymphadenopathy occur about 3 to 6 weeks after end of primary phase and eventually resolves.
- **Tertiary** (latent): Affects about 30% and includes CNS and cardiovascular symptoms 3 to 20 years after initial infection. Gummas (granulomatous lesions) may be widespread. Complications include dementia, meningitis, neuropathy, and thoracic aneurysm.

Diagnosis is by dark-field microscopy (primary or secondary) or serologic testing. The CDC provides treatment protocol for different populations.

Treatment includes:

- Primary, secondary, early tertiary: benzathine penicillin G 104 million units IM in 1 dose.
- Tertiary: benzathine penicillin G 2.4 million units IM weekly for 3 weeks.

CHLAMYDIA

Chlamydia is an STD caused by *Chlamydia trachomatis* and is often coinfected with gonorrhea. It may be transmitted by oral, anal, and vaginal sex. It is the most common STD in the United States. *Symptoms* of chlamydia include:

- **Males**: urethritis, epididymitis, proctitis, or Reiter syndrome (urethritis, rash, conjunctivitis). Many are asymptomatic.
- **Females**: Mild cervicitis with vaginal discharge and dysuria, but complications can lead to infertility and pelvic inflammatory disease (PID).

Diagnosis is most reliable from nucleic acid amplification test (NAAT) (*Amplicor, ProbeTEC*).

Treatment includes:

- Azithromycin 1 g orally in 1 dose OR
- Doxycycline 100 mg orally twice daily for 1 week.
- Avoidance of sexual contact for 1 week.
- Treatment of the infected person's sexual partner is very important to avoid reinfection after treatment.

GONORRHEA

Gonorrhea is caused by *Neisseria gonorrhoeae* and should be suspected with urinary infections. *Symptoms* include:

- **Males**: Dysuria and purulent discharge from the urethra, ependymitis, and prostatitis.
- **Females**: Many women are asymptomatic or may have lower abdominal pain, cystitis, or mucopurulent cervicitis, but untreated it can result in PID and chronic pain.
- **Rectal infections** are common in women and homosexual males. Untreated, gonorrhea can become a systemic infection, resulting in petechial or pustular skin lesions, arthralgias, tenosynovitis, fever and malaise, and septic arthritis.

Diagnosis is by cervical or urethral culture or NAAT. Gram stains of urethral smears are more accurate for males than females. Cultures of multiple sites may be needed to confirm disseminated disease.

Treatment includes dual therapy:

- Ceftriaxone 250 mg IM in 1 dose AND azithromycin 1 g orally in 1 dose

OR

- Ceftriaxone 250 mg IM in 1 dose AND doxycycline 100 mg twice daily for seven days

Hematopoietic

ANEMIA

Anemia results in a decrease in oxygen transportation and decreased perfusion throughout the body, causing the heart to compensate by increasing cardiac output. As the blood becomes less viscous, there is decreased peripheral resistance, so more blood is pumped to the heart, and this increased flow can cause turbulence that results in a heart murmur and, if severe or prolonged, heart failure. Anemia is commonly caused by hemorrhage, hemolysis, hematopoiesis, or dietary iron deficiency in women who are menstruating. Children can tolerate low oxygen levels better than adults; however, growth and sexual development may be delayed with chronic anemia.

Symptoms include:

- General malaise and weakness, poor feeding/anorexia.
- Pallor, shortness of breath on exertion.
- Headache, dizziness, apathy, depression, decreased attention span, slowed thought processes.
- Shock symptoms (with severe blood loss): tachycardia, hypotension, poor peripheral circulation, and pallor.

Treatment includes:

- Treatment of underlying cause.
- Blood or blood components as indicated.
- Supportive care: oxygen, IV fluids.
- Referral for splenectomy (hemolytic anemias).

SICKLE CELL DISEASE AND SICKLE CELL CRISIS

Sickle cell disease is a recessive genetic disorder of chromosome 11, causing hemoglobin to be defective so that red blood cells (RBCs) are sickle-shaped and inflexible, resulting in their accumulating in small vessels and causing painful blockage. While normal RBCs survive 120 days, sickled cells may survive only 10 to 20 days, stressing the bone marrow that cannot produce fast enough and resulting in severe anemia. There are 5 variations of sickle cell disease, with **sickle cell anemia** the most severe. Different types of crises occur (aplastic, hemolytic, vaso-occlusive, and sequestrating), which cause infarctions in organs, severe pain, damage to organs, and rapid enlargement of liver and spleen. Complications include anemia, acute chest syndrome, congestive heart failure, strokes, delayed growth, infections, pulmonary hypertension, liver and kidney disorders, retinopathy, seizures, and osteonecrosis. Sickle cell disease occurs almost exclusively in African Americans in the United States, with 8% to 10% carriers.

TREATMENT

Treatment for **sickle cell disease** includes:

- **Prophylactic penicillin** for children from 2 months to 5 years to prevent pneumonia.
- **IV fluids** to prevent dehydration.
- **Analgesics** (morphine) during painful crises.
- **Folic acid** for anemia.
- **Oxygen** for congestive heart failure or pulmonary disease.

- **Blood transfusions** with chelation therapy to remove excess iron OR erythropheresis, in which red cells are removed and replaced with healthy cells, either autologous or from a donor.
- **Hematopoietic stem cells transplantation** is the only curative treatment, but immunosuppressive drugs must be used and success rates are only about 85%, so the procedure is only used on those at high risk. It requires ablation of bone marrow, placing the patient at increased risk.
- **Partial chimerism** uses a mixture of the donor and the recipient's bone marrow stem cells and does not require ablation of bone marrow.

HEMOPHILIA

Hemophilia is an inherited disorder in which the person lacks adequate clotting factors. There are 3 types:

- **Type A**: lack of clotting factor VIII (90% of cases)
- **Type B**: lack of clotting factor IX
- **Type C**: lack of clotting factor XI (affects both sexes, rarely occurs in the United States).

Both Type A and B are usually **X-linked disorders**, affecting only males. The severity of the disease depends on the amount of clotting factor in the blood.

Symptoms include:

- Bleeding with severe trauma or stress (mild cases).
- Unexplained bruises, bleeding, swelling, joint pain.
- Spontaneous hemorrhage (severe cases), often in the joints but can be anywhere in the body.
- Epistaxis, mucosal bleeding.
- First symptoms often occur during infancy when the child becomes active, resulting in frequent bruises.

Treatment includes;

- Desmopressin acetate parenterally or nasally to stimulate production of clotting factor (mild cases).
- Infusions of clotting factor from donated blood or recombinant clotting factors (genetically engineered), utilizing guidelines for dosing.
- Infusions of plasma (Type C).

VON WILLEBRAND DISEASE

Von Willebrand disease is a group of congenital bleeding disorders (inherited from either parent) affecting 1% to 2% of the population, associated with deficiency or lack of vW factor (vWF), a glycoprotein that is synthesized, stored, and secreted by vascular endothelial cells. This protein interacts with thrombocytes to create a clot and prevent hemorrhage; however, with von Willebrand disease, this clotting mechanism is impaired. There are 3 types:

- **Type I**: Low levels of vWF and also sometimes factor VIII. (Dominant inheritance.)
- **Type II**: Abnormal vWF (subtypes a, b) may increase or decrease clotting. (Dominant inheritance.)
- **Type III**: Absence of vWF and less than 10% factor VIII. (Recessive inheritance.)

Symptoms vary in severity and include: bruising, menorrhagia, recurrent epistaxis, and hemorrhage.

Treatment includes:

- Desmopressin acetate parenterally or nasally to stimulate production of clotting factor (mild cases).
- Severe bleeding: factor VIII concentrates with vWF, such as *Humate-P*.

LEUKEMIA

PHYSIOLOGIC IMPACTS

Leukemia is a condition in which the proliferating cells compete with normal cells for nutrition. Leukemia affects all cells because the abnormal cells in the bone marrow depress the formation of all elements, resulting in several consequences, regardless of the type of leukemia:

- Decrease in production of **erythrocytes** (RBCs), resulting in anemia.
- Decrease in **neutrophils**, resulting in increased risk of infection.
- Decrease in **platelets**, with subsequent decrease in clotting factors and increased bleeding.
- Increased risk of **physiological fractures** because of invasion of bone marrow that weakens the periosteum.
- Infiltration of **liver, spleen, and lymph glands**, resulting in enlargement and fibrosis
- Infiltration of the **CNS**, resulting in increased intracranial pressure, ventricular dilation, and meningeal irritation with headaches, vomiting, papilledema, nuchal rigidity, and coma progressing to death.
- **Hypermetabolism** that deprives cells of nutrients, resulting in anorexia, weight loss, muscle atrophy, and fatigue.

TREATMENT OPTIONS

Leukemia treatment depends upon the protocol established for each type of leukemia. Chemotherapy usually includes 3 stages: Induction (4-6 weeks), consolidation (4-8 months), and maintenance (2-3 years):

- **Induction therapy**: The purpose is to induce remission to the point that the bone marrow is clear of disease and blood cell counts are normal. Chemotherapy is usually given for about 4 to 6 weeks, followed by transplantation or the next stage of chemotherapy. The chemotherapy is potent and suppresses blood elements, so high risk for serious infections/hemorrhage.
- **Consolidation therapy**: The goal is to kill any cells that may have escaped the induction stage. This stage lasts 4 to 8 months. Intrathecal chemotherapy may be coadministered as a prophylaxis to prevent CNS involvement.
- **Maintenance therapy**: Treatment may continue for another 2 to 3 years, but with less intense chemotherapy to maintain the patient's remission.

Other treatments include:

- **Intrathecal chemotherapy** with invasion of the CNS.
- **Radiation to the brain** may be indicated in addition to intrathecal chemotherapy with severe disease poses danger to brain.
- **Hematopoietic stem cell transplantation** (HCST) may be done if chemotherapy fails or after the first remission for (AML), which has a lower cure rate.

COMMON CHILDHOOD LEUKEMIAS

AML and **ALL** are the 2 most common types of leukemias that affect children.

- **AML** is also referred to as granulocytic, myelocytic, monocytic, myelogenous, monoblastic, and monomyeloblastic leukemia. It is caused by a defect in the stem cells that differentiate into all myeloid cells. It affects all ages, occurring in children and adults, and often has a genetic component. Survival rates with adequate treatment are about 50%.
- **ALL** is also referred to as lymphatic, lymphocytic, lymphoblastic, or lymphoblastoid leukemia, and is caused by a defect in the stem cells that differentiate into lymphocytes. This is the most common type of childhood leukemia, peaking between ages 2 to 5. The cause is not known. There are a number of different types of ALL, and treatment and survival relate to the type. Overall survival rates with adequate treatment are about 80%.

Some rare forms of leukemia are named for the cells involved, such as basophilic leukemia.

> **Review Video: Leukemia**
> Visit mometrix.com/academy and enter code: 940024

Autoimmune Disorders

JUVENILE ARTHRITIS

Juvenile arthritis (JA) is an autoimmune disorder that affects girls more than boys and may have involved a genetic predisposition. It may be triggered by an immune response to environmental agents, including viruses. It is most common in those <16 (often as young as 7 or 8), but more than half will have symptoms after 10 years. There are many sub-types of JA, depending upon the degree of joint involvement and other symptoms. The polyarticular form is similar to adult rheumatoid arthritis. The systemic form can cause inflammation of multiple organs. *Symptoms* of JA may include:

- Fever and rash may precede joint pain.
- Iridocyclitis may cause photophobia with pain and damage to eye.
- Painful swollen joints.
- Contractures and deformity.
- Impairment of growth.

Treatment includes:

- Nonsteroidal anti-inflammatory drugs (NSAIDs) such as ibuprofen.
- DMARDS (disease-modifying anti-rheumatic drugs) such as methotrexate or Azulfidine.
- Biologic agents (etanercept).
- Corticosteroids, especially if pericarditis occurs.
- Physical therapy to optimize mobility.
- Surgical repair may be indicated.

SYSTEMIC LUPUS ERYTHEMATOSUS

Systemic lupus erythematosus is a systemic reaction to collagen or connective tissue in the body, believed triggered by an antibody-antigen immune response to an environmental agent, resulting in widespread damage of **vessels and organs**, primarily in females. Onset is usually 9-15 and is more common in African American, Hispanic, and Asian girls than Caucasian. *Symptoms* vary widely and may include:

- "Butterfly" rash (scaly erythematous maculopapular patches) on face, chest, and arms.
- Arthritic-type pain, stiffness, and swelling of joints.
- Central nervous system (CNS) involvement with seizures, headache, and psychosis.
- Heart (pericarditis) and lung (pleurisy) inflammation.
- Kidney failure.
- Anemia (erythrocytopenia)
- Spleen, liver, and lymph nodes enlarged.
- Gastrointestinal (GI) symptoms: nausea, vomiting, pain, and hepatitis.

Treatment varies according to severity of disease and includes:

- Nonsteroidal anti-inflammatory drugs (NSAIDs) for pain and inflammation.
- Steroids for organ inflammation.
- Antimalarial drugs for skin involvement.
- Immunosuppressant agents if steroids not adequate.

> **Review Video: Lupus**
> Visit mometrix.com/academy and enter code: 657082

Endocrine

DIABETES MELLITUS

Diabetes mellitus, often simply referred to as diabetes, is a group of metabolic diseases which are characterized by dysfunctional use or production of **insulin**, resulting in elevated blood glucose levels. It is the most common metabolic disorder in children, affecting about 1.5 million children and adolescents with 70% to 85% with type I and the rest with type II.

Type I: Immune-mediated form with insufficient insulin production because of destruction of pancreatic beta cells.

Symptoms include:

- Pronounced polyuria and polydipsia.
- Short onset.
- May be overweight, or have recent weight loss.
- Ketoacidosis present on diagnosis.

Treatment includes:

- Insulin as needed to control blood sugars.
- Glucose monitoring 1-4 x daily.
- Diet control with carb control.
- Exercise.

Type II: Insulin-resistant with defect in insulin secretion. Symptoms include:

- Long onset.
- Obese with no weight loss or significant weight loss.
- Mild or absent polyuria and polydipsia.
- May have ketoacidosis or glycosuria without ketonuria.
- Androgen-mediated problems such a hirsutism and acne.
- Hypertension

Treatment includes diet and exercise, glucose monitoring, oral medications, and possibly insulin.

> **Review Video: <u>Diabetes Mellitus: Diet, Exercise, & Medications</u>**
> Visit mometrix.com/academy and enter code: 774388

HYPERGLYCEMIC HYPEROSMOLAR NONKETOTIC SYNDROME

Hyperosmolar hyperglycemic state (HHS), also known as hyperosmolar hyperglycemic nonketotic syndrome (HHNS), occurs in people without history of diabetes or with mild type 2 diabetes but with insulin resistance resulting in persistent hyperglycemia, which causes **osmotic diuresis**. Fluid shifts from intracellular to extracellular spaces to maintain osmotic equilibrium, but the increased glucosuria and dehydration results in hypernatremia and increased osmolarity. This condition is most common in those 50-70 years old and often is precipitated by an acute illness, such as a stroke, medications such as thiazides, or dialysis treatments. HHS differs from ketoacidosis because, while the insulin level is not adequate, it is high enough to prevent the breakdown of fat. Onset of symptoms often occurs over a few days.

SYMPTOMS

Symptoms include:

- Polyuria.
- Dehydration.
- Hypotension & Tachycardia.
- Blood glucose: >600 mg/dL.
- Serum osmolality >350 mOsm/L
- Increased BUN and creatinine
- Changes in mental status, seizures, hemiparesis.

TREATMENT

Treatment is similar to that for ketoacidosis:

- Insulin
- Intravenous fluids and electrolytes.
- Correct blood glucose and other labs.

Expect increased serum sodium, serum osmolality and urine osmolality.

DIABETIC KETOACIDOSIS

DKA is a complication of diabetes mellitus. Inadequate production of insulin results in glucose being unavailable for metabolism, so lipolysis (breakdown of fat) produces free fatty acids (FFAs) as an alternate fuel source. Glycerol in both fat cells and the liver is converted to ketone bodies (beta-hydroxybutyric acid, acetoacetic acid, and acetone), which are used for cellular metabolism

141

less efficiently than glucose. Excess ketone bodies are excreted in the urine (ketonuria) or exhalations. The ketone bodies lower serum pH, leading to ketoacidosis. *Symptoms* include:

- **Kussmaul respirations**: hyperventilation to eliminate buildup of carbon dioxide, associated with "ketone breath."
- **Fluid imbalance**, including loss of potassium and other electrolytes from cellular death, resulting in dehydration and diuresis with excess thirst.
- **Cardiac arrhythmias**, related to potassium loss, can lead to cardiac arrest.
- **Hyperglycemia**, with glucose levels above normal. Normal values:
  - Neonate: 40 to 60 mg/dL.
  - Younger than 12 months: 50 to 90 mg/dL.
  - Older than 12 months: 60 to 100 mg/dL.

Treatment includes:

- Insulin therapy by continuous infusion initially.
- Electrolyte replacement.

ACUTE HYPOGLYCEMIA

Acute hypoglycemia (hyperinsulinism) may result from pancreatic islet tumors or hyperplasia, increasing insulin production, or from the use of insulin to control diabetes mellitus. Hyperinsulinism can cause damage to the **central nervous and cardiopulmonary systems**, interfering with functioning of the brain and causing neurological impairment. Causes may include:

- Genetic defects in chromosome 11 (short arm)
- Severe infections, such as Gram-negative sepsis, endotoxic shock.
- Toxic ingestion of alcohol or drugs, such as salicylates.
- Too much insulin for body needs.
- Too little food or excessive exercise.

Symptoms include:

- Blood glucose <50-60 mg/dL.
- Central nervous system: seizures, altered consciousness, lethargy, and poor feeding with vomiting, myoclonus, respiratory distress, diaphoresis, hypothermia, and cyanosis.
- Adrenergic system: diaphoresis, tremor, tachycardia, palpitation, hunger, and anxiety.

Treatment depends on underlying cause and includes:

- Glucose/Glucagon administration to elevate blood glucose levels.
- Diazoxide (Hyperstat®) to inhibit release of insulin.
- Somatostatin (Sandostatin®) to suppress insulin production.
- Careful monitoring.

ACUTE PANCREATITIS

Acute pancreatitis is related to chronic alcoholism or cholelithiasis in 90% of patients. Pancreatitis may be triggered by a variety of drugs (tetracycline, thiazides, acetaminophen, oral contraceptives). Pain is usually acute and may be in mid-epigastric, left upper abdominal, or more generalized.

Nausea and vomiting as well as abdominal distention may be present. Complications may include shock, acute respiratory distress syndrome, and multi-organ failure. *Diagnostic* tests include:

- Serum lipase >2 X normal value.
- Serum amylase (less accurate than lipase).
- CT with contrast to determine if there is pancreatic necrosis.
- Ultrasound to check bile duct for obstruction.
- MR cholangiopancreatography may be used in place of CT and ultrasound where available.

Treatment is usually supportive with oral intake NPO or restricted to clear liquids to help manage vomiting, ileus, and aspiration. Rehydration with intravenous fluids may be needed or TPN. Hemodynamic support as needed. Biliary obstruction needs to be removed with cholecystectomy. Antibiotics are given if necrosis is related to infection. Analgesia may be indicated, but avoid morphine as it may cause spasms in the sphincter of Oddi.

HYPOTHYROIDISM

Hypothyroidism occurs when the thyroid produces inadequate levels of thyroid hormones. Conditions may range from mild to severe myxedema. There are a number of causes:

- Chronic lymphocytic thyroiditis (Hashimoto's thyroiditis).
- Excessive treatment for hyperthyroidism
- Atrophy of thyroid.
- Medications, such as lithium, iodine compounds
- Radiation to the area of the thyroid.
- Diseases that affect the thyroid, such as scleroderma
- Iodine imbalances.

Symptoms may include chronic fatigue, menstrual disturbances, hoarseness, subnormal temperature, low pulse rate, weight gain, thinning hair, thickening skin. Some dementia may occur with advanced conditions. Clinical findings may include increased cholesterol with associated atherosclerosis and coronary artery disease. Myxedema may be characterized by changes in respiration with hypoventilation and CO_2 retention resulting in coma. *Treatment* involves hormone replacement with synthetic levothyroxine (Synthroid®) based on TSH levels, but this increases the oxygen demand of the body, so careful monitoring of cardiac status must be done during early treatment to avoid myocardial infarction while reaching euthyroid (normal) level.

HYPERTHYROIDISM

Hyperthyroidism (thyrotoxicosis) usually results from excess production of thyroid hormones (Graves' disease) from immunoglobulins providing abnormal stimulation of the **thyroid gland**. Other causes include thyroiditis and excess thyroid medications.

Symptoms include:

- Hyperexcitability
- Tachycardia (90-160) and atrial fibrillation.
- Increased systolic (but not diastolic) BP.
- Poor heat tolerance, skin flushed and diaphoretic.
- Dry skin and pruritus (especially in the elderly).
- Hand tremor, progressive muscular weakness.

143

- Exophthalmos (bulging eyes).
- Increased appetite and intake but weight loss.

Treatment includes:

- Radioactive iodine to destroy the thyroid gland. Propranolol may be used to prevent thyroid storm. Thyroid hormones are given for resultant hypothyroidism.
- Antithyroid medications, such as Propacil® or Tapazole® to block conversion of T4 to T3.
- Surgical removal of thyroid is used if patients cannot tolerate other treatments or in special circumstances, such as large goiter. Usually one-sixth of the thyroid is left in place and antithyroid medications are given before surgery.

> **Review Video: 7 Symptoms of Hyperthyroidism**
> Visit mometrix.com/academy and enter code: 923159
>
> **Review Video: Graves' Disease**
> Visit mometrix.com/academy and enter code: 516655

THYROTOXIC STORM

Thyrotoxic storm is a severe type of hyperthyroidism with sudden onset, precipitated by stress, such as injury or surgery, in those un-treated or inadequately treated for hyperthyroidism. If not promptly diagnosed and treated, it is fatal. Incidence has decreased with the use of antithyroid medications but can still occur with medical emergencies or pregnancy. Diagnostic findings are similar to hyperthyroidism, and include increased T3 uptake and decreased TSH.

Symptoms include:

- Increase in symptoms of hyperthyroidism.
- Increased temperature >38.5°C.
- Tachycardia >130 with atrial fibrillation and heart failure.
- Gastrointestinal disorders, such as nausea, vomiting, diarrhea, and abdominal discomfort.
- Altered mental status with delirium progressing to coma.

Treatment includes:

- Controlling production of thyroid hormone through antithyroid medications, such as propylthiouracil and methimazole.
- Inhibiting release of thyroid hormone with iodine therapy (or lithium).
- Controlling peripheral activity of thyroid hormone with propranolol.
- Fluid and electrolyte replacement.
- Glucocorticoids, such as dexamethasone.
- Cooling blankets.
- Treatment of arrhythmias as needed with antiarrhythmics and anticoagulation.

PRECOCIOUS PUBERTY

Precocious puberty is onset of puberty before age 7 in girls and 9 in boys. It can result from disorders of the gonads, the adrenal gland, or the hypothalamic-pituitary-gonad axis, producing **gonadotropin-releasing hormone** (GnRH) that cause early maturing of secondary sexual characteristics. It is much more common in girls than boys. *Symptoms* of complete precocious puberty include:

- Breast development and menstruation in girls.
- Enlargement of testes and penis in boys with deepening of voice.
- Development of pubic and axillary hair in both and facial hair in boys.
- Acne.
- Rapid increase in height for age.
- Production of perspiration and odor.

Partial precocious puberty presents similarly but results from overproduction of sex hormones, often because of a tumor of the ovary or testes, hyperplasia of the adrenal gland, or exogenous sources of hormones:

Treatment includes:

- Identifying and treating underlying causes.
- If caused by GH, parenteral synthetic analog of luteinizing hormone-releasing hormone until puberty to slow development.

Hypopituitarism Related to Deficient Growth Hormone

Hypopituitarism may affect production of 1 or multiple hormones because of organic defects or idiopathic ideology, but deficiency in somatotropin, or growth hormone (GH), is the primary disorder, which may be associated with other disorders. A decrease in GH causes a condition known as **hypopituitary dwarfism**, with *symptoms* characterized by:

- Normal growth in the first year but below 5th percentile in 2nd year.
- Height retarded to a greater extent than weight.
- Well-nourished with proportional skeleton.
- Inactive as infants and children.
- Primary teeth normal but permanent teeth delayed and overcrowded because of lack of adequate development of the jaw.
- Sexual development delayed.

Treatment includes:

- Identifying any organic causes, such as tumors, and treating.
- Biosynthetic GH administration can more than double growth rate but the degree of benefit depends upon the age the treatments are started and the individual response.
- Sex hormone therapy during adolescence.

Psychological

Attention Deficit/Hyperactivity Disorder

Mental health problems can interfere with normal growth and development in children and adolescents. Studies indicate that about 10% of children suffer mental disorders that cause some degree of impairment. There are a number of different disorders that affect children. **ADHD** affects 2-3% of children. ADHD usually has 3 characteristics:

- Inattention
- Impulsivity
- Hyperactivity

These make it difficult for the child to pay attention in school and keep track of assignments and often results in behavioral and social problems. Additionally, ADHD may be accompanied by **learning disabilities**, such as dyslexia, as well as depression or other mood disorders. *Diagnosis* often includes observation and surveys of family and teachers to determine patterns of behavior. *Intervention* includes medications and coping and organizing skills. Studies of different treatments indicate that a combined approach with **medications and behavioral therapy** is more effective than either medication alone or behavioral therapy alone. The combined approach may allow lower medication dosages.

AUTISM SPECTRUM DISORDERS

Autism spectrum disorders (ASD), or **pervasive developmental disorders (PDD)**, affect 3.4 out of 1,000 children in the United States and present with a wide range of symptoms, including impairment in thinking and expressions of emotion, using language, and communicating and relating with others. Some children are profoundly impaired and are diagnosed early but more high functioning children, such as those with Asperger's, may go undiagnosed. All exhibit some degree of impairment in 3 areas:

- Social interaction
- Communication (verbal and non-verbal)
- Repetitive behavior

Because they lack social skills, children are often **isolated** and **bullied**. They may do well in school or have some degree of intellectual disability. About 25% suffer from seizure disorders as well. ASD may be identified through developmental screening, and/or specific screening instruments for autism. *Intervention* includes referrals to special education programs, including early intervention programs for children <3 and may include behavioral and speech therapy. *Early diagnosis* helps maximize the child's potential and may allow the child to live independently as an adult.

BORDERLINE PERSONALITY DISORDER

Borderline personality disorder (BPD) affects about 2% of adults, mostly young women, but symptoms may begin to develop slowly from about 9 and on into the teen years resulting in unstable moods and disordered thinking in relation to **self-image and behavior**. Self-injury, including self-mutilation, and suicide attempts are common as are drinking and drug use. Patients may perceive themselves as bad and suffer severe separation anxiety and fears. They often engage in impulsive high-risk behaviors, such as promiscuous sex and binge eating. Studies have linked BPD to **child and sexual abuse as children**, with 40-71% of young women diagnosed with BPD victims of sexual abuse during childhood. While definitive diagnosis is usually delayed until young adulthood, because of the associated social and behavioral problems, early recognition of the symptoms and intervention with medications and/or behavioral therapy may help the person to cope and develop better behavioral strategies. Medications include mood stabilizers, anticonvulsants, selective serotonin reuptake inhibitors (SSRIs), atypical antipsychotics, and opiate receptor antagonists.

BIPOLAR DISORDER

Bipolar disorder causes severe mood swings between **hyperactive states** and **depression**, accompanied by impaired judgment because of distorted thoughts. The hypomanic stage may allow for creativity and good functioning in some people, but it can develop into more severe mania, which may be associated with psychosis and hallucinations, and then into periods of profound depression. While most cases are diagnosed in late adolescents, there is increasing evidence that some children present with symptoms earlier, especially at risk are children with a bipolar parent. Bipolar disorder is associated with high rates of **suicide**, so early diagnosis and treatment is critical. *Symptoms* may be relatively mild or involve severe rapid cycling between mania and depression. *Intervention* includes both medications (usually given continually) to prevent cycling and control depression and psychosocial therapy, such as cognitive therapy, which helps patients control disordered thought patterns and behavior. Medications include anticonvulsants, mood stabilizers, antidepressants, atypical antipsychotics, and anti-anxiety medications. Family and group therapy are often useful.

DEPRESSION

Depression is increasingly recognized as a risk factor not only for adults but for **children**, manifesting in young children as pretending illness or refusal to go to school and in older children as behavioral problems, negativity, and difficulties at school rather than the more common withdrawal and overt depression of some adults. However, children may feel persistent anxiety and sadness and often have profound fears that something will happen to a parent. Usually **changes in behavior** become apparent. Both children and adults may have suicidal thoughts. Adults often have insomnia or sleep excessively, have trouble concentrating, and have feelings of hopelessness. They may become easily angered. While there is some concern about antidepressants and children, suicide is a leading cause of death in teenagers, so medications, such as selective serotonin reuptake inhibitors (SSRIs) and tricyclic antidepressants, with careful monitoring along with psychotherapy, such as cognitive behavioral therapy, similar to adult therapy, seem to provide the best form of treatment.

EATING DISORDERS

Eating disorders are a profound health risk, especially for young girls (although boys may also have eating disorders, often presenting as excessive exercise). Different types include:

- **Anorexia nervosa** affects 0.5-3.7% of females, characterized by profound fear of weight gain and severe restriction of food intake, often accompanied by abuse of diuretics and laxatives, which can cause electrolyte imbalances as well as kidney and bowel disorders and delay or cause cessation of menses. Anorexics may become emaciated and risk death.
- **Bulimia nervosa** affects 1.1-4.2% of females and includes binge eating followed by vomiting often along with diuretics, enemas, and laxatives. Gastric acids can damage the throat and teeth. While bulimics may maintain a normal weight, they are at risk for severe electrolyte imbalances that can be life threatening.
- **Binge eating** affects 2-5% of females and includes grossly overeating, often resulting in obesity, depression, and shame.

Early *intervention* can prevent physical damage but hospitalization and intense therapy may be required for long periods of time to change altered thinking.

Pain

NUMERICAL PAIN SCALE

Pain is subjective and may be influenced by the individual's pain threshold (the smallest stimulus that produces the sensation of pain) and pain tolerance (the maximum degree of pain that a person can tolerate). The most common current pain assessment tool is the **1-10 scale**:

$$0 = \text{no pain}$$
$$1 - 2 = \text{mild pain}$$
$$3 - 5 = \text{moderate pain}$$
$$6 - 7 = \text{severe pain}$$
$$8 - 9 = \text{very severe pain}$$
$$10 = \text{excruciating pain}$$

However, there is more to pain assessment than a number on a scale. Assessment includes information about onset, duration, and intensity. Identifying what triggers pain and what relieves it can be very useful when developing a plan for pain management. Patients may show very different behavior when they are in pain: some may cry and moan with minor pain and others may exhibit little difference in behavior when truly suffering; thus, judging pain by behavior can lead to the wrong conclusions.

PAIN ASSESSMENT OF NEONATES/INFANTS

Pain assessment of neonates and infants depends on careful observation of a number of different characteristics. NIPS assesses 6 areas with a score >3 indicating pain. Five areas are scored 0-1, depending upon the degree of stress. Crying, which is often the most indicative of pain, is scored 0-2:

Characteristic	0	1	2
Facial expression	Rested, normal	Negative, tightened muscles, grimace	
Crying	None	Intermittent, moaning, whimper	Loud, shrill continuous crying
Respiratory patterns	Relaxed, normal	irregular breathing, tachypnea, holding breath, gagging	
Upper extremities	Relaxed, random movement	Tense, rigid or rapid extending and flexing.	
Lower extremities	Relaxed, random movement	Tense, rigid or rapid extending and flexing.	
Arousal state	Quiet, awake or asleep with random leg movements	Restless, fussing, thrashing about.	

CHEOPS Pain Assessment of Children Ages 1-7

The **Children's Hospital Eastern Ontario Pain Scale (CHEOPS)** is used for children 1-7 and is based on scores of 6 different characteristics with scores of 0-2 except for crying, which is scored 0-3. A score >4 indicates pain.

Characteristic	0	1	2	3
Crying		Not crying	Silent crying, moans or whimpers	Sobs/ Scream
Facial expression	Smiling positive	Neutral	Grimaces, negative	
Verbalization	Positive	No talking/ complaining	Complains about pain or other things.	
Torso		Inactive, at rest, relaxed	Tense, moves, shudders, shivers, sits upright or restrained.	
Upper extremities		No touching/ reaching for injury.	Reach for, touches gently, grabs wound, injury, arms restrained.	
Lower extremities		Relaxed, random movement	Restless or tense, moves, legs flexed, kicks, crouches, kneels, legs restrained.	

Assessment of Pain for Patients with Cognitive Impairment or Inability to Verbalize Pain

Patients with cognitive impairment or inability to verbalize pain may not be able to indicate the degree of pain, even by using a face scale with pictures of smiling to crying faces. The **Pain Assessment in Advanced Dementia (PAINAD)** scale may be helpful. Careful observation of non-verbal behavior can indicate that the patient is in pain:

- **Respirations**: Patients often have more rapid and labored breathing as pain increases with short periods of hyperventilation or Cheyne-Stokes respirations.
- **Vocalization**: Patients may remain negative in speech or speak quietly and reluctantly. They may moan or groan. As pain increases, they may call out, moan or groan loudly, or cry.
- **Facial expression**: Patients may appear sad or frightened, may frown or grimace, especially on activities that increase pain.
- **Body language**: Patients may be tense, fidgeting, pacing and as pain increases may become rigid, clench fists, or lie in fetal position. They may become increasingly combative.
- **Consolability**: Patients are less distractible or consolable with increased pain.

Differential Diagnosis

Differential Diagnosis Process

The **differential diagnosis** is an important tool that allows the clinician to familiarize him or herself with the patient's condition, understand the condition, create an effective treatment plan, and follow the progress of the patient. To start, thoroughly examine the patient's chart, making a list of all of the abnormal test results and laboratory values. Add to this list all of the patient's complaints. Once this list is complete, organize the test results, labs, and complaints by anatomic location or organ system. After breaking the list down by organ site, look for any relationships between symptoms and/or results. Create another list of those data that seem to be related, and list all of the diseases or conditions that explain the findings, eliminating any that do not fit.

CREATION OF PROBLEM LIST AS PART OF DOCUMENTATION AND DIAGNOSIS

Once the history is complete and objective data, such as laboratory findings and physical information (such as height, weight, blood pressure) is completed, the nurse practitioner should carefully review the **documentation** to observe for patterns that may relate to a particular **diagnosis**. Isolated information (laboratory tests) provides only part of the picture, so each element of the assessment (including functional and developmental information) must be evaluated in terms of others. The nurse practitioner reviews the record and identifies conditions that match findings and eliminates others, gradually building a **problem list** of possible causes. All items on the problem list should be related to subjective or objective data. This problem list then is used to determine whether further assessment, such as history taking, laboratory tests, or radiography is needed to arrive at a clinical diagnosis. Once a diagnosis is established, intervention is planned based on this diagnosis, and then the treatment is evaluated.

FACTORS INFLUENCING THE CLINICAL DECISION-MAKING PROCESS

Although one would like to think that there isn't much variation in the **clinical decision-making process**, this simply is not true. The process, of course, will differ depending on the patient, the differential diagnosis, and the clinician. First, let's start with the clinician. The way that the clinician conducts the clinical decision-making process is influenced by the knowledge base of the clinician, as well as the level of his experience, the ability he possesses to think both critically and creatively, and the confidence that he has in his ability to make educated decisions. The acuity level of the patient is also a factor in the clinical decision-making process, as is the length of the differential. A time stressor is placed on the clinician when the condition of the patient is critical, and when there are more diseases that must be eliminated from the differential. An element of stress may also exist if the clinician has a high number of patients, especially if he has multiple high-acuity patients.

Test Selection and Evaluation

UNIVERSAL PRINCIPLES OF DIAGNOSTIC TESTING

First, it is important to remember that the positive and negative predictive values of a test are not **absolute**. For example, if an NP tests a high-risk population for diabetes (say 180 out of 200 have the disease), and then tests a low-risk population (20 out of 200 have the disease), the sensitivity and specificity of the test will stay the same, but the predictive values will change. Also, a test that has less than 100% sensitivity and specificity is most useful for the patient with an equivocal or intermediate probability of disease, rather than a high-risk patient or a low-risk patient. One other important point to remember is that sensitivity and specificity are inversely related. If a diagnostic test is modified in order to increase its sensitivity, the specificity of the test will decrease, and vice versa.

SENSITIVITY AND SPECIFICITY IN RELATION TO DIAGNOSTIC TESTING

Some **degree of error** is inherent in almost all diagnostic testing. When ordering a diagnostic test for a patient, how confident should the NP be that the result will be accurate? The terms sensitivity and specificity are used to illustrate the accuracy of diagnostic tests. The **sensitivity** of a test refers to its ability to correctly identify patients who do have the disease. If a test is administered to 100 patients with diabetes, and all 100 patients test positive, the test is considered to have a sensitivity of 100%. If only 85 of those tested have a positive result, however, that means that the test has a false-negative rate of 15%, and a sensitivity of 85%. On the other hand, the **specificity** of a diagnostic test refers to its ability to identify patients who do not have the disease. If 100 nondiabetic patients are tested for diabetes, and 50 of them have a positive result, the test has a specificity of only 50%.

TESTING NUTRITIONAL STATUS
TOTAL PROTEIN AND ALBUMIN

Total protein levels can be influenced by many factors, including stress and infection, but it may be monitored as part of an overall nutritional assessment. Protein is critical for wound healing, and because metabolic rate increases in response to a wound, protein needs increase:

- Normal values: 5-9 g/kg per day.
- Diet requirements for wound healing: 1.25-1.5 g/kg per day.

Albumin is a protein that is produced by the liver and is a necessary component for cells and tissues. Levels decrease with renal disease, malnutrition, and severe burns. Albumin levels are the most common screening to determine protein levels. Albumin has a half-life of 18-20 days, so it is sensitive to long-term protein deficiencies more than short-term.

- **Normal values**: 3.5-5.5 g/dL
- Mild deficiency: 3-3.5 g/dL
- Moderate deficiency: 2.5-3.0 g/dL
- Severe deficiency: <2.5 g/dL.

Levels below 3.2 correlate with increased morbidity and death. Dehydration (poor intake, diarrhea, or vomiting) elevates levels, so adequate hydration is important to ensure meaningful results.

PREALBUMIN

Prealbumin (transthyretin) is most commonly monitored for acute changes in nutritional status because it has a half-life of only 2-3 days. Prealbumin is a protein produced in the liver, so it is often decreased with liver disease. Oral contraceptives and estrogen can also decrease levels. Levels may rise with Hodgkin's disease or the use of steroids or nonsteroidal inflammatory drugs (NSAIDs). Prealbumin is necessary for transportation of both thyroxine and vitamin A throughout the body, so if levels fall, both thyroxine and vitamin A utilization are also affected.

- **Normal values**: 16-40 mg/dL.
- Mild deficiency: 10-15 mg/dL
- Moderate deficiency: 5-9 mg/dL
- Severe deficiency: <5 mg/dL.

Prealbumin is a good measurement because it quickly decreases when nutrition is inadequate and rises quickly in response to increased protein intake. Protein intake must be adequate to maintain levels of prealbumin. Death rates increase with any decrease in prealbumin levels.

TLC

The immune system responds quickly to changes in protein intake because proteins are critical to antibody and lymphocyte production. T lymphocytes develop in the thymus gland and are a part of the cell-mediated immune response. B-lymphocytes develop in the bone marrow and are part of the humoral (antibody-mediated) immune response. **Total Lymphocyte Count (TLC)** can reflect changes in nutritional status because a decrease in protein causes decreased immunity. Lymphocytes are expressed on a differential as a percentage of the white blood count. The TLC is calculated by multiplying the percentage by the total white blood count and then dividing by 100.

- **Normal values**: 2000 cells/mm^3.
- **Mild deficiency**: 1500-1800 cells/mm^3.

151

- **Moderate deficiency**: 900-1500 cells/mm³.
- **Severe deficiency**: <900 cells/mm³.

While low levels may be indicative of malnutrition, levels are also depressed with stress, autoimmune diseases, chemotherapy, infection, and human immunodeficiency virus (HIV).

TRANSFERRIN

Transferrin, which transports about one-third of the body's iron, is a protein produced by the liver. It transports iron from the intestines to the bone marrow where it is used to produce hemoglobin. The half-life of transferrin is about 8-10 days. It is sometimes used as a measure of nutritional status; however, transferrin levels are sensitive to many different things. Levels rapidly decrease with protein malnutrition. Liver disease and anemia can also depress levels, but a decrease in iron, commonly found with inadequate protein, stimulates the liver to produce more transferrin, which increases levels but also decreases production of albumin and prealbumin. Levels may also increase with pregnancy, use of oral contraceptives, and polycythemia. Thus, transferrin levels alone are not always reliable measurements of nutritional status:

- **Normal values**: 200-400 mg/dL.
- **Mild deficiency**: 150-200 mg/dL.
- Moderate deficiency: 100-150 mg/dL.
- Severe deficiency: <100 mg/dL.

> **Review Video: Transferrin**
> Visit mometrix.com/academy and enter code: 267479

RENAL FUNCTION AND HYDRATION TESTS

A number of different tests can be used to diagnose **renal conditions and hydration**:

- **BUN**, a protein by-product, is excreted by the kidneys. An elevation of both BUN and creatinine indicates kidney disease, but elevated BUN alone may indicate dehydration:
  - **Normal values**: 7-23 mg/dL.
  - **Dehydration**: >23 mg/dL.
- **BUN-creatinine ratio** monitors renal failure, where there is enhanced reabsorption in the proximal tubules, causing the urea level to rise. Dehydration or conditions that limit fluid into the kidneys increases urea. Increased urea is also an indication of an upper GI bleed where the proteins in the blood are broken down and reabsorbed in the lower intestinal tract.
  - Normal value: 10:1
  - Dehydration: >25:1
- **Specific gravity/urine** measures the ability of the kidneys to concentrate or dilute the urine according to changes in serum. The most common cause of an increased specific gravity is dehydration. It may also increase with an increased secretion of anti-diuretic hormone (ADH).
  - **Normal value**: 1.003-1.028
  - Dehydration: >1.028

Hydration is essential for proper healing and for meaningful results of laboratory measures of nutrition. A number of different tests can be used to monitor hydration:

- **Serum sodium** measures the sodium level in the blood. Some drugs, such as steroids, laxatives, contraceptives, nonsteroidal inflammatory drugs (NSAIDs), and IV fluids containing sodium can elevate levels. Other drugs, such as diuretics and vasopressin can reduce levels.
  - **Normal values**: 135-150 mEq/L.
  - **Dehydration**: >150 mEq/L.
- **Serum osmolality** measures the concentration of ions, such as sodium, chloride, potassium, glucose, and urea in the blood. Levels increase with dehydration, which stimulates the antidiuretic hormone (AD), resulting in increased water reabsorption and more concentrated urine in an effort to compensate. Changes in osmolality can affect normal cell functioning, eventually destroying the cells if levels remain high.
  - **Normal levels**: 285-295 mOsm per kilogram/H2O.
  - **Dehydration**: >295 mOsm/kg H2O.

DIAGNOSTIC TESTING
COMPLETE BLOOD COUNT WITH RBCS, PLATELETS, HGB, AND HCT

The **complete blood count** with differential and platelet (thrombocyte) count provides information about the blood and other body systems. Red blood cell (RBC) (erythrocyte) counts and concentrations may vary with anemia, hemorrhage, or various disorders and decrease may affect healing because of less oxygen to tissues:

- **Hemoglobin (Hgb)**, a protein found in erythrocytes, uses iron to bind and transport oxygen. Deficiencies of amino acids, vitamins or minerals can cause a decrease, impacting healing by reducing oxygen to tissue. Dehydration and severe burns can cause increase. Normal values include:
  - **Neonates**: 14.5-24.5g/dL; 1-6 years: 9.5-14.1 g/dL; men >18: 13-18 g/dL; women >18:12-16 g/dL.
- **Hematocrit (Hct)**measures the percentage of packed RBCs in 100 mL of blood. Decrease can indicate blood loss and anemia. Increase may indicate dehydration. Normal values include:
  - **Neonates**: 44-64%; 1-6 years: 30-40%, men >18: 42-52%; women >18: 37-48%.
- **Platelet** normal values of 140-300,000 at birth stabilize at 150,000-400,000 for adults but may increase to over a million during acute infection.

WBCS AND DIFFERENTIAL

White blood cell (WBC) (leukocyte) count is used as an indicator of bacterial and viral infection. WBC count is reported as the total number of all WBCs:

- **0-2 weeks**: 9,000-30,000/mL
- 2 months to 6 years: 5,000-19,000/mL
- **6-18 years**: 4800-10,800/mL
- **>18 years**: 4,500-11,000/mL
- **Acute infection**: 10,000+ (30,000 indicates a severe infection)
- **Viral infection**: 4,000 and below

The **differential** provides the percentage of each different type of leukocyte. An increase in the white blood cell count is usually related to an increase in 1 type and often an increase in immature neutrophils, known as bands, referred to as a "shift to the left, an indication of an infectious process:

- **Normal immature neutrophils** (bands): 10-18% at birth but decrease to 5-11% at one year and 3-6% in adults. Increase with infection.
- **Normal segmented neutrophils** (segs) for adults: 32-62% at birth but decrease to 13-33% at 1 year and, 34-64% at 16-18, and 50-62% for adults. Increase with acute, localized, or systemic bacterial infections.
- **Normal eosinophils**: 0-3% (all ages). Decrease with stress and acute infection.
- **Normal basophils**: 0-1% (all ages). Decrease during acute stage of infection.
- **Normal lymphocytes**; 26-36% at birth, 46-76% at 1 year and 25-40% for adults. Increase in some viral and bacterial infections.
- **Normal monocytes**: 0-6% at birth, 0-9% at 2-4 weeks, 0-5% by 6 months and 3-7% for adults. Increase during recovery stage of acute infection.

Leukemia occurs when 1 type of WBC proliferates with immature cells, with the defect occurring in the hematopoietic stem cell, either lymphoid (lympho-) or myeloid (myelo-). Usually leukemias classified as blast cell or stem cell refer to lymphoid defects. With acute leukemia, WBC count remains low because the cells are halted at the blast stage and the disease progresses rapidly. Chronic leukemia progresses more slowly and most cells are mature.

GLUCOSE AND HEMOGLOBIN A1C

Glucose is manufactured by the liver from ingested carbohydrates and is stored as glycogen for use by the cells. If intake is inadequate, glucose can be produced from muscle and fat tissue, leading to increased wasting. High levels of glucose are indicative of **diabetes mellitus**, which predisposes people to skin injuries, slow healing, and infection. Fasting blood glucose levels are used to diagnose and monitor:

- **Normal values**: 70-99 mg/dL.
- **Impaired**: 100-125 mg/dL.
- **Diabetes**: >126 mg/dL.

There are a number of different conditions that can increase glucose levels: stress, renal failure, Cushing syndrome, hyperthyroidism, and pancreas disorders. Medications, such as steroids, estrogens, lithium, phenytoin, diuretics, tricyclic antidepressants, may increase glucose levels. Other conditions, such as adrenal insufficiency, liver disease, hypothyroidism, and starvation can decrease glucose levels.

Hemoglobin A1C comprises hemoglobin A with a glucose molecule because hemoglobin holds onto excess blood glucose, so it shows the average blood glucose levels over a 2-3-month period and is used primarily to monitor long-term diabetic therapy.

- Normal value: <6%
- Elevation: >7%

Review Video: Glucose Testing
Visit mometrix.com/academy and enter code: 887714

Review Video: Glucose Tolerance Test
Visit mometrix.com/academy and enter code: 539108

URINALYSIS

Routine **urinary screening** measures these components of urine to determine if there is an abnormality:

- **pH** should range from 4.5 to 8.0. An alkaline (high) pH can be caused by urinary tract infections, diarrhea, or kidney infection. An acidic (low) pH may reflect lung disease, severe diabetes, diarrhea with dehydration, excessive alcohol intake, or starvation.
- **Glucose** should not be found in the urine and may indicate uncontrolled diabetes mellitus but may also indicate liver damage, brain injury, and some kinds of kidney disease.
- **Nitrites** in the urine are indicative of a urinary tract infection.
- **Leukocyte esterase** indicates that there are white blood cells in the urine, probably from a urinary tract infection.
- **Ketones** should not be found in urine and can indicate uncontrolled diabetes, a low carbohydrate diet, anorexia or bulimia, excessive alcohol intake, or fasting for 18 hours or more.

MICROSCOPIC ANALYSES OF URINE

Microscopic analyses of urine involve placing the urine specimen in a centrifuge to separate out the **sediment**, which is then examined under a microscope:

- **Erythrocytes** should not be in the urine and may indicate inflammation, injury, or slight bleeding from strenuous exercise.
- **Leukocytes** in the urine usually are indicative of infection, cancer, or kidney disorders.
- **Casts** are caused from kidney disease that causes tiny tube-like plugs of material (red or white cells, protein, fatty substances) to be flushed from the kidneys to the urine. The type of cast may help with diagnosis.
- **Crystals** should appear in small numbers. Some types of crystals or large numbers of crystals may be a sign of kidney stones or a metabolic disorder.
- **Bacteria** in the urine indicate an infection.
- **Fungi** in the urine indicate a yeast infection.
- **Parasites** may migrate to the urinary system in some types of infestation.

ERYTHROCYTE SEDIMENTATION RATE

Erythrocyte sedimentation rate (sed rate) measures the distance erythrocytes fall in a vertical tube of anticoagulated blood in 1 hour. Because fibrinogen, which increases in response to infection, slows the fall, the sed rate can be used as a non-specific test for **inflammation** when infection is suspected. The sed rate is sensitive to osteomyelitis and may be used to monitor treatment response. Values vary according to gender and age:

- **Neonate**: Men 0-2 mm/hr. Women 0-2 mm/hr.
- **<50**: Men 0-15 mm/hr. Women 0-25 mm/hr.
- **>50**: Men 0-20 mm/hr. Women 0-30 mm/hr.

The sed rate increases with many disorders, including collagen disease, acute myocardial infarction (MI), carcinoma, pregnancy, rheumatic fever, rheumatoid arthritis, lymphoma, heavy metal poisoning, Crohn's disease, anemia, infections, pulmonary embolism, temporal arteritis, and tuberculosis (TB). It decreases with high blood glucose or conditions causing increased red blood cells (RBC) or hemoglobin count. Rates may be falsely elevated during menses.

ELECTROLYTE IMBALANCES
SODIUM

Sodium (Na) regulates fluid volume, osmolality, acid-base balance, and activity in the muscles, nerves and myocardium. It is the primary cation (positive ion) in extracellular fluid (ECF), necessary to maintain ECF levels that are needed for tissue perfusion:

- **Normal value**: 135-145 mEq/L.
- **Hyponatremia**: <135 mEq/L.
- **Hypernatremia**: >145 mEq/L.

Hyponatremia may result from inadequate sodium intake or excess loss, through diarrhea, vomiting, nasogastric (NG) suctioning. It can occur as the result of illness, such as severe burns, fever, syndrome of inappropriate antidiuretic hormone secretion (SIADH), and ketoacidosis. *Symptoms* vary:

- Irritability to lethargy to lethargy and alterations in consciousness.
- Cerebral edema with seizures and coma.
- Dyspnea to respiratory failure.

Treatment: Identify and treat underlying cause and replace sodium. **Hypernatremia** may result from renal disease, diabetes insipidus, and fluid depletion. *Symptoms* include:

- Irritability to lethargy to confusion to coma, seizures.
- Flushing.
- Muscle weakness, spasms.
- High-pitching crying (infants).
- Thirst.

Treatment: Identify and treat underlying cause, monitor Na levels, and provide IV fluid replacement.

HYPERKALEMIA

Hyperkalemia is caused by renal disease, adrenal insufficiency, metabolic acidosis, severe dehydration, burns, hemolysis, and trauma. It rarely occurs without renal disease but may be induced by treatment (such as nonsteroidal anti-inflammatory drugs [NSAIDs] and potassium-sparing diuretics). Untreated renal failure results in reduced excretion. Those with Addison's disease and deficient adrenal hormones suffer sodium loss that results in potassium retention:

- **Hyperkalemia**: >5.5 mEq/L.

The primary *symptoms* relate to the effect on the cardiac muscle and include ventricular arrhythmias with increasing changes in electrocardiogram (ECG) leading to cardiac and respiratory arrest, weakness with ascending paralysis and hyperreflexia, diarrhea, and increasing confusion.

Treatment includes identifying underlying cause and discontinuing sources of increased K:

- **Calcium gluconate** to decrease cardiac effects.
- **Sodium bicarbonate** shifts K into the cells temporarily.
- **Insulin and hypertonic dextrose** shift K into the cells temporarily.
- **Cation exchange resin** (Kayexalate®) to decrease K.
- Peritoneal dialysis or hemodialysis.

156

HYPOKALEMIA

Potassium (K) is the primary electrolyte in intracellular fluid (ICF) with about 98% inside cells and only 2% in extracellular fluid (ECF), although this small amount is important for neuromuscular activity. K influences activity of the skeletal and cardiac muscles. K level is dependent upon adequate renal functioning because 80% is excreted through the kidneys and 20% through the bowels and sweat.

- **Normal values**: 3.5-5.5 mEq/L.
- **Hypokalemia**: <3.5 mEq/L.

Hypokalemia is caused by loss of K through diarrhea, vomiting, gastric suction, and diuresis, alkalosis, decreased K intake with starvation, and nephritis. *Symptoms* include:

- Lethargy and weakness.
- Nausea and vomiting.
- Paresthesias.
- Dysrhythmias with electrocardiogram (ECG) abnormalities: premature ventricular contractions (PVCs), flattened T waves.
- Muscle cramps with hyporeflexia.
- Hypotension.
- Tetany.

Treatment: Identify and treat underlying cause and replace K.

> **Review Video: Fluid and Electrolytes**
> Visit mometrix.com/academy and enter code: 384389

PHOSPHORUS

Phosphorus (PO_4) is necessary for neuromuscular and red blood cell function, the maintenance of acid-base balance, and provides structure for teeth and bones. About 85% is in the bones, 14% in soft tissue, and <1% in extracellular fluid (ECF). Children have higher levels of phosphorus because of high rate of skeletal growth.

- **Normal values**: Neonates: 4.6-8.0 mg/dL; Children 4-6 years: 4.0-5.4 mg/dL; Adult: 2.5-4.5 mg/dL.
- **Hypophosphatemia**: varies with age, but critical value <1.0 mg/dL
- **Hyperphosphatemia**: > varies with age

Hypophosphatemia occurs with severe protein-calorie malnutrition, excess antacids with magnesium, calcium or albumin, hyperventilation, severe burns, and diabetic ketoacidosis. *Symptoms* include irritability, tremors, seizures to coma, hemolytic anemia, decreased myocardial function, and respiratory failure.

Treatment: Identify and treat underlying cause and replace phosphorus. **Hyperphosphatemia** occurs with renal failure, hypoparathyroidism, excessive intake, and neoplastic disease, diabetic ketoacidosis, muscle necrosis, pulmonary embolism and chemotherapy. *Symptoms* include tachycardia, muscle cramping, hyperreflexia, tetany, nausea, and diarrhea,

Treatment: Identify and treat underlying cause, correct imbalance, calcium, and dialysis.

CALCIUM

More than 99% of **calcium** (Ca) is in the skeletal system with 1% in serum, but it is important for transmitting nerve impulses and regulating muscle contraction and relaxation, including the myocardium. Calcium activates enzymes that stimulate chemical reactions and has a role in coagulation of blood:

- **Normal values**: 1.15-1.34 mg/dL.
- **Hypocalcemia**: <1.15 mg/dL.
- **Hypercalcemia**: >1.34 mg/dL.

Hypocalcemia may be caused by hypoparathyroidism and occurs after thyroid and parathyroid surgery, pancreatitis, renal failure, inadequate vitamin D, alkalosis, magnesium deficiency and low serum albumin. *Symptoms* include tetany, tingling, altered mental status, seizures, and ventricular tachycardia.

Treatment: Calcium replacement and vitamin D.

Hypercalcemia may be caused by acidosis, kidney disease, hyperparathyroidism, prolonged immobilization, and malignancies. Crisis carries a 50% mortality rate. *Symptoms* include increasing muscle weakness with hypotonicity, anorexia, constipation, nausea and vomiting, bradycardia and cardiac arrest. *Treatment*: Identify and treat underlying cause, give loop diuretics and IV fluids.

MAGNESIUM

Magnesium (Mg) is the second most common intracellular electrolyte (after potassium) and activates many intracellular enzyme systems. It is important for carbohydrate and protein metabolism, neuromuscular function, and cardiovascular function, producing vasodilation and directly affecting the peripheral arterial system:

- **Normal values**: Neonate: 1.23-1.81 mEq/L; Children: 1.4-1.73 mEq/L; Adults: 1.32-2.14 mEq/L.
- Hypomagnesemia: <1.4 mEq/L.
- Hypermagnesemia: >1.73 mEq/L.

Hypomagnesemia occurs with chronic diarrhea, chronic renal disease, chronic pancreatitis, excess diuretic or laxative use, hyperthyroidism, hypoparathyroidism, severe burns, pancreatitis, and diaphoresis. *Symptoms* include neuromuscular excitability/ tetany, confusion, headaches, dizziness, seizure, coma, tachycardia with ventricular arrhythmias, and respiratory depression. *Treatment*: Identify and treat underlying cause and replace magnesium.

Hypermagnesemia occurs with renal failure or inadequate renal function, diabetic ketoacidosis, dehydration, hypothyroidism, and Addison's disease. *Symptoms* include muscle weakness, dysphagia with ↓ gag reflex, seizures, and tachycardia with hypotension. *Treatment*: Identify and treat underlying cause, IV hydration with calcium, and dialysis.

Clinical Management

Teaching Caregivers

ENVIRONMENT AND MEDICATIONS

Too often, family/caregivers are left to care for **Alzheimer's/cognitively impaired patients** with little information about dealing with problems that arise, so the FNP should provide **guidance**:

- **Environment**: Clutter and unnecessary items from dressers, drawers, and bookshelves should be removed and signs and labels (if the person can still read) made—such as a label on the patient's bedroom door or drawer. Alternately, one can post pictures of actions or people. All dangerous items, such as knives, scissors, and matches, should be removed and secured. Child safety gates can be used if patient is unable to climb over a gate.
- **Medications**: In the early stages, patients may be able to manage medications if they are prepared in medication containers, but use should be monitored as patients may stop taking medications, take extra, or throw them away. If any problems arise, the caregiver should dispense medications. Medications may need to be ground or replaced by liquid formulations and disguised in food, such as applesauce, as patients often refuse medications.

TOILETING

Urinary and fecal incontinence are usually inevitable over time, but scheduled toileting (every 2-4 hours), monitoring fluid, food, and fiber intake, and reducing fluids after dinner can help in earlier stages. Stool softeners may help bowel function, but laxatives should be avoided. Diet may need to be monitored carefully to avoid constipation or diarrhea. Protective coverings should be placed over the mattress and seat cushions. In time, the patient may need to use disposable pads or adult diapers. Patients may be resistive, and the caregiver should be advised to persist and try different products, as some feel more like regular undergarments than others. Inappropriate "toilets" such as wastebaskets may need to be removed. A commode may be placed close to a chair or the bed if the person urinates on the floor on the way to the toilet.

SUNDOWNER'S SYNDROME AND SLEEP-WAKE CYCLE DISRUPTION

Some patients get up and wander about the house during the night or go through drawers or closets, moving things about or tying them up in packages. Caregivers can attempt to keep the patient awake during the daytime by engaging the person in activities and turning on bright lights in the evening. Reestablishing the sleep-wake cycle may take 1-2 weeks of concerted effort, and some people simply resist or get up at night to urinate and forget to go back to bed. If the patient gets up to urinate, restricting fluids in the evening or scheduling toileting at a specific time (midnight) and putting the patient back to bed may help. Any method that soothes and relaxes a patient (and this is very individual) should be used at bedtime to calm the patient. Some patients will not stay in bed but get up and fall asleep in a chair. In that case, sometimes placing a comfortable recliner in the room may encourage the patient to sit down and fall asleep.

WANDERING

Some patients tend to wander for reasons that are not clear. They may have tried to go to the bathroom and got lost or may have wanted to go to the store or visit someone, but they soon become very confused and frightened and may compound the problem by hiding. Patients should be registered with the Alzheimer's Association MedicAlert, Safe Return program and wear the

MedicAlert bracelet at all times. Alarms, latches, and locks may be necessary, but alarms may frighten the patient, so it is best that they ring in another room (such as the caregiver's). Latches at the top or bottom of a door are usually adequate because patients don't think to look. Sometimes just hanging a sheet or curtain over a doorway will keep patients inside as they forget the door was there. Baby monitors may be used to monitor the patient's activities.

GENERAL MANAGEMENT

Patients should be kept to a regular schedule if possible because changes increase confusion. Caregivers should avoid having the patient make unnecessary choices, as something as simple as "Do you want apple or orange juice?" may be overwhelming. Directions should be given with only 1 or 2 simple steps. Simple clothes without zippers or buttons may be easiest for patient and caregivers to manage. If patients are resistive to bathing, Comfort Bath® disposable cloths may be used and 1 part of the body done at a time (such as the face and arms in the morning, trunk and legs at night). Some patients pace obsessively and when possible, the patients should be allowed to do so as attempting to stop them is rarely successful and only causes distress. If possible, it is good to take patients outside for a walk rather than having them pace back and forth in a room or hallway.

SUPPORTIVE CARE

Caregivers often need to be reminded that patients are not doing disturbing things purposely, as caregivers may become very resentful, exhausted, and angry. Often patients are disruptive because they need or want something and are unable to express what they need, but careful observation can often give clues. Some patients, especially women, are comforted by holding dolls or stuffed animals, and there are often simple activities (such as folding clothes, throwing balls, or coloring) that they enjoy. It is important to continue to engage the person in activities and conversation even if the person is confused, but caregivers should not try to "fix" the person's confused perceptions, as it serves little purpose. Holding the patient's hand or arm while walking provides security and prevents the patient from bolting if something frightens him/her (such as a loud noise). Many patients become very agitated and nervous in confusing environments, such as large department stores, so these places are best avoided.

Developmental Guidance

NORMAL GROWTH AND DEVELOPMENT DURING INFANCY
FIRST MONTH

Newborn infants sleep about 16 hr/d during the **first month** but are growing and developing:

- **Growth:** Infants lose 5%-7% of their birth weight and then gain 4-7 oz/wk (about 2 lb/mo). Both length and head circumference increase 1.5 cm/mo.
- **Mobility:** Infants make a fist and flex their arms and legs. Reflexes such as Moro, sucking, grasping, startle, rooting, and asymmetric tonic neck are present.
- **Feeding:** Infants breastfeed and bottle-feed about every 2-3 hours.
- **Urine/Feces:** Urination occurs about eight times a day. Breastfed infants may have frequent loose stools or may skip 2-3 days. If infants are bottle-fed, stools are usually firm. Color varies (yellow, tan, green, brown).

- **Sensory:** Infants can follow items in their line of vision and often prefer faces and contrasting geometric designs. Vision is somewhat blurry, but they are able to focus at about 8-15 inches. Color distinction is poor. Infants can hear well and respond with the startle reflex (Moro). Their sense of smell is strong.
- **Communication:** Infants signal distress by crying, gagging, and arching the body, but they are also quick to respond to comfort measures.

2-4 MONTHS

During the first **2-4 months**, infants continue to sleep much of the time but are often awake for periods in the morning, afternoon, and evening:

- **Growth:** Infants gain 4-7 oz/wk; both length and head circumference increase 1.5 cm/mo. The posterior fontanelle closes.
- **Mobility:** Infants lose the grasp reflex, and the hands begin to stay open and grasp. Infants are able to lift the head while prone or supine and turn from side to side. They can roll easily from stomach to back by 4 months. The Moro reflex fades. Infants often play with their hands. They can be pulled to a standing position.
- **Feeding:** Infants need about 2 oz/lb/24 hr of milk, usually feeding every 4 hours.
- **Urine/Feces:** Urination occurs about five to six times a day. Stools occur variously from one after each feeding to one every 2-3 days; they are usually firm and regular.
- **Sensory:** Infants can focus at about 12 inches and follow objects 180 degrees with their eyes.
- **Communication:** Crying is differentiated to show hunger, pain, and frustration. Infants can smile indiscriminately by 2 months and have a socially responsive smile by 3 months. Infants often show a preference for their mother and may turn from strangers.

4-6 MONTHS

During the first **4-6 months**, the infant sleeps about 10-11 hours at night, with two to three daytime naps, often sleeping a total of 15 hours:

- **Growth:** Infants double their weight by 5-6 months, gaining 5-7 oz/wk.
- **Mobility:** Infants roll over and roll from back to side by 6 months; they hold their head up at 90 degrees and turn their head in both directions when sitting or lying down. Infants sit with support for 10-15 minutes. Grasp improves, and they may hold their bottle and play with their feet. By 6 months, infants pick up items and move items from one hand to the other. They manipulate and mouth objects and they like to watch objects fall.
- **Feeding:** Infants still need about two feedings at night and every 4 hours during the day (i.e., 1.5 oz/lb/24 hr).
- **Urine/Feces:** Urination and defecation begin to occur regularly.
- **Sensory:** Eyes begin to focus well, and infants can follow items or people with their eyes.
- **Communication:** Infants begin to vocalize more and mimic tones. They often squeal and laugh as well as yell with anger. Infants vocalize to get attention and recognize family members.

161

6-8 MONTHS

During the first **6-8 months**, the child begins to have more waking hours, sleeping 10-11 hours with two naps:

- **Growth:** Growth begins to slow with infants gaining 3-5 oz/wk and 1 cm/mo in length.
- **Mobility:** Infants sit without support by 8 months. They can stand supported and bounce on their legs. They start to use the pincer grasp and can easily manipulate objects. Most birth reflexes have faded. Infants regularly bang objects together and mouth objects freely.
- **Feeding:** Infants start to take solid foods (i.e., cereal, vegetables, fruit) two to three times daily as well as breastfeed or bottle-feed three to five times daily. Teething biscuits, graham crackers, and Melba toast may be introduced during this time.
- **Urine/Feces:** Stools are larger with solid foods. Urination occurs five to six times daily.
- **Sensory:** Infants watch and listen actively, turning their head to sounds and to follow objects.
- **Communication:** Infants increase their babbling and mimicking sounds, including two syllable sounds, such as "mama" or "dada," but they do not use words intentionally. Infants have babbling conversations and may be fearful of strangers.

8-10 MONTHS

During the first **8-10 months**, children sleep about 10-11 hours at night, usually sleeping through the night, with two naps during the day:

- **Growth:** Children gain 3-5 oz/wk and 1 cm/mo in length.
- **Mobility:** Children use the pincer grasp well and can pick up small objects. They crawl or creep readily. They sit up and by 10 months pull themselves to a standing position by holding onto furniture.
- **Feeding:** Meat can be introduced at this time. Children may breastfeed or bottle-feed three to four times daily with three meals. Egg yolks only may be introduced. Children enjoy finger foods, such as meat sticks.
- **Urine/Feces:** Urination and stools are fairly regular.
- **Sensory:** Children are attentive and watch and listen actively.
- **Communication:** Children continue to babble and may be able to say one or two words besides "mama" or "dada." They understand basic vocabulary, such as "no" and "cookie." Babbling follows a speech-like rhythm when "talking."

10-12 MONTHS

During the first **10-12 months**, children sleep 10-11 hours a night with two naps during the day:

- **Growth:** Children gain 3-5 oz/wk and 1 cm/mo in length. Head and chest circumference are equal. Birth weight triples by 12 months.
- **Mobility:** Most children are able to make marks on paper with pens or crayon and to fit objects through holes. They stand alone and walk holding onto furniture. They sit from a standing position.
- **Feeding:** Children breastfeed or bottle-feed three to four times daily; they may begin using a "sippy" cup. Children eat solid foods, both prepared baby foods and soft home-cooked foods. They enjoy finger food and may resist being fed.
- **Urine/Feces:** Children begin to hold urine for longer periods of time, especially girls. They may smear feces.

- **Sensory:** Children actively watch and listen as well as engage in activities.
- **Communication:** Children understand many words and now use "mama" and "dada" intentionally. They play patty-cake and peek-a-boo games and enjoy repetition.

1-2 YEARS

Between **1 and 2**, children grow in size and independence:

- **Growth:** Toddlers gain 8 oz/mo and 3-5 in/yr. The anterior fontanelle closes.
- **Mobility:** Toddlers begin with first steps and by 2 years of age walk, run, and go up and down stairs. They scribble on paper, throw toys, and stack blocks. They begin independent exploration of their environment.
- **Diet:** Toddlers eat three meals, two or three snacks, and two to three cups of whole cow's milk (after 1 year) daily. Some toddlers may still breastfeed, but they consume a wide range of foods.
- **Toileting:** Between 18-24 months, some toddlers show an interest in potty training.
- **Communication:** Toddlers begin with one word and continue to add words. They learn the names of common objects and begin to communicate with simple words, leading to short sentences around 2 years of age with a vocabulary of 30-50 words. They may demonstrate apprehension with strangers and anger with temper tantrums.

2-3 YEARS

Between **2-3 years of age**, children make significant changes over the course of a year:

- **Growth:** Toddlers gain 3-5 lb/yr and 3.5-5 in/yr.
- **Mobility:** Toddlers run steadily, jump on two feet, and climb. Scribbling becomes more intentional, and they can draw simple shapes and often make an effort to color in the lines. Toddlers are able to undress at 2 years of age and dress at 3 years of age. They are able to throw a ball overhand. While they often parallel play, they begin to interact with others.
- **Diet:** Toddlers can be switched to low-fat milk, 2-3 cups daily, along with a regular well-balanced meal of meat, fruits, vegetables, and grains. Fruit juice should be limited to 2-4 oz/d because of the high sugar content. Bottle feedings should be stopped.
- **Toileting:** Most children become potty-trained some time during this time.
- **Communication/Cognition:** Toddlers begin to talk in short three-word sentences and to understand rules. They begin to use the pronouns I, me, and you and can talk about their feelings. They usually know at least five body parts and colors and can categorize objects by size (e.g., big, little).

NORMAL GROWTH AND DEVELOPMENT DURING PRESCHOOL YEARS

Around **3-6 years of age**, children move from being a toddler to a young child:

- **Growth:** Preschoolers gain 3-5 lb/yr and 1.5-2.5 in/yr. Most growth occurs in the long bones as children increase in stature, and proportionate head size decreases.
- **Mobility:** Preschoolers become increasingly adept, drawing various shapes easily, coloring in the lines, and using scissors to cut along lines. They are able to brush their teeth, and by 6 years of age, they are able to tie their shoes. Young children are able to climb, run, jump, balance, and ride a tricycle or a bicycle with training wheels. They interact with others.
- **Diet:** Preschoolers eat three meals and snacks in the morning and afternoon; they can manage a spoon, fork, and knife independently by 6 years of age.

- **Communication/Cognition:** Preschoolers become increasingly verbal and social and command a large complex vocabulary by age 6. They are able to understand concepts of right and wrong, good and bad, and they can lie. By age 6, preschoolers learn letters and numbers and begin to read. They may focus on one thing to the exclusion of others.

GROWTH AND DEVELOPMENT PROBLEMS DURING SCHOOL-AGE YEARS
AGES 6-12

During the school years **(6-12 years of age)**, children go through many changes:

- **Dental:** School-age children lose deciduous teeth and begin acquiring permanent teeth.
- **Height and Weight:** Both height and weight progress slowly and steadily, with children gaining an average of 2 in/yr, beginning at about 45 inches at age 6 and 59 inches at age 12. Weight usually doubles during this time from 46 pounds at age 6 to 88 pounds at age 12. Boys and girls are similar in size, but by age 12, some girls undergo pubertal changes and may gain height and weight over boys.
- **Proportions:** The body becomes slimmer and better proportioned with an increase in muscle mass and a decrease in fat. In relation to height, head circumference decreases, leg length increases, and waist circumference decreases. Facial characteristics change.
- **Body Systems:** Systems mature with respirations and heart rate decreasing. Bladder capacity is usually better in girls than boys. Muscles strengthen, and bones begin to ossify. Physical variation increases with age.

AGES 11-14

Early adolescence (11-14 years of age) is a transitional time for children as their hormones and their bodies go through changes. Adolescents mature at varying rates, so there are wide differences. Emotions may be labile, and the adolescent may feel isolated and confused, trying to find an identity. Peers become more influential, and the adolescent may challenge the values of the family. Adolescents may have anxiety about their bodies and sexuality as secondary sexual characteristics develop. **Developmental concerns** include:

- Delayed maturation.
- Short stature (female).
- Spinal curvature (females).
- Poor dental status (caries, malocclusion).
- Chronic illnesses, such as diabetes.
- Lack of adequate physical activity/ Obesity.
- Poor nutrition or anorexia.
- Concerns about sexual identity.
- Negative self-image.
- Depression.
- Lack of close friends, fighting, or violent episodes.
- Poor academic progress with truancy and failure to complete assignments.
- Lack of impulse control.

NORMAL GROWTH AND DEVELOPMENT ISSUES FOR MIDDLE ADOLESCENCE

In **middle adolescence (15-17 years of age)** most body changes have occurred; there is less concern about this but more concern about the image that is projected to others. Girls may worry about weight, and boys may worry about muscle development. Adolescents are interested in sexuality, and many begin sexual experimentation. There is strong identification with peer groups, including codes of dress and behavior, often putting them at odds with their families. **Developmental concerns** include:

- Spinal curvature (females) and short stature (males).
- Lack of testicular maturation or persistent gynecomastia.
- Acne.
- Anorexia or obesity.
- Sexual experimentation, multiple partners, and unprotected sex.
- Sexual identification concerns.
- Depression and poor self-image.
- Lack of adequate exercise, poor nutrition, and poor dental health.
- Chronic diseases.
- Experimentation with drugs and alcohol and problems with authority figures.
- Lack of peer group identification or gang associations.
- Poor academic progress, failing classes, truancy, attention deficits, disruptive class behavior, poor judgment, and impulse control.

NORMAL GROWTH AND DEVELOPMENT ISSUES FOR LATE ADOLESCENCE (18-21)

Late adolescence (18-21 years of age) is the time when adolescents begin to take on adult roles and responsibilities, enter the work world, or go to college. Most adolescents have come to terms with their sexuality and have a more mature understanding of people's motivations. Some young people continue to engage in high-risk behaviors. Many of the problems associated with middle adolescence may continue if unresolved, interfering with the transition to adulthood. **Developmental concerns** include:

- Failure to take on adult roles or having no life goals or future plans.
- Low self-esteem.
- Lack of intimate relationships or sexual-identification concerns.
- Gang association.
- Continued identification with peer group or dependence on parents.
- High-risk sexual behavior, multiple partners, and unprotected sex.
- Poor academic progress or ability.
- Psychosomatic complaints or depression.
- Lack of impulse control.
- Poor nutrition, obesity, or anorexia.
- Poor dental health.
- Chronic disease.
- Lack of exercise.

Behavioral Guidance

LEADING CAUSES OF DEATH

For the **birth to 10-year** age group, the US Preventive Services Task Force has assembled a list of the **5 leading causes of death**. The number 1 cause of death in this age group is actually a group of conditions that arise in the time period surrounding birth (the "**perinatal period**"). There are a number of conditions that arise surrounding birth that are fatal, including placental problems (premature separation, abruption), umbilical cord problems (cord prolapse, nuchal cord, single umbilical artery), infections (chorioamnionitis, congenital pneumonia), trauma during the birthing process (nerve damage, intracranial hemorrhage), and hemolytic disease of the newborn. The second leading cause of death is attributed to **congenital defects**, including tetralogy of Fallot, transposition of the great arteries, spina bifida, and anencephaly. Other leading causes of death include **sudden infant death syndrome (SIDS), motor vehicle injuries, and other unintentional injuries**.

INJURY PREVENTION COUNSELING

Injury prevention counseling is a strong recommendation for the **birth to 10-year** age group, owing to the fact that motor vehicle accidents and other unintentional accidents are leading causes of death for this population. Children (and their parents) should be advised to use car safety seats until the age of 5 (this is subject to state law, however, as some states require the use of booster seats until a certain height or age is reached). After the age of 5, standard safety belts should always be used. When biking, skating, or skateboarding, a helmet should always be worn; these activities should not take place in the street. Parents should be advised to become CPR certified. They should also be advised to keep drugs, poisons, guns and other weapons, and matches out of the reach of children; to install smoke detectors and plan an escape route in the event of fire; and to make sure that stairs, windows, and pools are safe for children.

11 TO 24-YEAR AGE POPULATION
LEADING CAUSES OF DEATH

The list of the top 5 leading causes of death in the **11-24** age population differs significantly from the leading causes of death in the birth to 10-year age population. Leading the list for age 11-24 are deaths caused by either **motor vehicle accidents or other unintentional accidents**. Second on the list is **homicide**, followed by **suicide** as the third leading cause of death. The fourth leading cause of death in the 11-24 age population is **cancer**; the most common fatal cancers in this age group include leukemia (acute lymphocytic leukemia and acute myeloid leukemia), brain tumors (medulloblastoma, astrocytoma, and brainstem glioma), rhabdomyosarcoma, neuroblastoma, Wilms tumor, Ewing sarcoma, and Hodgkin lymphoma. The fifth leading cause of death in this age population is due to **general heart diseases**, which may include cardiomyopathies and faulty valves.

COUNSELING FOR INDIVIDUALS

Individuals in the **11-24** age group should be provided counseling in the following areas: injury prevention, substance use, sexual behavior, diet and exercise, and dental health. Regarding injury prevention, these individuals should be advised about the use of seat belts and helmets. Counseling about the dangers of drug, alcohol, and tobacco use is also important. This age group should be educated regarding safe sex practices and sexually transmitted disease prevention, including abstinence, condoms, and other contraceptive devices. Education should also be provided concerning the importance of a balanced diet (avoiding too much fat and cholesterol, eating a variety of grains, fruits, and vegetables, limiting sugar intake) and regular exercise. The clinician may also advise that the individual schedule regular dental checkups, and brush and floss on a daily basis.

25 TO 64-YEAR AGE POPULATION
LEADING CAUSES OF DEATH

In the **25-64** age population, the leading cause of death is **cancer**. For adult women, the leading causes of cancer deaths are lung cancer, breast cancer, colorectal cancer, pancreatic cancer, and ovarian cancer. For adult men, the leading causes of cancer deaths are lung cancer, prostate cancer, colorectal cancer, pancreatic cancer, and liver cancer. The next leading cause of death in this age group is **heart disease** (coronary artery disease, congestive heart failure, acute myocardial

166

infarction), followed by **motor vehicle accidents and other unintentional accidents**. The fourth leading cause of death in adults age 25 to 64 is **infection with HIV** and its complications. **Suicides and homicides** account for the fifth leading cause of death.

RECOMMENDED COUNSELING

For the **25-64** age population, counseling should be available or provided in the following areas: substance use, diet and exercise, injury prevention, and sexual behavior. Regarding substance abuse, the patient should be commended for not smoking, or, if the patient does smoke, he or she should be advised to stop smoking. The clinician should provide the smoker with some smoking cessation tips. The patient should also be advised of the ill effects of excessive alcohol use, as well as the dangers of drinking and driving. The importance of a proper, balanced diet and regular physical activity should be stressed as well. Injury prevention includes advising the patient to wear a safety belt, keep weapons in a safe place, and check smoke detectors regularly. Ways to prevent sexually transmitted disease and pregnancy can also be discussed during an intervention.

POPULATION OLDER THAN 65 YEARS OF AGE

LEADING CAUSES OF DEATH

For adults **older than 65** years of age, **heart disease** is the leading cause of death. In fact, heart disease is the number 1 cause of death overall in the United States. Heart disease is actually a general term for a group of diseases including cardiomyopathy, cardiovascular disease (which includes atherosclerosis and coronary artery disease), ischemic heart disease, heart failure, valvular heart disease, and hypertensive heart disease. **Cancer** is the second leading cause of death, with the top 3 offenders being lung cancer, breast cancer, and colorectal cancer. **Cerebrovascular disease**, or stroke, is the third leading cause, and is followed by or **chronic obstructive pulmonary disease** (COPD) as number four. The fifth leading cause of death in adults older than 65 years of age is **pneumonia and influenza**.

RECOMMENDED COUNSELING

Recommended counseling for the population **older than 65** is largely similar to that of the 25-64 age population (advice regarding smoking cessation, excess alcohol abuse, diet and exercise, and sexual behavior). However, some additions should be noted regarding injury prevention, as this age group is at greater risk for injury. The standard counseling regarding seat belts, helmets, and smoke detectors is recommended; the clinician should also advise family members of the patient to become CPR certified in case of emergency. The patient (and his or her family members) should be counseled regarding fall prevention (confining the patient to one floor of the house, making sure that the stairs are free of clutter, placing hand rails in the bathroom).

SLEEP PATTERNS FOR INFANTS AND CHILDREN

While **sleeping patterns** may vary considerably for older children and teenagers, who often get insufficient sleep, the patterns of sleep for infants are fairly predictable:

- **Neonates** sleep about 16 hours a day, awakening to eat every 2-3 hours around the clock. Usually infants in the first 1-2 months should not sleep more than 4 hours at a time because they may become dehydrated. By 3 months, daytime sleep decreases to 5.5 hours with 9.5 at night.
- By **6 months**, most infants can sleep through the night (10-11 hours) and take 2 naps during the day (3.5-4 hours).

- Children slowly increase nighttime sleep and average 11-11.5 hours until about **age 4-5**. Naps, decreasing in duration, usually continue until about age 3 when 1-hour naps are common.
- **6- to 9-year-old children** need 10-11 hours of sleep, decreasing to about 9 in the teen years and 8-9 by age 18.

HEALTH PROMOTION EFFORTS SURROUNDING CO-SLEEPING

While **co-sleeping** (bed sharing) has been the norm for thousands of years and remains so in many cultures, it has been proven to increase the risk for SIDS, suffocation, and breathing difficulties. For this reason, the American Academy of Pediatrics (AAP) does not recommend co-sleeping, but does acknowledge that many parents unintentionally fall asleep with their baby in the bed, most often when a sleep-deprived mother breastfeeds her child in bed at night. While breastfeeding in bed poses this risk, the AAP feels that this option is safer than many of the alternatives (getting up to feed the infant in a chair or on the couch), and therefore continues to recommend breastfeeding in bed overnight. Parents should be advised to keep the bed clear of loose bedding or pillows that could pose the risk of suffocation if mother and baby fall asleep. Additionally, if the mother falls asleep with the baby during or after nighttime feeding, the AAP recommends that she return the infant to its crib as soon as she wakes up.

The **ABC's of infant sleeping** are that the infant should sleep **alone**, on their **back,** in a **crib**, but the AAP advises pediatricians to withhold judgment when supporting parents who are struggling to implement this guidance. In addition to these ABC's, the AAP now recommends that newborns through 6 months should sleep on their own bed/crib in the same room as the parents. This arrangement, called **room sharing**, has been found to reduce the risk of SIDS.

PROVIDING ANTICIPATORY GUIDANCE
CHILDREN/FAMILIES

Providing **anticipatory guidance** to children/families is an important role for the nurse practitioner, who is guided by knowledge about risk factors and growth and development. As the child moves from 1 stage of development to another, the nurse should provide information first to the parents and then to the parents and child about what to expect in terms of development, both physically and emotionally, as well as how to minimize risk factors. **Guidance** may be related to a number of different areas of concern:

- **Diet and nutrition**, especially for those children at risk for obesity or eating disorders.
- **Safety measures**, including information about common types of childhood injuries.
- **Sexual development** and normal related changes and behaviors.
- **Sports activities** and exercise that is age-appropriate,
- General growth and development.
- **Academic progress** and advice about testing and intervention for learning disabilities.
- Peer influence.
- Drug and alcohol abuse.

EARLY ADOLESCENCE

Children during **early adolescence** (11-14) are undergoing many changes in their bodies and emotions. Relationships with family and peers may begin to change, and the child may be very self-conscious and concerned that they are normal. **Anticipatory guidance** helps the child to navigate changes in his/her life and to negotiate changes in relationships as the child seeks more autonomy:

- **Physical changes**: Outline what the child should expect in terms of bodily changes, such as development of secondary sexual characteristics, including normal variations, and height and weight changes.
- **Cognitive changes**: Allow the child to express changes in thought patterns and awareness and discuss how that relates to developing maturity and stress the importance of maintaining academic responsibilities.
- **Sociobehavioral changes**: Ask the child about peer groups and pressures at school and discuss methods to avoid gangs, tobacco, drugs, alcohol, and abusive relationships.

MIDDLE ADOLESCENCE

Middle adolescence (15-17) is a time of conflict for many young people as they strive to establish an identity separate from their parents and at the same time fit in and find acceptance with their peers. For many, this is the most difficult time of adolescence, and the nurse practitioner should provide **anticipatory guidance** to the adolescent through this time, even if the adolescent appears uninterested. Adolescents want respect and often respond when treated with respect. Encouraging the adolescent to discuss issues is more productive that providing direct guidance:

- **Physical changes**: Discuss the responsibilities that come with sexual maturity, including abstinence or birth control. Demonstrate breast and testicular self-examinations.
- **Cognitive changes**: Discuss future goals, both life plans and academic plans, providing guidance in relation to steps the adolescent needs to take in order to meet those goals.
- **Sociobehavioral changes**: Discuss relationships and risk-taking behavior while focusing on means to increase safety.

IMPORTANCE OF COUNSELING A COUPLE TOGETHER REGARDING LIFESTYLE MODIFICATIONS

In some situations, the clinician may find him or herself counseling a patient to stop smoking, eat healthier, and begin an exercise routine, because the patient has developed a number of health problems related to these areas. The clinician may find the patient receptive, but notices that there is no change in behavior from one visit to the next. In this case, it may be beneficial for the clinician to speak to the patient and his or her spouse. Perhaps the patient has good intentions, but has a spouse that enables him or her, or is not supportive of their lifestyle change, and so the patient does not change. By speaking to both the patient and the spouse together, the clinician may be able to get both to realize the importance of changing their habits. By committing to a change together, they may have a greater chance of succeeding.

> **Review Video: Basic Skills of a Counselor**
> Visit mometrix.com/academy and enter code: 965456

HEALTH PROMOTION EFFORTS SURROUNDING SUN EXPOSURE

For many years, parents were advised to protect children from all **sun exposure** in order to prevent skin damage that could lead to skin cancer, but this, and a decrease in milk drinking, has resulted in increasing evidence of **vitamin D deficiency** and even an increase in cases of rickets. This is fueling a debate between physicians who believe that some sun exposure is warranted for children and others who insist that all exposure is harmful. Recent guidelines suggest that approximately 20 minutes of sun exposure daily with arms exposed, avoiding direct mid-day sun from 10-2 PM and burns, is a safe amount of time and will prevent vitamin D deficiency. Dark-skinned children may tolerate more time in the sun without burning. For longer periods of time,

sunscreen should be applied to all exposed areas of skin, especially in children who are fair and prone to burning.

AMERICAN GERIATRICS SOCIETY GUIDELINE FOR THE PREVENTION OF FALLS IN OLDER PERSONS

The American Geriatrics Society Guideline for the **Prevention of Falls** in Older Persons includes:

- All geriatric patients should be asked if they have had falls in the past **year**.
- If **no falls**, no intervention is needed.
- If **1 fall**, the patient should be assessed for gait and balance, including the get-up-and-go test in which the patient stands up form a chair without using arms to assist, walks across the room and returns. If the patient is steady, no further assessment is needed. If the patient demonstrates unsteadiness, further assessment to determine the cause is necessary.
- If **multiple falls**, a full assessment should be completed: history, vision, neurological status, muscle strength, joint function, mental status, reflexes, cardiovascular status, including rate and rhythm), postural pulse, and blood pressure. Referral to a geriatric specialist may be appropriate.
- **Long-term exercise** focusing on strength and balance training. Tai chi has been found to be helpful for some people.
- **Modification of home environment** (remove throw rugs, install grab bars, provide easy access to bathroom).
- **Review of medications** to determine if the number can be reduced, especially if the patient is taking >4 medications or psychotropic medications, as many medications or medication interactions can cause dizziness and instability.
- **Assistive devices**, such as walkers and crab canes to improve stability.
- **Control of cardiovascular conditions**, such as heart block or fibrillation, which may cause dizziness/syncope and precipitate falls.
- Remediation of visual deficits when possible (glasses).
- **Footwear** providing adequate support.

SAFETY WITH REGARDS TO CRUTCH WALKING

Crutches should be properly fitted before patient attempts ambulation. Correct height is one hand-width below axillae. The handgrips should be adjusted so the patient supports the body weight comfortably with elbows slightly flexed rather than locked in place. The patient should be cautioned not to bear weight under the axillae as this can cause nerve damage but to hold the crutches tight against the side of the chest wall. The type of **gait** that the patient uses depends on the type of injury. Typical gaits include:

- **Two-point** in which both crutches are placed forward and then the well leg advances to the crutches.
- **Three-point** in which the injured extremity and both crutches are advanced together and then the well leg advances to the crutches.
- The patient should be advised whether there is partial or no weight bearing and demonstration provided. **Stair climbing** should be practiced:
  - **Ascending**: well foot goes first and then crutches and injured extremity.
  - **Descending**: Crutches go first and then the well foot.

TOBACCO USE IN CHILDREN AND ADOLESCENTS

The CDC conducts the Youth Risk Surveillance System to determine health-risk behaviors that contribute to significant morbidity in adolescents. **Tobacco,** often thought of as an adult issue, is a cause of concern for children and teenagers. Tobacco use is one of the leading preventable causes of death in the United States, but about 70% of children have tried smoking before high school, often beginning by age 12, putting themselves at risk for heart and lung disease as adults. Additionally, many teenagers use chewing tobacco or cigars, which can cause mouth cancer. Those most at risk are **males in low-income families with parents who smoke**. Male adolescents may smoke to be rebellious, but females often smoke to lose weight. Other factors include the desire to be part of a group, lack of supervision, and accessibility of tobacco. *Intervention* includes identifying those smoking, providing information about the dangers of smoking beginning with children at about 9 years old, and providing programs to help teenagers quit smoking.

LIFESTYLE CHANGES TO REDUCE WEIGHT

While the 7th and 8th Reports of the Joint National Committee on Prevention, Detection, Evaluation, and Treatment of High Blood Pressure have slightly different guidelines regarding hypertension, both recommended a number of **lifestyle changes to reduce weight**:

- **Decrease sedentary behaviors**: Avoid long periods watching television, searching the Internet, playing video games, and instant messaging. Establish time limits, especially for children.
- **Increase exercise and physical activity**: Engage in exercise at least 40 minutes daily if possible. Walking, biking, aerobic dancing, weight lifting, tennis, soccer, basketball, baseball, and exercise and dance classes are beneficial. Group activities, such as hiking, can encourage participation.
- **Modify diet**: Decrease portions and reduce fat and simple carbohydrates as well as avoid snacking between meals or substitute healthy snacks (such as celery sticks).
- **Modify beverage intake**: Reduce consumption of high-caloric, high carbohydrate beverages, such as sodas, juices, flavored and sweetened water.

DIETARY MANAGEMENT OF OBESITY IN CHILDREN

Obesity in children and teenagers is increasing with 16-33% classified as overweight. While there is no clear agreement about weight standards for children, excess weight is having a profound effect on children's health. However, helping the child to lose weight can be difficult:

- Dieting is best approached as a healthier **change in eating habits** for the whole family so that the child does not eat differently from others.
- No more than 30% of nutrition should be **fats**.
- Carbohydrates should be **complex** rather than simple sugars, decreasing consumption of white flour and sugar.
- **Healthy snacks**, such as fruit, air-popped popcorn, and nonfat yogurt, should be provided with high-caloric snacks (chips, candy) not available.
- The child should eat **3 meals daily**, served adequate but not large portions, and not be forced to "clean the plate."
- Television viewing or other **sedentary activities** should be progressively limited over time and exercise activities encouraged.

171

Crisis Management

DISASTER MANAGEMENT PLANS

TYPES

There are several different types of **disaster management plans**, some more specific than others. They are listed and briefly described below:

1. **Emergency Action Plan** – OSHA required, evacuation plans and emergency drills.
2. **Business Continuity Plan** – Business operation-specific, aimed at reducing losses and resuming productivity.
3. **Risk Management Plan** – Off-site effects of chemical exposures.
4. **Emergency Response Plan** – Immediate response to disasters.
5. **Contingency Plan** – General, designed to handle events not covered in other plans.
6. **Federal Response Plan** – Coordinates federal resources.
7. **Spill Prevention, Control, and Countermeasures Plan** – Deals with the prevention, control, and clean-up of oil spills.
8. **Mutual Aid Plan** – Plan for shared resources between other companies/firms.
9. **Recovery Plan** – Deals with repair and rebuilding post-disaster.
10. **Emergency Management Plan** – Plan for healthcare facilities.
11. **All-Hazard Disaster Management Plan** – General plan that is not hazard-specific.

STEPS FOR DEVELOPMENT

There are many different types of **disaster management plans**. Regardless of the type, however, there are several basic steps for its development. To begin with, a **planning team** must be established that includes representatives from all levels within the organization. The planning team is responsible for putting together a timeline for completion of the plan as well as an estimation of the costs, fees, and resources necessary to complete the plan. Once this is done, an **analysis of potential disasters** can begin. In this step, potential hazards are identified and vulnerability of the organization to disasters is assessed. A disaster response plan is established that includes the reduction/removal of hazardous situations. The final steps are **plan implementation and review**. The plan can be tested for efficacy through drills and mock disaster situations. It is critical to review and update the plan yearly.

MANAGEMENT OF SUICIDAL PATIENTS

Patients may attempt **suicide** for many reasons, including severe depression, social isolation, situational crisis (job loss, divorce), bereavement, or psychotic disorder (such as schizophrenia). It is important that the FNP provide **support** and not negative attitude, which may further depress the patient's self-esteem, increasing the risk of further attempts. Suicidal patients should be referred for psychiatric evaluation. Initial treatment depends upon the type of suicide attempt. Antidotes for ingestion of common drugs include:

- **Opiates**: Naloxone (Narcan®).
- **Acetaminophen**: N-acetylcysteine.

The patient should be assessed for suicide risk after initial treatment. Those at high risk should be hospitalized. High-risk findings include:

- Violent suicide attempt (knives, gunshots).
- Suicide attempt with low chance of rescue.
- Ongoing psychosis or disordered thinking.

172

- Ongoing severe depression and feeling of helplessness.
- History of previous suicide attempts.
- Lack of social support system.

Helping Smokers Quit

The US Department of Health and Human Services guidelines for **helping smokers quit** includes:

- Ask about and record **smoking status** at every visit.
- Advise all smokers to quit and explain **health reasons**.
- Assess **readiness** to quit by questioning and if willing, provide resources. If patient is not willing, provide support and attempt to motivate the person to quit with information.
- Assist smokers with a **plan** that sets a date (within 2 weeks), removes cigarettes, enlists family and friends, reviews past attempts, and anticipates challenges during the withdrawal period. The FNP must give advice about the need for abstinence and discuss the association of smoking with drinking. Medications to help control the urge to smoke (patches, gum, lozenge, prescriptions) and resources should be provided.
- **Follow-up** monitoring should be done to evaluate progress and reinforce the program.

Iatrogenic Illness

An **iatrogenic illness** is defined as any illness or symptoms that occur as a **result of treatment**. Of course, treatment is administered with the intent to make the patient better, not worse, but sometimes treatments do have adverse effects; aging adults are especially at risk of developing an iatrogenic illness. Individuals with multisystem diseases or failures, those who take multiple medications, and those who tend toward atypical disease presentation are especially at risk. The longer a patient remains hospitalized, the more likely he or she is to develop an iatrogenic illness as well. Common iatrogenic illnesses include urinary and fecal incontinence, decubital ulcers (bedsores), muscle wasting, drug reactions, electrolyte imbalance, fluid imbalance, and even heart failure. Nosocomial (hospital-acquired) infections may also be considered iatrogenic; pneumonia and wound infections are common nosocomial infections in the older adult.

Age-Appropriate Prevention

Primary, Secondary, and Tertiary Prevention

Risk assessment can be divided into 3 different prevention strategies; for the nurse practitioner, this depends largely on the point at which he or she **intervenes** with the patient. Nurses that work in community health clinics, public health, urgent care, and primary care, for example, will most often be focused on primary and secondary prevention; an acute care nurse practitioner, on the other hand, is typically concerned with secondary and tertiary prevention. **Primary prevention** involves patient education concerning stressors, allowing the patient to identify and defend against them; the focus in this case is on illness prevention. If an illness is identified, **secondary prevention** focuses on immediate treatment and alleviation of symptoms. **Tertiary prevention** focuses on the reduction of future stressors, as well as preparation of the patient to readapt to the environment.

Nutrition in Infants

1-6 Months

Breast milk provides the best **nutrition** for infants and breastfeeding should be encouraged for all mothers during the child's **first year**, with solid food added during the last 6 months. If formula is used, it should be iron-fortified for the first year. Cow's milk must be avoided until after 1 year because it can cause bleeding and anemia because of immaturity of the digestive tract

- **First month**: Eats about every 2-3 hours, taking 60-90 ml per feeding.
- **2-4 months**: Eats about every 3-4 hours, taking 90-120 ml per feeding.
- **4-6 months**: Eats 4-5 times daily, taking 100-150 ml per feeding. Often begins rice cereal at 4 months, 1-2 tablespoons 1-2 times daily before formula or breastfeeding, increasing to 1/4 cup 2 times daily by 6 months. Rice cereal contains iron, has low allergic potential, and is easy to digest.

6-12 MONTHS

As the child begins to eat other foods at **6-12 months**, milk must remain part of the **nutrition**, either breast milk or iron-fortified formula:

- **6-8 months**: Eats 4 times daily, 160-225 ml per feeding. Now having rice cereal, fruits, and vegetables with meals, with foods introduced one at a time about ≥3 days apart to observe for allergies.
- **8-10 months**: Eats 4 times daily, taking 160 ml per feeding. Meats may gradually be added at this time, but are harder to digest and may cause indigestion in some children. Eats finger foods, such as soft pieces of vegetables, cheese, tofu, cereals and meat sticks.
- **10-12 months**: Eats 4 times daily, taking about 160-225 ml per feeding. Usually weaning from breast or bottle and begins using "sippy" cup with lid. Is able to eat most soft foods with rest of the family and continues to enjoy finger foods. Makes attempts to self-feed with spoon.

NUTRITION FOR TODDLERS AND PRESCHOOLERS

Growth begins to slow for the **toddler and preschooler**, but nutritional demands remain high because of the child's increased size and activity. During these years, children still need milk, but intake should not exceed 1 quart daily. Children usually eat 3 meals and 2 snacks, the same foods as the rest of the family, learning eating habits from parents. Two different phenomena may occur:

- **Physiologic anorexia** occurs when high metabolic demands of infancy slow and toddlers may have periods when they eat little, but if intake is averaged over days or weeks, it is adequate.
- **Food jags** are common with preschoolers, days or even weeks when they refuse all but one or two foods. Studies have indicated that children seem to suffer no ill effects, so forcing the child to eat other food isn't necessary, but other foods should be offered until child resumes a more normal diet.

COMMON DIET DEFICIENCIES IN INFANTS AND CHILDREN

While poor nutritional intake can result in a number of different **dietary deficiencies**, some are more common in infants and children:

- **Calcium**: Calcium is essential for the growth and development of bones, but children, especially teenagers, are increasingly substituting fruit juice and sodas for milk. This can cause fractures and osteomalacia with eventual osteoporosis as an adult. Recommended daily intake for adolescents is 1500mg.
- **Folic acid**: Intake is often low among teenagers, resulting in high rates of congenital abnormalities if they get pregnant. Cereals and breads are fortified with folic acid to combat this.

- **Iron**: Newborns deplete their maternally-supplied iron by about 4 months and may become anemic if breast-fed without supplementary rice cereal. Formula is iron-fortified. Teenage girls are also often iron-deficient because of menses and poor dietary intake.
- **Vitamin D**: Deficiencies are on the rise because of judicious use of sunscreen and protecting children from all sun exposure. Breast-fed infants may need Vitamin D supplements.

EXERCISE NEEDS AT DIFFERENT AGES

Daily **exercise** is an important component of good health practices but should be age-appropriate, and some health conditions may pose restrictions on types of activities. Toddlers and young children usually get exercise by running and playing and do not need organized activities, but older children and teenagers may benefit from activities such as biking or other sports:

- **4- to 5-year-olds** may participate in dancing, skating and other supervised activities but lack coordination and judgment about safety.
- **6- to 12-year-olds** are still growing and muscles are short, so they do best with non-competitive sports, such as bicycling and swimming, until about age 10. Team sports should be supervised to ensure children are not straining muscles. Weight lifting may be done at 11 to build strength. Gymnastics may begin but children should be monitored for eating disorders.
- **12- to 18-year-olds** can participate in any sports activity unless limited by illness or disability. Exercise should be done at least 3 times weekly for 30 minutes.

Immunizations

TYPES OF VACCINES

There are a number of different **types of vaccines**:

- **Conjugated forms**: An organism is altered and then joined (conjugated) with another substance, such as a protein, to potentiate immune response (such as conjugated Hib).
- **Killed virus vaccines**: The virus has been killed but can still cause an immune response (such as inactivated poliovirus).
- **Live virus vaccines**: The virus is live but in a weakened (attenuated) form so that it doesn't cause the disease but confers immunity (such as measles vaccine).
- **Recombinant forms**: The organism is genetically altered and for example, may use proteins rather than the whole cell to stimulate immunity (such as hepatitis B and acellular pertussis vaccine).
- **Toxoid**: A toxin (antigen) that has been weakened by the use of heat or chemicals so it is too weak to cause disease but stimulates antibodies.

RECOMMENDATIONS FOR THE BIRTH TO 10-YEAR AGE POPULATION

There are a number of immunizations that are recommended for children in the **birth to 10-year** age group; it is important that parents are informed of these immunizations and know at what age each should be administered. The **diphtheria-tetanus-pertussis series** of immunizations (DTP) are administered in 5 doses, to be given between the ages of 2 months and 6 years; the recommended progression is one dose at 2 months, followed by a dose at 4 months, 6 months, between 12 and 18 months, and again between the ages of 4 and 6 years. The **oral poliovirus** vaccine (OPV) is also given in 5 doses, with the same recommended progression as the DTP series. The **measles-mumps-rubella** vaccine (MMR) is given twice; once between the ages of 12 and 15 months, and again between 4 and 6 years of age. The **H. influenzae type B** vaccine is given at 2 and

175

4 months and again between 12 and 15 months, and the **varicella** vaccine between 12 and 18 months.

RECOMMENDATIONS FOR THE 11 TO 24-YEAR AGE POPULATION

For the **11 to 24-year** age population, **tetanus** and **diphtheria** booster immunizations are recommended between the ages of 11 and 16 years. If the individual has not previously been immunized against the **hepatitis B virus**, it is recommended that he or she be immunized during this time. This immunization is administered in a series of 3, with 1 shot during the initial visit, the next shot 1 month later, and the third shot 6 months after the initial shot. If the patient did not receive his or her second **MMR** dose (which should have been administered between the ages of 4 and 6 years), it is advised that they be provided with the second dose between the ages of 11 and 12. If the child is susceptible to **chicken pox** (having not had the disease yet, and having not been previously immunized), he or she should be immunized between the ages of 11 and 12 as well.

ISSUES RELATED TO IMMUNIZATION

Immunization is the best means to protect children from a number of communicable diseases. Educating parents about the need for vaccinations is an important role for the nurse practitioner. While parents must be advised of potential **side effects**, many of the major concerns of parents in relation to thimerosal (which is about 50% mercury by weight) and autism and other disorders have not been supported by studies. Since 2000, vaccines have been thimerosal-free except for influenza although some may still contain trace amounts. Despite that, the benefits outweigh perceived risks. Vaccines promote 2 types of immunity:

- **Active immunity**: Antigens are given to promote production of antibodies.
- **Passive immunity**: Antibodies derived from another person with resistance are given to the child.

Some vaccines provide immunity throughout life, but others require periodic **booster injections**. If a child has a severe allergic reaction to 1 injection in a series, the rest of the series is contraindicated.

ROTAVIRUS VACCINE

Rotavirus is a cause of significant morbidity and mortality in children, especially in developing countries. Most children, without vaccination, will suffer from severe diarrhea caused by rotavirus within the first 5 years of life. Three doses are required:

- 2 months (between 6-12 weeks)
- 4 months
- 6 months

The **new rotavirus vaccine** is advised for all infants, but the 1st dose should not be initiated after 12 weeks and the 3rd dose should not be administered after 32 weeks, so there is a narrow window of opportunity. An earlier vaccine was withdrawn from the market because it was associated with an increase in intussusception, a disorder in which part of the intestine telescopes inside another. However, rates of intussusception in those receiving the current (RotaTeq®) vaccine have been investigated, and incidence of intussusception was within the range of normal occurrences with no evidence linking the occurrences to the vaccine.

HEPATITIS A VACCINE

Hepatitis A is the cause of a serious liver disease that can cause serious morbidity and death. It is spread through the feces of a person who is infected and often causes contamination of food and water. It is now recommended for all children at 1 year of age. It is not licensed for use in younger infants. Two doses are needed:

- 12 months (12-23 months).
- 18 months (or 6 months after previous dose).

Older children, teenagers, and adults may receive the two-injection series if they are considered at risk, depending upon lifestyle, such as men who have sex with other men, illegal drug users, chronic liver disease, those receiving clotting factor concentrates, and those working in experimental labs. It is also recommended if outbreaks occur. Adverse reactions are mild and include soreness, headache, anorexia, and malaise although severe allergic reactions can occur as with all vaccines.

A vaccine is available for the **hepatitis A virus,** and should be administered to those individuals who are deemed to be at high risk of contracting the disease. Individuals who are planning to travel to or have recently traveled to an area where hepatitis A is endemic (including Africa, South America, Mexico, and Eastern Europe) should be immunized against the virus. Other high-risk populations include drug abusers, homosexual men, and individuals who work in areas where they may come into contact with infected individuals (such as health care workers and child care workers). Those in the military should also be immunized in the event that they are stationed in an endemic country. Hepatitis A outbreaks may also occur in the food service industry when an individual does not wash his or her hands and then prepares food. In these cases, immunization is recommended for anyone who may have been exposed.

HEPATITIS B VACCINE

Hepatitis B is transmitted through blood and body fluids, including during birth; therefore, it is now recommended for all newborns as well as those <18 and those in high-risk groups >18 (drug users, men having sex with men, those with multiple sex partners, partners of those with hepatitis B, and healthcare workers). Hepatitis B can cause serious liver disease leading to liver cancer. Three injections of **monovalent HepB** are required to confer immunity:

- Birth (within 12 hours)
- Between 1-2 months
- ≥24 weeks
- Note: if combination vaccines are given after the birth dose then a dose at 4 months can be given.

If the mother is hepatitis B positive, the child should be given both the monovalent HepB vaccination as well as HepB immune globulin within 12 hours of birth. Adolescents (11-15) who have not been vaccinated require 2 doses, 4-6 months apart. Adverse reactions include local irritation and fever. Severe allergic reactions can occur to those allergic to baker's yeast.

DIPHTHERIA, TETANUS, AND PERTUSSIS (DTAP) VACCINE

Diphtheria and pertussis (whooping cough) are highly contagious bacterial diseases of the upper respiratory tract. Cases of diphtheria are now rare in the United States although it still occurs in some developing countries. There have, however, been recent outbreaks of pertussis in the United States. **Tetanus** is a bacterial infection contracted through cuts, wounds, and scratches. The diphtheria, tetanus, and pertussis (DTaP) vaccine is recommended for all children. DTaP is a newer and safer version of the older DTP vaccine, which is no longer used in the United States. **DTaP** requires 5 doses:

- 2 months
- 4 months
- 6 months
- 5-18 months
- 4-6 years (or at 11-12 years if booster missed between 4-6)

This vaccine is not licensed for use for children over 7 years old, but a different vaccine (**Tdap**) is given to those 11-64 in 1 dose. Adverse reactions can occur, but they are usually mild soreness, fever, and/or nausea. About 1 in 100 children will have high fever (>105°) and may develop seizures. Severe allergic responses can occur.

INACTIVATED POLIOVIRUS VACCINE

Poliomyelitis is a serious viral infection that can cause paralysis and death. Prior to introduction of a vaccine in 1955, polio was responsible for >20,000 cases in the United States each year. There have been no cases of polio caused by the poliovirus for >20 years in the United States, but it still occurs in some third world countries, so continuing vaccinations is very important. **Oral polio vaccine** (OPV) is no longer recommended in the United States because it carries a very slight risk of causing the disease (1:2.4 million). Children require 4 doses of **injectable polio vaccine** (IPV):

- 2 months
- 4 months
- 6-18 months
- 4-6 years (booster dose)

IPV is contraindicated for those who have had a severe reaction to neomycin, streptomycin, or polymyxin B. Rare allergic reactions can occur, but there are almost no serious problems caused by this vaccine.

VARICELLA VACCINE

Varicella (chickenpox) is a common infectious childhood disease caused by the varicella zoster virus, resulting in fever, rash, and itching, but it can cause skin infections, pneumonia, and neurological damage. After infection, the virus retreats to the nerves by the spinal cord and can reactivate years later, causing herpes zoster (shingles), a significant cause of morbidity in adults. Infection with varicella conveys immunity, but because of associated problems, it is recommended that all children receive **varicella vaccine**. Two doses are needed:

- 12-15 months
- 4-6 years (or at least 3 months after 1st dose)

Children ≥13 years and adults who have never had chickenpox or previously received the vaccine should receive 2 doses at least 28 days apart. Children should not receive the vaccine if they have had a serious allergic reaction to gelatin or neomycin. Most reactions are mild and include soreness, fever, and rash. About 1:1000 may experience febrile seizures. Pneumonia is a very rare reaction.

HERPES ZOSTER VACCINE

Adults who have had chicken pox as children or adults retain the **varicella zoster virus** in the nerve cells, and the virus can become reactivated and cause herpes zoster ("shingles"). Herpes zoster is most common in those ≥50 with chronic medical conditions and those who are immunocompromised. Since 2006, the **herpes zoster vaccine** has been recommended for those ≥60 years old. A single dose of the vaccine is needed. Studies indicate that it prevents about 50% of herpes zoster cases and decreases the pain and severity of those who still develop the disease. It is contraindicated in those with an allergy to gelatin or neomycin and those who are immunocompromised because of human immunodeficiency virus (HIV)/acquired immunodeficiency syndrome (AIDS), chemotherapy, radiation, steroid use, history of leukemia or lymphoma, and active tuberculosis (TB). Adverse reactions are rare and include allergic response, local inflammation, and headache.

MMR Vaccine

Measles is a viral disease characterized by fever and rash but can cause pneumonia, seizures, severe neurological damage, and death. **Mumps** is a viral disease that causes fever and swollen glands but can cause deafness, meningitis, and swelling of the testicles. **Rubella**, also known as German measles is also a viral disease that can cause rash, fever, and arthritis, but the big danger is that it can cause a woman who is pregnant to miscarry or deliver a child with serious birth defects. The measles, mumps, and rubella (**MMR**) vaccine is given in 2 doses:

- 12-15 months
- 4-6 years

Children can get the injections at any age if they have missed them, but there must be at least 28 days between injections. Children with severe allergic reactions to gelatin or neomycin should not get the injection. Severe adverse reactions are rare, but fever and mild rash are common. Teenagers may have pain and stiffness in joints. Occasional seizures (1:3,000) and thrombocytopenia (1:30,000) occur.

HPV Vaccine

Human papilloma virus (HPV) comprises >100 viruses. About 40 are sexually transmitted and invade mucosal tissue, causing genital warts, which carry low risk for cancer, or changes in the mucosa, which can lead to cervical cancer. Most HPVs cause few or no symptoms, but they are very common, especially in those 15-25 years. Over 99% of cervical cancers are caused by HPV, and 70% are related to HPVs 16 and 18. The HPV vaccine, **Gardasil®**, protects against HPVs 6, 11 (which cause genital warts), 16, and 18, which causes cancer. Protection is only conveyed if the female has not yet been infected with these strains. The vaccine is currently recommended for females <26 years of age. Studies are determining the benefit for men and women over 18. A series of 3 injections are required over a 6-month period:

- Initial dose 11-12 years (but may be given as young as 9 or ≥18).
- 2 months after 1st dose.
- 6 months after 1st dose.

INFLUENZA VACCINE

A different **influenza ("flu") vaccine** is formulated each year, and administration begins in September prior to flu season. There are two types of flu vaccine:

- **Trivalent inactivated influenza vaccine** (TIV) (injectable) is available for use in those over 6 months old, including older people who are healthy or have chronic medical conditions.
- **Live attenuated influenza vaccine** (LAIV) is a nasal spray for use in those 2 to 49 years of age. It is not for use in pregnant women and is not used for older adults.

Antibodies against the viruses used to formulate the vaccines develop in about 2 weeks. Vaccination is recommended for all people over six months of age.

Flu vaccine is contraindicated in individuals with an allergy to eggs, a history of reaction to flu vaccine, and a history of Guillain-Barré. The vaccine should not be administered 6 weeks or less after a previous flu vaccine. Adverse effects include infection with local inflammation, fever, and aching.

HEPTAVALENT PNEUMOCOCCAL CONJUGATE VACCINE

Heptavalent pneumococcal conjugate vaccine (PCV-7) (Prevnar®) was released for use in the United States in 2001 for treatment of children under 2 years old. It provides immunity to 7 serotypes of Streptococcus pneumoniae to protect against **invasive pneumococcal disease**, such as pneumonia, otitis media, bacteremia, and meningitis. Because children are most at risk <1, vaccinations begin early:

Administration:

- 1st dose: 6-8 weeks.
- 2nd dose: 4 months.
- 3rd dose: 6 months.
- 4th dose: 12-18 months.

Although less effective for older children, PCV-7 has been approved for children between 2 and 5 years of age who are at high risk because of the following conditions:

- **Chronic diseases**: sickle cell disease, heart disease, lung disease, liver disease.
- Damaged or missing **spleen**.
- Immunosuppressive disorders: diabetes, cancer.
- **Drug therapy**: chemotherapy, steroids.

PCV-7 may also be considered for all children <5, especially those <3 and in group day care and in some ethnic groups (Native American, Alaska Natives, and African Americans).

MENINGOCOCCAL VACCINE

Meningitis is severe bacterial meningitis that can result in severe neurological compromise or death. A number of different serotypes of meningococci can cause meningitis and current vaccines protect against 4 types although not against subtype B, which causes about 65% of meningitis cases in children. However, the vaccines provide 85-100% protection against sub-types A, C, Y, and W-135. There are 2 types of vaccine:

- **Meningococcal polysaccharide vaccine** (MPSV4) is made from the outer capsule of the bacteria and is used for children 2-10.
  - One dose is given at 2 years although those at high risk may receive 2 doses, 3 months apart.
  - Under special circumstances, children 3-24 months may receive 2 doses, 3 months apart.
- **Meningococcal conjugate vaccine** (MCV4) is used for children ≥11 (who have not received MPSV4). One dose is required:
  - 11-12, all children should receive the vaccine.
  - If not previously vaccinated, high school and college freshmen should be vaccinated.

Side effects are usually only local tenderness.

HIB VACCINE

Haemophilus influenzae type b (HIB) vaccine (HibTITER® and PedavaxHIB®) protects against infection with Haemophilus influenzae, which can cause serious respiratory infections, pneumonia, meningitis, bacteremia, and pericarditis in children <5 years old. Administration:

- 1st dose: 2 months
- 2nd dose: 4 months
- 3rd dose: 6 months (may be required, depending upon the brand of vaccine)
- Last dose: 12-15 months (this booster dose must be given at least 2 months after the earlier doses for those who start at a later age than 2 months.

Children over age 6 usually do not require HIB, but it is recommended for older children and some adults with conditions that place them **at risk**:

- Sickle cell disease.
- Human immunodeficiency virus (HIV)/acquired immunodeficiency syndrome (AIDS).
- Bone marrow transplant.
- Chemotherapy for cancer.
- Damaged or missing spleen.

Some chemotherapy drugs, corticosteroids, and other immunosuppressive drugs may interact with the vaccine.

PPV VACCINE

Pneumococcal polysaccharide-23 vaccine (PPV; Pneumovax® and Pnu-Immune®) protects against 23 types pneumococcal bacteria. It is given to adults ≥65 and those with increased risk, such as those with chronic disease (sickle cell, asplenia, Hodgkin's, cardiopulmonary and liver disease, diabetes), and children ≥2 years in high-risk groups (similar to adults) that include:

- Children with chronic heart, lung, sickle cell disease, diabetes, cirrhosis, alcoholism, and leaks of cerebrospinal fluid.
- Children with lowered immunity from Hodgkin's disease, lymphoma, leukemia, kidney failure, multiple myeloma, nephrotic syndrome, HIV/AIDS, damaged or missing spleen, and organ transplant.

181

Children <2 may not respond to this vaccine and should take PCV-7. Administration:

- One dose is usually all that is required although a second dose may be advised for children with some conditions, such as cancer or organ/bone marrow transplantations, and for those >65 years, 5 years after 1st vaccination (if given <65 years).
- If needed, a second dose is given 3 years after the first dose for children <10 and 5 years after the first for those ≥10 years.

CHEMOPROPHYLAXIS

Chemoprophylaxis refers to the administration of a drug or other pharmaceutical treatment with the intention of **preventing disease or infection**. The initiation of chemoprophylaxis treatment may be recommended by a clinician, although the patient can refuse treatment. These recommendations may be based on age populations that are determined to be at greater risk. It is important for the clinician (and the patient) to weigh the risks and benefits of chemoprophylaxis. Examples of chemoprophylaxis include treatment for exposed individuals during outbreaks of influenza type A and influenza type B; hepatitis B immunization for health care workers, babies born to positive mothers, and individuals who have had sexual contact with a positive person; prophylactic rabies treatment for individuals who have been bitten by an animal suspected to have rabies; and rifampin prophylaxis for individuals who have been exposed to tuberculosis.

Wellness Visit

NORMAL HEART RATE, RESPIRATORY RATE, AND BLOOD PRESSURE FOR CHILDREN

When evaluating the **vital signs** of children, it is important to take the **age** of the child into account, for what is normal for a child of 2 years may not be considered normal for a child of 12. Because children grow so rapidly in such a short period of time, these numbers will change rapidly as well. For a newborn baby, the normal heart rate is between 100 and 170 bpm, the normal respiratory rate is between 30 and 80 respirations per minute, and the normal blood pressure is 73/55. For a 6-month-old child, the normal ranges are 90 to 130, 24 to 36, and 80/53, respectively. Normal vitals for a 1-year-old are 90 to 130, 20 to 40, and 90/56; a 3-year-old 80 to 120, 20 to 30, and 92/55; a 6-year-old 70 to 110, 16 to 22, and 96/57; and a 10-year-old 60 to 100, 16 to 20, and 100/60.

ADOLESCENT CHECK-UPS

Adolescent (ages 12-19 years) check-ups – According to the American Medical Association (AMA), an adolescent also needs 3 regular checks at ages 11-14, 15-17, then 18-21 years, except when more visits are needed. When there is a big chance, give advice and assess for HIV and VDRL, and check understanding of birth control and condoms. Immunizations include Tetanus-diphtheria booster and more when necessary. Be aware of indications of depression or suicide. Get a dental exam every year. For girls, instruct about self-breast exam, identify **Tanner stage** (regarding puberty), and do Pap smear if the patient is having sex or is over the age of 18 years. Tanner stages include:

- **Stage I** – Growth spurt (average age 10).
- **Stage II** – Breast bud; slight pubic hair.
- **Stages III-IV** – Breasts grow.
- **Stage V** – Mature.

For boys, educate regarding self-testicular exam and find Tanner stage:

- **Stage I** – Growth spurt (average 12 ½).
- **Stage II** – Minimal pubic hair.
- **Stages III-IV** – Penis grows larger.
- **Stage V** – Mature.

ADOLESCENTS (AGE 12-19)

EXPECTATIONS FOR ADOLESCENTS

Expect alterations in the body with puberty and a necessity for taking responsibility for well-being, diet, physical activity, getting enough sleep, and staying out of danger. Eat a range of food and eat breakfast, good snacks, and restrict sugar and fast food. Take care of the skin. Take care of the dental needs, including using fluoride and going to the dentist (6-12 months apart). Keep safe: wear protective gear when doing sports, seat belts, gun safety, defensive driving, coaching about driving, and stay away from aggressive actions or gangs. The adolescent will need habitual exercise with sports, social life, and being active in school and/or church. Do not smoke or stop smoking, and make a point about how it makes the patient become unattractive (teeth and nails, bad breath, clothes smell) and do worse in sports (cannot go as long; lose breath easily). Sexuality issues include dating, being accountable for sex life, abstinence, birth control, and chances of STDs or unplanned pregnancy.

PHYSICAL

Utilize anthropometric chart for height and weight. Assess for an eating disorder when needed. Evaluate the patient's point of view about eating and body weight. Check the skin. Look for gingivitis, caries, and problems with alignment. Check for indications of abuse or neglect. If the patient has been near a lot of noise, check the hearing. Check sight. Check the blood pressure (2 years apart) to see normal at 120/80 mm Hg or lower. Do a TB skin assessment (2 years apart), if there has been any contact or if the patient has a chance of getting TB.

YOUNG ADULTS (AGES 20-39 YEARS)

EXPECTATIONS

Top reasons for death include car wrecks, murder, suicide, harm to the body, heart disease, and AIDS. As far as eating and physical activity, the patient needs to maintain a healthy weight (even with adjustments in the basal metabolic rate) and choose a routine of physical activity. Get proper dental work. Regarding sexuality, make arrangements for planning for a family or birth control and avoiding STDs. Educate regarding signs of cancer and taking care of the skin. Stop smoking as the main way to prevent problems, and educate regarding drinking alcohol or using other substances. The patient needs to keep safe by using protective gear in sports or exercise, seat belts, helmets, practicing gun safety, driving carefully, and avoiding aggressive actions. The patient will need coping mechanisms for stress and family and parenting abilities. Be aware of personal well-being with regard to protection and the surroundings.

CHECK-UPS

Do a total physical at 20 (5-6-year increments). Check blood pressure (2 years apart) to look for normal systolic: 110-130 mm Hg and diastolic 60-80 mm Hg. Check total cholesterol in 5-year increments and do more when it is higher than 200 mg/dL. Do PPD when patient had contact with TB, get Td immunization in 10-year increments, teach self-skin assessment, and dental check-up should occur every year. Men need to perform self- testicular exam every month. Women need self-breast exam every month, Pap and pelvic assessments in 3-year increments, GC and Chlamydia assessments, and clinical breast exam in 3-year increments.

MIDDLE-AGE PATIENTS (AGES 40-59)

EXPECTATIONS

Top reasons for death include heart disease, accidents, lung cancer, cerebrovascular disease, breast cancer, colorectal cancer, and obstructive lung disease. As far as eating and physical activity, the patient needs to maintain a healthy weight (even with adjustments in the basal metabolic rate) and choose a routine of physical activity. Get proper dental work. Deal with menopause, sexual alterations that come with getting older, STDs, indications of cancer, and taking care of the skin. The main way to prevent problems is to stop smoking, and educate regarding drinking alcohol or using other substances. The patient needs to keep safe by using protective gear in sports or exercise, seat belts, helmets, practicing gun safety, driving carefully, and avoiding aggressive actions. Deal with mid-life issues, including children leaving home, becoming grandparents, getting ready for retirement, and coping with stress. Be aware of personal well-being with regard to protection and the surroundings.

CHECK-UPS

Get a total physical (5-6 years apart), check blood pressure (2 years apart) to see normal systolic: 110-130 mm Hg and diastolic 60-80 mm Hg. The aim is < 120/80 if the patient has diabetes or ongoing renal problem. Check cholesterol (5 years apart) and do more when it is > 200 mg/dL. Do ECG at 40 years and older when there is a chance of cardiac problems. Women need self-breast exam every month, clinical breast exam every year, ACS says mammogram every year (USPSTF says 1-2 years apart), and Pap and pelvic assessment (3 years apart when there are not any other risks). Men need STE every month. All middle-age adults need colorectal screen at age 50 (yearly), glaucoma screen (yearly), dental assessment and cleaning (6-12 months apart), cancer screen (every year) and tetanus (10 years apart).

ELDERLY POPULATION (AGES 60 AND OLDER)

EXPECTATIONS

Top reasons for death include heart disease, cerebrovascular disease, obstructive lung disease, pneumonia and/or influenza, lung cancer, and colorectal cancer. As far as eating and physical activity, the patient needs to maintain a healthy weight (even with adjustments in the basal metabolic rate) and choose a routine of physical activity. Get proper dental work. Deal with sexual differences that occur because of getting older and any STDs. Look for cancer indications and take care of the skin. Stop smoking as the main way to prevent problems, and educate regarding drinking alcohol or using other substances. The patient needs to keep safe by using protective gear in sports or exercise, seat belts, helmets, practicing gun safety, driving carefully, and avoiding aggressive actions. Deal with differences in the way life is, including retirement, losing a husband, wife, or friends, and dealing with differences in the body (sight, hearing, responses, bowel/bladder routines). Be aware of personal well-being with regard to protection and the surroundings.

CHECK-UPS

Get a total physical (2 years apart) including lab tests, check blood pressure (2 years apart) to see: normal systolic 110-120 mm Hg, diastolic 60-80mm Hg. Check total cholesterol (5 years apart) and do more when it is over 200 mg/dL. Do ECG every year when there are cardiac risks. Women need self-breast exam every month, mammogram (ACS says every year; USPSTF says 1-2 years apart), and Pap and pelvic assessment (3 years apart). Men need self-testicular exam every month. Everyone needs colorectal screen (fecal occult or sigmoidoscopy) at age 50 (yearly), glaucoma test (yearly), dental exam and cleaning (6-12 months apart), tetanus shot (10 years apart) pneumococcal vaccine (one time) and influenza vaccine (every year). Top reasons elderly die include: heart disease, cerebrovascular disease, obstructive lung disease, pneumonia and/or influenza, lung cancer, colorectal cancer.

Pharmacologic Interventions

PHARMACOKINETICS

Pharmacokinetics relates to the effects that the body has on a drug, while pharmacodynamics relates to the effects that a drug has on the body. Both must be considered to ensure adequate dosing to achieve the optimal response from medications. With all drugs there is an **intake** (dose) and a **response**. Pharmacokinetics relates to the route of administration, the absorption, the dosage, the frequency of administration, the distribution, and the serum levels achieved over time. The drug's rate of clearance (elimination) and doses needed to ensure therapeutic benefit must be considered. Most drugs are cleared through the kidneys, with water-soluble compounds excreted more readily than protein-soluble compounds. Volume of distribution (intravenous drug dose divided by plasma concentration) determines the rate at which the drug passes into tissue. Drug distribution depends on the degree of protein binding and ion trapping that takes place. Elimination half time is the time needed to reduce plasma concentrations to 50% during elimination.

ELEMENTS OF PHARMACOKINETICS

Usually the equivalent of 5 **half-lives** is needed to completely eliminate a drug. Five half-lives are also needed to achieve steady-state plasma concentrations if giving doses intermittently. Context-sensitive half-life, in contrast, is the time needed to reach a specific amount of decrease (50%, 60%) after stopping administration of a drug.

Recovery time is the length of time it takes for plasma levels to decrease to the point that the person awakens. This is affected by plasma concentration.

Effect-site equilibrium is the time between administration of a drug and clinical effect (the point at which the drug reaches the appropriate receptors) and must be considered when determining dose, time, and frequency of anesthetic agents.

The **bioavailability** of drugs may vary, depending upon the degree of metabolism that takes place before the drug reaches its site of action.

PHARMACODYNAMICS

Pharmacodynamics relates to **biological effects** (therapeutic or adverse) of drug administration over time. Drug transport, absorption, means of elimination, and half-life must all be considered when determining effects. Responses may include continuous responses, such as blood pressure variations, or dichotomous response in which an event either occurs or does not (such as death). Information from pharmacodynamics provides feedback to **modify medication dosage** (pharmacokinetics). Drugs provide biological effects primarily by interacting with **receptor sites** (specific protein molecules) in the cell membrane. Receptors include voltage-sensitive ion channels (sodium, chloride, potassium, and calcium channels), ligand-gated ion channels, and transmembrane receptors. Agonist drugs exert effects after binding with a receptor while antagonist drugs bind with a receptor but have no effects, so they can block agonists from binding. The total number of receptors may vary, upregulating or downregulating in response to stimuli (such as drug administration). Dose-response curves show the relationship between the amount of drug given and the resultant plasma concentration and biological effects.

PHARMACOTHERAPEUTICS

COST OF DRUGS

The **cost of drugs** is one of the most expensive aspects of medical care for patients. Even those with insurance drug coverage or Medicare D may have considerable costs, especially with non-generic drugs. There is much pressure from drug representatives to prescribe new drugs, and patients are often influenced by direct-to-consumer advertising, but the FNP must ensure that drugs are prescribed based on evidence. Additionally, the cost versus benefit of drugs must always be considered. It is the responsibility of the FNP to act in the best interests of the patient and to educate the patient about drugs. The FNP should evaluate the costs of drugs when determining which drug to prescribe. If a less expensive drug is as effective as a more expensive or newer drug, then the less expensive drug should be prescribed. The FNP should educate people about the use of generic drugs as a cost-saving measure, as—in most cases—these are as effective as non-generic.

LIFE SPAN CONCERNS

Prescribing drugs across the life span requires an understanding of differences in types of medications used and dosages according to age and gender.

- Dosage and administration of **pediatric medications** is weight and age related, and only pediatric medications should be prescribed if possible. Adult pills, for example, should not be cut for use for a child, as even small variations in dosage may have adverse effects. Dosage should always be checked. The Broselow® tape can be used to measure the child to guide medication dosage.
- **Geriatric patients** often have decreased renal and hepatic function that affects clearance of drugs so that action is prolonged or the drug may accumulate and cause an overdose. Patients may have increased sensitivity to drugs and require a smaller dose than younger adults. In many cases, beginning with a small dose and then increasing if needed is a safe approach.

Respiratory Pharmacology

PHARMACOLOGICAL AGENTS USED FOR ASTHMA TO RELIEVE BRONCHOSPASM

Numerous pharmacological agents are used for control of **asthma/bronchospasm**, some long acting to prevent attacks and others short-acting to provide relief for acute episodes:

- **β-Adrenergic agonists** include both long-acting and short-acting preparations used for relaxation of smooth muscles and bronchodilation, reducing edema and aiding clearance of mucus. Medications include salmeterol (Serevent), sustained release albuterol (Volmax ER®), and short-acting albuterol (Proventil®) and levalbuterol (Xopenex®).
- **Anticholinergics** aid in preventing bronchial constriction and potentiate the bronchodilating action of β-Adrenergic agonists. The most-commonly used medication is ipratropium bromide (Atrovent®).
- **Corticosteroids** provide anti-inflammatory action by inhibiting immune responses, decreasing edema, mucus, and hyper-responsiveness. Because of numerous side effects, glucocorticosteroid are usually administered orally or parentally for 5 days (prednisone, prednisolone, methylprednisolone) and then switched to inhaled steroids. If a patient receives glucocorticoids for more than 5 days, then dosages are tapered. Inhaled corticosteroids include beclomethasone (Vanceril®), budesonide (Pulmicort®), and fluticasone propionate (Flovent®).

- **Methylxanthines** are generally contraindicated in children unless the child is critically ill, in which case they appear to have a role in improving pulmonary function and decreasing need for mechanical ventilation. Medications include aminophylline and theophylline.
- **Magnesium sulfate** is used to relax smooth muscles and decrease inflammation. If administered intravenously, it must be given slowly to prevent hypotension and bradycardia. Inhaled, it potentiates the action of albuterol.
- **Heliox** (helium-oxygen) is administered to decrease airway resistance with airway obstruction, thereby decreasing respiratory effort. Heliox improves oxygenation of those on mechanical ventilation.
- **Leukotriene inhibitors** are used to inhibit inflammation and bronchospasm for long-term management. Medications include montelukast (Singulair®).

SMOKING CESSATION MEDICATIONS

Smoking cessation is critical to the prevention of many diseases, and there are a number of medical treatments that can assist patients through the withdrawal period, during which the person may experience anxiety, irritability, and nicotine craving. Most of the medications contain **nicotine**, but it is released in a slower manner to avoid the sudden increase in nicotine ("rush") associated with smoking. Additionally, these products help the smoker avoid other toxins, such as tar and carbon monoxide:

- **Nicotine patch**: This is available over the counter and by prescription and are used in decreasing doses for about 8 weeks: 21 mg/24 hours for 4 weeks, 14 mg/24 hours for 2 weeks, and then 7 mg/24 hours for 2 weeks. Side effects include insomnia, nervousness, and local skin irritation.
- **Nicotine inhaler**: This is available only by prescription. Six to 16 cartridges per day may be used for <6 months. Side effects include irritation of the mouth and throat.
- **Bupropion SR (Zyban®)**: This is available by prescription and may be for 7-12 weeks with maintenance for < 6 months. Treatment begins 2 weeks before quitting with 150 mg in AM for 3 days and then 150 mg BID. It is contraindicated with history of seizure, eating disorder, or monoamine oxidase (MAO) inhibitor use (within 14 days). Side effects include insomnia and dry mouth.
- **Varenicline**: This is available by prescription. It is begun about 5-7 days prior to quitting at 0.5 mg daily and increased to 0.5 mg BID 1-4 days before quitting. On the day of quitting, the dose is increased to 1 mg daily. The patient must be monitored for mood or behavioral changes, psychiatric manifestations and suicidal thoughts. Side effects include insomnia and nausea.
- **Nicotine gum**: This is available over the counter in 2 mg and 4 mg dosages for use up to 12 weeks. If people smoke <24 cigarettes daily, they may use up to 24 pieces of 2 mg gum daily. If they smoke ≥25 cigarettes daily, they may use up to 24 pieces of 4 mg gum. Side effects include mouth irritation and dyspepsia.
- **Nicotine lozenge**: This 2 or 4 mg lozenge is available OTC and may be used for 12 weeks. If patients usually have the first cigarette >30 minutes of awakening, they may use up to 10 2-mg lozenges daily. If the first cigarette is usually <30 minutes of awakening, patients may use up to 5 4-mg lozenges daily. Side effects include irritation of throat, hiccups, nausea, indigestion, and heartburn.
- **Nicotine nasal spray**: This is available by prescription only and may be used for 3-6 months with 8-40 doses per day. Side effects include local nasal irritation.

Cardiac Pharmacology

TREATMENT FOR HYPERTENSION AND HEART FAILURE

There are a number of different types of medications used for the treatment of heart failure and hypertension:

- **ACE inhibitors**, such as captopril (Capoten®), enalapril (Vasotec®), and lisinopril (Prinivil®), decrease afterload and preload and reverse ventricular remodeling but may cause hypotension initially and are contraindicated with renal insufficiency.
- **β-Blockers**, such as metoprolol (Lopressor®), carvedilol (Coreg®), and esmolol (Brevibloc®), slow the heart rate, reduce hypertension, prevent dysrhythmias, and reverse ventricular remodeling, but should not be used during decompensation and should be monitored carefully for those with airway disease, uncontrolled diabetes, slow irregular pulse, or heart block.
- **Aldosterone agonists**, such as spironolactone (Aldactone®), decreases preload and myocardial hypertrophy and reduces edema and sodium retention but may increase serum potassium.

VASODILATORS

Vasodilators may be used for arterial dilation or venous dilation in order to improve cardiac function. These drugs may be used to treat pulmonary hypertension or generalized systemic hypertension. They may be used for those who cannot tolerate angiotensin-converting enzyme (ACE) inhibitors or angiotensin receptor blockers. Vasodilators may dilate arteries, veins, or both.

- **Arterial dilation** reduces afterload, improving cardiac output.
- **Venous dilation** reduces preload, reducing filling pressures.
- **Smooth muscle relaxants** decrease peripheral vascular resistance but may cause hypotension and headaches:
  - Sodium nitroprusside (Nipride®) dilates both arteries and veins and is rapid in action and used for reduction of hypertension and afterload reduction for heart failure.
  - Nitroglycerin (Tridil®) primarily dilates veins and is used intravenously to reduce preload for acute heart failure, unstable angina, and acute myocardial infarction. Nitroglycerin may also be prophylactically after PCIs to prevent vasospasm.
  - Hydralazine (Apresoline®) dilates arteries and is given intermittently to reduce hypertension.
- **Calcium channel blockers** are primarily arterial vasodilators that may affect the peripheral and/or coronary arteries. Side effects include lethargy, flushing, abdominal and peripheral edema, and indigestion:
  - Dihydropyridine, such as nifedipine (Procardia®) and nicardipine (Cardene®) are primarily arterial vasodilators affecting both coronary and peripheral arteries, used to treat acute hypertension.
  - Benzothiazine, such as diltiazem (Cardizem®) and phenylalkylamine, such as verapamil (Calan®, Isoptin®) dilate primarily coronary arteries and are used for angina and supraventricular tachycardias.
- **BNP (B-type natriuretic peptide)**, such as nesiritide (Natrecor®), is a new type of vasodilator, which is a recombinant form of a peptide of the human brain. It decreases filling pressure, vascular resistance, and increases urinary output but may cause hypotension, headache, bradycardia, and nausea.

- **Alpha-adrenergic blockers** block alpha receptors in arteries and veins, causing vasodilation but may cause orthostatic hypotension and edema from fluid retention:
  - Labetalol (Normodyne®) is a combination peripheral alpha-blocker and cardiac β-blocker and is used to treat acute hypertension, acute stroke, and acute aortic dissection.
  - Phentolamine (Regitine®) is a peripheral arterial dilator that reduces afterload and is used for pheochromocytoma.
- **Selective specific dopamine DA-1-receptor agonists**, such as fenoldopam (Corlopam®) is a peripheral dilator affecting renal and mesenteric arteries and can be used for patients with renal dysfunction or those at risk of renal insufficiency.

> **Review Video: Calcium Channel Blockers**
> Visit mometrix.com/academy and enter code: 942825

ANTIDYSRHYTHMICS

Antidysrhythmics include a number of drugs that act on the conduction system, the ventricles and/or the atria to control dysrhythmias. There are 4 classes of drugs that are used as well as some that are unclassified:

- **Class I**: 3 subtypes of sodium channel blockers (quinidine, lidocaine, procainamide)
- **Class II**: β-receptor blockers (Esmolol, propranolol)
- **Class III**: Slows repolarization (amiodarone, ibutilide)
- **Class IV**: Calcium channel blockers (diltiazem, verapamil)
- **Unclassified** (Adenosine)

TREATMENT FOR SUPRAVENTRICULAR TACHYCARDIA

Certain specific drugs are used to treat **supraventricular tachycardia**:

- **Adenosine** affects conduction system and may cause transient flushing, ↓ blood pressure (BP), and shortness of breath.
- **Diltiazem** (Cardizem®, Tiazac®) affects conduction system and may cause bradycardia, AV block, and ↓BP.
- **Esmolol** (Brevibloc®) affects the conduction system and may cause ↓BP, bradycardia, and heart failure.
- **Propranolol** (Inderal®) affects conduction system and may cause bradycardia, heart block, and heart failure.
- **Procainamide** affects the atria and ventricles and may cause ↓BP and electrocardiogram abnormalities (widening of QRS and QT).

ANTIDYSRHYTHMICS USED TO TREAT PAROXYSMAL SUPRAVENTRICULAR TACHYCARDIA

The following are antidysrhythmics used to treat paroxysmal supraventricular tachycardia:

- **Paroxysmal supraventricular tachycardia**: Adenosine; Digoxin (Lanoxin®) affects the conduction system and may cause bradycardia, heart block, nausea and vomiting, and CNS depression; Verapamil (Calan®, Verelan®) affects the conduction system and may cause ↓BP, bradycardia, and heart failure.

- **Atrial fibrillation**: Digoxin (Lanoxin®), Diltiazem (Cardizem®, Tiazac®); Ibutilide (Corvert®) affects the conduction system and rarely has side effects; Amiodarone (Cordarone®) affects the atria and ventricles and may cause ↓BP, and adverse hepatic effects.
- **Atrial flutter**: Digoxin (Lanoxin®), Diltiazem (Cardizem®, Tiazac®), Ibutilide (Corvert®), Verapamil (Calan®, Verelan®), Amiodarone (Cordarone®), Procainamide.
- **Sinus tachycardia**: Esmolol (Brevibloc®)
- **Premature ventricular contractions**: Lidocaine affects the ventricles and may cause CNS toxicity with nausea and vomiting; Procainamide.
- **Ventricular tachycardia**: Lidocaine, Amiodarone (Cardizem®, Tiazac®), Procainamide
- Ventricular fibrillation: Lidocaine

LOOP DIURETICS

Diuretics increase renal perfusion and filtration, thereby reducing preload and decreasing peripheral and pulmonary edema, hypertension, congestive heart failure (CHF), POS, diabetes insipidus, and osteoporosis. There are different types of diuretics: loop, potassium-sparing, and thiazide.

Loop diuretics inhibit the reabsorption of sodium and chloride (primarily) in the ascending loop of Henle. They also cause increased secretion of other electrolytes, such as calcium, magnesium, and potassium, and this can result in imbalances that cause dysrhythmias. Other side effects include frequent urination, postural hypotension, and increased blood sugar and uric acid levels. They are short-acting so are less effective than other diuretics for control of hypertension:

- **Bumetanide** (Bumex®) is given intravenously after surgery to reduce preload or orally to treat heart failure.
- **Ethacrynic acid** (Edecrin®) is given intravenously after surgery to reduce preload.
- **Furosemide** (Lasix®) is used for the control of congestive heart failure as well as renal insufficiency. It is used after surgery to decrease preload and to reduce the inflammatory response caused by cardiopulmonary bypass (post-perfusion syndrome).

> **Review Video: Diuretics**
> Visit mometrix.com/academy and enter code: 373276

POTASSIUM-SPARING DIURETICS

Potassium-sparing diuretics inhibit the reabsorption of sodium in the late distal tubule and collecting duct. They are weaker than thiazide or loop diuretics, but do not cause a reduction in potassium level; however, if used alone, they may cause an increase in potassium, which can cause weakness, irregular pulse, and cardiac arrest. Because potassium-sparing diuretics are less effective alone, they are often given in a combined form with a thiazide diuretic (usually chlorothiazide), which mitigates the potassium imbalance. Typical side effects include dehydration, blurred vision, nausea, insomnia, and nasal congestion, especially in the first few days of treatment:

- **Spironolactone** (Aldactone®) is a synthetic steroid diuretic that increases the secretion of both water and sodium and is used to treat congestive heart failure. It may be given orally or intravenously.
- **Eplerenone** is similar to spironolactone but has fewer side effects so it may be used with patients who can't tolerate the other drug.

THIAZIDE DIURETICS

Thiazide diuretics inhibit the reabsorption of sodium and chloride primarily in the early distal tubules, forcing more sodium and water to be excreted. Thiazide diuretics increase secretion of potassium and bicarbonate, so they are often given with supplementary potassium or in combination with potassium-sparing diuretics. Thiazide diuretics are the first line of drugs for treatment of hypertension. They have a long duration of action (12-72 hours, depending on the drug) so they are able to maintain control of hypertension better than short-acting drugs. They may be given daily or 3-5 days per week. There are numerous thiazide diuretics, including:

- Chlorothiazide (Diuril®)
- Bendroflumethiazide (Naturetin®)
- Chlorthalidone (Hygroton®)
- Trichlormethiazide (Naqua®)

Side effects include dizziness, lightheadedness, postural hypotension, headache, blurred vision, and itching, especially during initial treatment. Thiazide diuretics cause sensitivity to sun exposure, so people should be counseled to use sunscreen.

ANTI-LIPIDS

Anti-lipid medications are frequently used to **lower cholesterol levels** if dietary modifications are unsuccessful in order to decrease coronary artery disease. There are 5 primary types of medications:

- **Statins** (3-hydroxy-3-methylglutaryl coenzyme A reductase inhibitors), such as atorvastatin (Lipitor®), rosuvastatin (Crestor®), fluvastatin (Lescol®), lovastatin (Mevacor®), pravastatin (Pravachol®), and simvastatin (Zocor®), inhibit the liver enzyme that produces cholesterol, but different statins vary in the ability to reduce cholesterol and in drug/other interactions (protease inhibitors, erythromycin, grapefruit juice, niacin, and fibric acids). Adverse effects include rhabdomyolysis (which causes severe muscle pain and weakness), headache, rash, weakness, and gastrointestinal disorders.
- **Nicotinic acid** (Niacor®, Niaspan®) decreases synthesis of lipoprotein, lowers low-density lipoprotein (LDL) and triglycerides, and increases high-density lipoprotein (HDL). It is used for low elevations of cholesterol and may be combined with statins. Adverse effects include flushing, hyperglycemia, gout, upper gastrointestinal disorders, and hepatotoxicity. Liver function must be monitored.
- **Fibric acids**, or fibrates, such as gemfibrozil (Lopid®), fenofibrate (TriCor®, Fenoglide®, Lofibra®, Triglide®), decrease low-density lipoprotein (LDL), increase high-density lipoprotein (HDL), and decrease triglycerides. They inhibit production of very low-density lipoprotein in the liver and decrease triglycerides in the blood, so they are primarily used for elevated triglycerides. Fibric acids are usually given in combination with other drugs as studies have indicated they do not lower risk of death if used alone. Adverse effects include indigestion, cholelithiasis, and myopathy. Contraindicated with renal or hepatic disease.
- **Bile acid sequestrants,** such as cholestyramine (LoCholest®, Questran®, Prevalite®) colesevelam (WelChol®) and colestipol HCL (Colestid®), decrease LDL, increase HDL, and do not affect triglyceride levels. They bind to bile acids in the intestines so that more are excreted in the stool rather than returned to the liver, so the liver has to produce bile acids by converting cholesterol. Adverse effects include gastrointestinal disorders and decrease in absorption of other drugs.

Gastrointestinal/Genitourinary Pharmacology

HISTAMINE RECEPTOR ANTAGONISTS

Histamine receptor antagonists (actually **reverse agonists**) are used to treat conditions in which excessive stomach acid causes heartburn and GERD. They block histamine 2 (H2) (parietal) cell receptors in the stomach, thereby decreasing acid production. These drugs are used less commonly now than proton-pump inhibitors. Smoking decreases effect. These drugs pass into breast milk, so they should not be taken by women who are breastfeeding. They should be used with caution in women who are pregnant. Children usually tolerate the medications well, but geriatric patients may experience confusion and dizziness. Side effects are uncommon although cimetidine has the most frequent adverse effects, which include male gynecomastia, impotence, and decreased libido. Side effects for other drugs include hypotension, headache, diarrhea, constipation, confusion, and dizziness. A number of drug interactions can occur (primarily with cimetidine and ranitidine) with warfarin, phenytoin, lidocaine, tricyclic antidepressants, and other drugs.

Common histamine receptor antagonists include:

- **Cimetidine** (Tagamet®): The first H_2 antagonist, it is used less frequently than others because of inhibition of enzymes that result in drug interactions, especially with contraceptive agents and estrogen.
- **Ranitidine** (Zantac®): This was developed to decrease drug interactions and improve patient tolerance. Its activity is about 10 times that of cimetidine. It may be used in combination with other drugs to treat ulcers.
- **Famotidine** (Pepcid®): This may be combined with an antacid to increase the speed of effects as it has a slow onset. It may be used pre-surgically to reduce post-operative nausea.
- **Nizatidine** (Axid®): The last H_2 antagonist developed, it is about equal in potency and action to ranitidine.

ANTACIDS

Antacids are medications used to reduce stomach acids by raising the pH and neutralizing the acids present. They are commonly used to treat heartburn or indigestion. Adverse reactions are relatively rare unless taken to excess or with renal impairment. Drugs include:

- **Aluminum hydroxide** (Amphojel®) may cause constipation and with renal impairment, hypophosphatemia and osteomalacia.
- **Magnesium hydroxide** (Milk of Magnesia®) may cause diarrhea and with renal impairment can cause hypermagnesemia.
- **Aluminum hydroxide** with magnesium hydroxide (Maalox®, Mylanta®).
- **Calcium carbonate** (TUMS®, Rolaids®, and Titralac®) may cause gastric distention. Excess calcium intake may cause toxic reactions, including kidney stones and renal failure; so excess intake should be avoided.
- **Alka-Seltzer®** combines sodium bicarbonate with aspirin and citric acid so this compound may cause gastric irritation, nausea and vomiting, and tarry stools.
- **Bismuth subsalicylate** (Pepto-Bismol®). Pepto-Bismol® may react with sulfur in the body to create a black tongue and black stools, but this is temporary. Pepto-Bismol® has been associated with Reye's syndrome in children with influenza or chickenpox.

LAXATIVE PRODUCTS

Different types of **laxatives**:

- **Bulk formers** have high fiber content and both soften stool and create more formed stools. These include products such as Metamucil®, Citrucel®, and FiberCon®, which are usually added to liquids because without adequate fluids, they can increase constipation.
- **Lubricants** include both oral mineral oil and glycerin suppositories. They coat the stool, preventing fluid absorption and keeping the stool soft. Mineral oil absorbs fat soluble vitamins and should be used only temporarily
- **Saline**, such as Milk of Magnesia® and Epsom Salt, contain ions, such as magnesium phosphate, magnesium hydroxide, and citrate, which are not absorbed through the intestines and draw more fluid into the stool. The magnesium in the preparations also stimulates the bowel. People with impairment of kidney function should avoid magnesium products, and saline laxatives should be used infrequently to avoid dependence. Epsom Salt often has a purging effect and is rarely used.
- **Stool softeners** (emollients, such as Colace®, and Philip's Liqui-Gels®) use wetting agents, such as docusate sodium, to increase liquid in the stool, thereby softening it. They should not be used with mineral oil because of increased absorption of the oil through the intestines.
- **Hyperosmotics** (available by prescription) contain materials that are not digestible and serve to retain fluid in the stool. Products, such as Kristalose® and MiraLAX® soften the stool but may result in increased abdominal distention and flatus, especially initially. There are 3 types of hyperosmolar laxatives: lactulose, polymer, and saline. Lactulose types use a form of sugar and work similarly to saline laxatives, but more slowly, and may be used for long-term treatment. The salines empty the bowels quickly and are used short-term. The polymers contain polyethylene glycol, which retains fluid in the stool and is used short-term.
- **Combinations** use 2 or more types, such as stool softener with stimulant and should be used only short-term.

STIMULANTS

Stimulants increase intestinal motility, moving the stool through the bowel faster and reducing the absorption of fluids so that the stool remains softer. Common ingredients include cascara in Castor oil®, senna in Senokot® and sennosides in Ex-lax®. Stimulants work quickly and are effective but can result in electrolyte imbalance, abdominal distention and cramping. Chronic use may cause a cycle of constipation and diarrhea. Stimulant suppositories, such as Dulcolax® are also available. Tegaserod, marketed as Zelnorm® (by prescription), is a laxative specifically targeting irritable bowel syndrome, increasing contractions of the muscles of the bowel by blocking serotonin. Lubiprostone, marketed as Amitiza® (by prescription) taken twice daily increases chloride, sodium and water secretion from the intestinal lining, and is a new treatment that softens stools and increases frequency of defecation.

URINARY INCONTINENCE TREATMENT

Pharmacological treatments, both oral and topical medications, that help control **urinary incontinence**:

- **Adrenergic agents**, such as Ornade® or Sudafed®, increase pressure on urethra and prevent stress incontinence.
- **Antibiotics**, such as Bactrim®, treat urinary infections that exacerbate incontinence.

- **Anticholinergics**, such as Ditropan® and Detrol® serve to relax detrusor and pelvic floor muscles and reduce frequency. They may also increase bladder capacity and are useful for overactive bladder because they block the chemicals that stimulate bladder nerves.
- **Estrogens**, such as Premarin® (oral) and Estrace® (topical) improve muscles tone and prevent atrophic changes of the mucosa.
- **Serotonin norepinephrine reuptake inhibitor** (Cymbalta®) increases urethral sphincter contraction during storage phase.
- **Smooth muscle relaxants**, such as Pro-Banthine®, relieve bladder spasms.
- **Tricyclic antidepressants**, such as Tofranil®, increase urinary sphincter tone and decrease bladder spasms.
- **Urinary analgesics**, such as Pyridium®, alleviate spasms and discomfort caused by urinary infections.

Pharmacology for Pain

COX INHIBITORS

Cyclooxygenase (COX) inhibitors are NSAIDs that block COX enzymes that develop with inflammation and with precancerous/cancerous tissues. COX enzymes form prostanoids:

- **Prostaglandins**: Cell growth, inflammatory reactions, sensitivity to pain, platelet aggregation/disaggregation, hormone and calcium regulation.
- **Prostacyclin**: Platelet aggregation and vasodilation.
- **Thromboxane**: Platelet aggregation and vasoconstriction.

COX inhibitors are used as anti-inflammatory analgesics and antiplatelet drugs. Some drugs, such as ibuprofen and aspirin, block both COX-1 and COX-2 enzymes (non-selective inhibitors). Non-selective NSAIDs are associated with irritation of gastric mucosa because of inhibition of COX-1, which has a protective effect on gastrointestinal mucosa. Other drugs, such as celecoxib, block only COX-2 enzymes (selective inhibitors) and these tend to have fewer gastrointestinal adverse effects, but they have been implicated in increased risk for cardiovascular disease and thrombus formation. COX-2 NSAIDs specifically target inflammation. A third COX enzyme, COX-3, has been identified and some speculate acetaminophen (which has no anti-inflammatory properties) may target this, but research is inconclusive.

ACETYLSALICYLIC ACID

Acetylsalicylic acid (aspirin, ASA) is a nonspecific COX inhibitor nonsteroidal anti-inflammatory drugs (NSAID) used to treat fever, pain, and inflammation, and to reduce clotting. Long-term low doses are used to reduce the incidence of thrombus formation because ASA interferes with platelet aggregation, but this can increase clotting time, so aspirin is usually discontinued 10-14 days prior to elective surgery. **Routine aspirin treatment** is used for those who have had heart attack (myocardial infarction [MI]), unstable angina, cerebrovascular accident [CVA], ischemic), and/or transient ischemic accidents (TIAs) to reduce recurrence. Aspirin is given immediately after an MI (but not a CVA). Aspirin may be given post-operatively in some cases, such as orthopedic surgery, to prevent thrombus formation. Aspirin is associated with irritation of the gastrointestinal mucosa (from inhibition of COX-1), and can cause ulcerations and bleeding. Aspirin should not be given to children with fevers, especially related to viruses, as they may develop **Reye's syndrome**. Other side effects include tinnitus, swelling, nausea and vomiting, and headache. Aspirin should be avoided with other salicylates or anticoagulants.

Neurological Pharmacology

ANTICONVULSANTS

Anticonvulsant drugs are used to control seizure disorders. Usually treatment is started with 1 medication, but this may need to be changed or adjusted until the seizures are under control or to avoid adverse effects, which include allergic reactions, especially skin irritations, and acute or chronic toxicity. Milder reactions often subside with time or adjustment in doses. Toxic reactions may vary considerably, depending upon the medication and duration of use, so close monitoring is essential. Severe rash and hepatotoxicity are common toxic reactions that occur with many of the antiepileptic drugs. Dosages of drugs may need to be adjusted during times of stress, such as during illness or surgery. Most drugs cross the placenta and may result in birth defects. Antiepileptic agents include:

- **Carbamazepine** (Tegretol®) used for partial seizures, tonic-clonic, and absence seizures as well as analgesia for trigeminal neuralgia, can cause dizziness, drowsiness, nausea, and vomiting. Toxic reactions include severe skin rash, agranulocytosis, aplastic anemia, and hepatitis.

ANTICONVULSANTS INCLUDE:

- **Lamotrigine** (Lamictal®), used for partial seizures, Lennox-Gastaut syndrome, and primary generalized tonic-clonic seizures can cause tremor, ataxia, weight gain, dizziness, headache, and drowsiness. Toxic reactions include severe rash, which may require hospitalization.
- **Levetiracetam** (Keppra®), used for partial onset seizures, myoclonic seizures, generalized tonic-clonic seizures, and idiopathic generalized epilepsy, can cause dizziness, somnolence, and fatigue.
- **Oxcarbazepine** (Trileptal®), used for partial seizures, can cause double or abnormal vision, tremor, abnormal gait, gastrointestinal disorders, dizziness, and fatigue. Toxic reactions include hepatotoxicity.
- **Phenobarbital** (Luminal®), used for tonic-clonic, cortical local seizures, and acute convulsive episodes and as a hypnotic sedative for insomnia, can cause sedation, double vision, agitation, and ataxia. Toxic reactions include anemia and skin rash.
- **Phenytoin** (Dilantin®), used for tonic-clonic and complex partial seizures, can cause nystagmus, vision disorders, gingival hyperplasia, hirsutism, dysrhythmias, and dysarthria. Toxic reactions include rash, peripheral neuropathy, drowsiness, and blood dyscrasias.
- **Clonazepam** (Klonopin®) used for Lennox-Gastaut syndrome, akinetic, absence, and myoclonic seizure, can cause behavioral changes, hirsutism or alopecia, headaches, and drowsiness. Toxic reactions include hepatotoxicity, thrombocytopenia, ataxia, and bone marrow failure.
- **Ethosuximide** (Zarontin®), used for absence seizures, can cause headaches and gastrointestinal disorders. Toxic reactions include skin rash, blood dyscrasias (sometimes fatal), hepatitis, and lupus erythematosus.
- **Felbamate** (Felbatol®), used for Lennox-Gastaut syndrome, can cause headache, fatigue, insomnia, and cognitive impairment. Toxic reactions include aplastic anemia and hepatic failure. It is recommended only if other medications have failed.
- **Gabapentin** (Neurontin®), used for partial seizures as well as post-herpetic neuralgia, can cause dizziness, somnolence, drowsiness, ataxia, weight gain, and nausea. Toxic reactions include hepatotoxicity and leukopenia.

195

- **Primidone** (Mysoline®), used to treat grand mal, psychomotor, and focal seizures, can cause double vision, ataxia, impotence, lethargy, and irritability. Toxic reactions include skin rash.
- **Tiagabine** (Gabitril®), used for partial seizures, can cause concentration problems, weak knees, dysarthria, abdominal pain, tremor, dizziness, fatigue, and agitation.
- **Topiramate** (Topamax®), used for partial seizures and tonic-clonic seizures, is also used to treat migraines and can cause anorexia, weight loss, somnolence, confusion, ataxia, and confusion. Toxic reactions include kidney stones.
- **Valproate/valproic acid** (Depakote®, Depakene®), used for complex partial seizures and simple and complex absence seizures, can cause weight gain, alopecia, tremor, menstrual disorders, nausea, and vomiting. It is also used to treat bipolar disorder. Toxic reactions include hepatotoxicity, severe pancreatitis, rash, blood dyscrasias, and nephritis.
- **Zonisamide** (Zonegran®, Excegran®), used for partial seizures, can cause anorexia, nausea, agitation, rash, headache, dizziness, and somnolence. Toxic reactions include leukopenia and hepatotoxicity.

ANTIPARKINSONIAN DRUGS

Medications are used to manage symptoms of **Parkinson's disease** in order to maintain function:

- **Levodopa** (Dopar®) is the primary medication. Levodopa is converted to dopamine in the basal ganglia by dopa decarboxylase (an enzyme), relieving symptoms. However, levodopa may cause oxidation, which can damage the substantia nigra over time, worsening the motor symptoms (dyskinesia), so onset of treatment may be delayed as long as possible. Levodopa is most effective in the first few years, but can cause confusion, hallucination, insomnia, and depression.
- **Carbidopa** (Sinemet®) is usually given with levodopa to inhibit dopa decarboxylase to help prevent levodopa breakdown and allow more levodopa to reach the brain.
- **Anticholinergics**, such as benztropine mesylate (Cogentin®), biperiden (Akineton®), cycrimine (Pagitane®), and trihexyphenidyl (Artane®), and diphenhydramine (Benadryl®) reduce the action of acetylcholine to counteract decreased dopamine activity. Anticholinergics are used with levodopa to control tremors but may be poorly tolerated in the elderly, and intraocular pressure must be monitored.
- **Catechol-O-methyl transferase (COMT) inhibitors**, such as entacapone (Comtan®) and tolcapone (Tasman®), inhibit the COMT enzyme. Because the COMT enzyme metabolizes levodopa, inhibiting its action allows increased levodopa to reach the brain and become dopamine. COMT inhibitors are ineffective alone but may prolong the effectiveness of levodopa/carbidopa.
- **Antidepressants**, such as the tricyclic antidepressant amitriptyline (Elavil®), may be used to treat Parkinson-associated depression but the dosage is usually one-third to one-half of a normal dose. Selective serotonin reuptake inhibitors (SSRIs) are also effective in treating depression but may increase symptoms of Parkinson's disease.
- **Centrally acting acetylcholinesterase inhibitors**, such as rivastigmine (Exelon®), donepezil (Aricept®), and galantamine (Reminyl®) may be used to treat Parkinson-associated dementia, but response, as with much dementia treatment, is often mild and short acting.
- **Amantadine hydrochloride (Symmetrel®)**, an antiviral medication, releases dopamine from neuronal storage and may decrease levodopa-induced dyskinesia. It is used to reduce rigidity, tremor, and bradykinesia, usually in early stages of Parkinson's; however, it loses effectiveness within a few months.

- **Dopamine agonists**, such as bromocriptine (Parlodel®), Pramipexole (Mirapex®), ropinirole (Requip®), and rotigotine (Neupro®), are dopamine receptor agonists used in early Parkinson's disease to delay onset of levodopa/carbidopa therapy. They mimic the function of dopamine. They are also useful later in the disease when levodopa/carbidopa lose effectiveness.
- **Monoamine oxidase (MOA) inhibitors**, such as selegiline (Carbex®) inhibit MAO-B, which oxidizes dopamine, increasing the amount of dopamine available to the brain. MAO inhibitors may be used with levodopa or with dopamine agonists to delay treatment with levodopa.

ALZHEIMER'S DRUGS

Treatment for Alzheimer's disease is aimed at slowing the progression of the disease and ensuring patient safety. Two types of drugs are FDA approved, but many clinical trials are taking place. In some cases, 2 drugs (such as Aricept® and Namenda®) may be given. Patients must take medication daily and be monitored carefully as some drugs may worsen symptoms in some patients, so different drugs may need to be tried.

Type of Drug	Drug and Indication	Adverse Effects
Cholinesterase inhibitors (Prevents breakdown of acetylcholine, needed for learning and memory)	Donepezil (Aricept®): All stages of Alzheimer's. Rivastigmine (Exelon®): Mild to moderate disease. Galantamine (Razadyne): Mild to moderate disease.	Nausea, vomiting, loss of appetite, and frequent bowel movements.
	Tacrine (Cognex®): Mild to moderate disease.	Nausea, vomiting, & may damage the liver.
Memantine (Targets gluta-mate, involved in learning and memory)	Namenda®: Moderate to severe	Headache, confusion, dizziness, and constipation.

Endocrine Pharmacology

ORAL HYPOGLYCEMIC AGENTS

Oral hypoglycemic agents, also known as sulfonylureas, are used to treat diabetes mellitus, type II. These drugs are derived from sulfonamide and bind to potassium channel receptors, preventing potassium efflux, allowing influx of calcium and release of insulin from pancreatic islets. They are effective in decreasing serum levels of glucagon and potentiating the production of insulin. There are both first-generation drugs and second-generation drugs, which have shorter half-lives and increased potency over first-generation. First generation drugs include:

- **Acetohexamide** with half-life of 6-8 hours and duration of 12-18 hours.
- **Chlorpropamide** with half-life of 36 hours and duration of 60 hours.
- **Tolazamide** with half-life of 7 hours and duration of 12-14 hours.
- **Tolbutamide** with half-life of 4.5-6.5 hours and duration of 6-12 hours.

Second generation drugs include:

- **Glipizide** with half-life of 4 hours and duration of 24 hours.
- **Glyburide** with half-life of 1.5-3.0 hours and duration of 24 hours.

197

INSULIN

There are a number of different types of insulin with varying action times. **Insulin** is used to metabolize glucose for those whose pancreases do not produce insulin. People may need to take a combination of insulins (short and long-acting) to maintain glucose control. Duration of action may vary according to the individual's metabolism, intake, and level of activity:

- **Humalog** (Lispro H) is a fast acting, short duration insulin that acts within 5-15 minutes, peaking between 45-90 minutes and lasting 3-4 hours.
- **Regular** (R) is a relatively fast acting, 30 minutes, insulin that peaks in 2-5 hours and last 5-8 hours.
- **NPH** (N) or **Lente** (L)) insulin is intermediate acting with onset in 1-3 hours, peaking at 6-12 hours and lasting 16-24 hours.
- **Ultralente** (U) is long-acting insulin with onset in 4-6 hours, peaking at 8-20 hours, and lasting 24-28 hours.
- **Combined NPH/Regular** (70/30 or 50/50) has an onset of 30 minutes, peaks at 7-12 hours, and lasts 16-24 hours.

CORTICOSTEROIDS

The adrenal cortex, triggered by adrenocorticotropic hormone (ACTH) produced by the pituitary gland, produces 3 types of **steroids** from cholesterol: **Glucocorticoids** (such as cortisol and hydrocortisone), **mineralocorticoids** (aldosterone), and **androgens** (testosterone). Glucocorticoids, especially cortisol, have a powerful anti-inflammatory effect, inhibiting cell-mediated immune response, and have been synthesized into a number of corticosteroids, which are steroids that resemble cortisol. Replacement therapy for Addison's disease, however, is usually done with natural hydrocortisone and cortisone. Synthetic **corticosteroids** are used to treat many disorders, including arthritis, lupus erythematosus, inflammatory bowel disease, asthma, and cancer, but they have severe side effects, such as increased fatty deposits and weight gain, osteoporosis, sodium retention, adrenal suppression, diabetes mellitus, depression, mood swings, gastric ulcers, acne, thinning of skin, and impaired healing, so use must be carefully monitored.

Corticosteroids include:

- **Betamethasone** (Celestone®) is moderately potent and does not cause fluid retention. Topical preparations treat eczema and itching. It may be used IM for treatment of allergic reactions to poison oak/poison ivy. Oral preparations are used for a wide range of disorders, including allergies, dermatologic diseases, endocrine disorders, lymphomas and leukemias, multiple sclerosis (MS), cerebral edema, temporal arteritis, and rheumatoid disorders. It is also used to accelerate maturation of fetal lungs.
- **Budesonide** (Entocort EC®), with strong glucocorticoid and mild mineralocorticoid effect, is used to treat mild-moderate Crohn's disease involving the ileum and/or ascending colon for up to 8 weeks with repeated courses if necessary.
- **Cortisone** (Cortone®) is used for a wide range of disorders, including primary or secondary adrenocortical insufficiency, rheumatic disorders, collagen disease, allergic responses, ophthalmic disorders, respiratory diseases, blood diseases, gastrointestinal disorders, and neoplasms
- **Dexamethasone** (Decadron®) is used to treat the same disorders as cortisone but is also used for treatment of MS and cerebral edema related to brain tumor, craniotomy, and traumatic head injury.

- **Hydrocortisone** (Cortef®) is frequently used as topical preparations for relief of itching and in enemas (Cortenema®) for treatment of ulcerative colitis. Hydrocortisone is used IM and IV (Solu-Cortef®) for a wide range of disorders, similar to cortisone, and including MS and trichinosis.
- **Methylprednisolone** (Medrol®, Depo-Medrol®) has similar uses as hydrocortisone.
- **Prednisolone** (Prelone®) has similar uses as hydrocortisone and methylprednisolone.
- **Prednisone** (Deltasone®) has similar uses as hydrocortisone, methylprednisolone, and methylprednisolone. Prednisone, in oral preparation, is of the most commonly used corticosteroids.

Hematologic Pharmacology

ANTICOAGULANTS

Anticoagulants are used to prevent thrombo-emboli. Commonly used anticoagulants include:

- **Aspirin** is often used prophylactically to prevent clots and poses less danger of bleeding than other drugs.
- **Warfarin** (Coumadin®) blocks utilization of vitamin K and decreases production of clotting factors and is used orally for those at risk of developing blood clots, such as those with mechanical heart valves, atrial fibrillation, and clotting disorders.
- **Heparin** is the primary intravenous anticoagulant and increases the activity of antithrombin III. It is used for those with myocardial infarction (MI) and those undergoing PCI or other cardiac surgery.
- **Dalteparin** (Fragmin®) and **Enoxaparin** (Lovenox®) are low-molecular weight heparins that increase activity of antithrombin III, used for unstable angina, MI, and cardiac surgery.
- **Lepirudin** (Refludan®) and **bivalirudin** (Angiomax®) are direct thrombin inhibitors used for unstable angina, PCI, and for prophylaxis and treatment for thrombosis in heparin-induced thrombocytopenia (allergic response to heparin that causes a platelet count drop <150,000, usually to 30-50% of baseline and occurring 5-14 days after beginning heparin).

> **Review Video: Heparin – An Injectable Anti-Coagulant**
> Visit mometrix.com/academy and enter code: 127426
>
> **Review Video: Warfarin: Most Popular Anticoagulant?**
> Visit mometrix.com/academy and enter code: 844117

Psychological Pharmacology

TRICYCLIC ANTIDEPRESSANTS

Tricyclic antidepressants (named for the 3-ring chemical structure of the first of this group) inhibit the uptake of neurotransmitters, primarily norepinephrine and serotonin, and serve as antagonists to dopamine and histamine. Tricyclic antidepressants usually target **2 or 3 of these neurotransmitters** while newer antidepressants, such as selective serotonin reuptake inhibitors (SSRIs), target only one. Tricyclic antidepressants treat depression, attention deficit/hyperactivity disorder (ADHD), nocturnal enuresis, and pain (migraine). They are sometimes referred to as cyclic antidepressants because newer drugs have a 4-ring structure. Tricyclic antidepressants are **lipophilic and highly protein-bound**, so they absorb rapidly. Drugs include amitriptyline (Elavil®), imipramine (Tofranil®), and nortriptyline (Aventyl®, Pamelor®). They have long half-lives, which increases toxic affects with overdose, and anticholinergic (primarily muscarinic)

199

effects. Because of this, cyclic antidepressants tend to have more side effects than newer antidepressants: dry mouth, blurring vision, cardiac abnormalities, constipation, urinary retention, and hyperthermia. Alterations in memory and cognition, drowsiness, anxiety, muscle twitches, gynecomastia, and breast enlargement may occur. They are contraindicated with monoamine oxidase (MAO) inhibitors and cimetidine.

SSRIs

Selective serotonin reuptake inhibitors (SSRIs) are antidepressant medications that block reuptake of serotonin (neurotransmitter) in the brain, increasing the extracellular level of the neurotransmitter and improving transmission. Drugs include citalopram (Celexa®), escitalopram (Lexapro®), fluoxetine (Prozac®), and paroxetine (Paxil). All SSRIs have similar action but may have different chemical properties that cause various side effects, so some people tolerate one better than others. Side effects include nausea, weight gain, sexual dysfunction, excitation and agitation, and insomnia, drowsiness, increased perspiration, headache, and diarrhea. In rare cases, serotonin syndrome may occur from high levels of serotonin from overdose or combination with monoamine oxidase (MAO) inhibitors, so SSRIs must not be taken within 2 weeks of each other. *Symptoms* include severe anxiety and agitation, hallucinations, confusion, blood pressure swings, fever, tachycardia, seizures, and coma. SSRIs are not addictive but abrupt cessation may trigger discontinuation syndrome (flu-like symptoms).

LITHIUM

Lithium carbonate (Eskalith®, Lithobid®) is used to control the manic episodes associated with bipolar disorder. It may also sometimes be used in conjunction with antidepressants to treat depression. Lithium has properties similar to sodium and potassium and interferes with the action of sodium in neuromuscular cells, reducing agitation. It also interferes with the production and action of neurotransmitters and affects levels of tryptophan and serotonin in the central nervous system. It can also cause an increase in leukocyte production. Lithium crosses the placenta, so it should not be taken during pregnancy or while nursing. Overdosing can cause severe side effects so blood levels must be routinely monitored. Side effects include hand tremors, twitching, nausea, diarrhea, seizures, confusion, and increase in urinary output. About 1 patient in 25 develops goiter from lithium-induced hypothyroidism. Nonsteroidal anti-inflammatory drugs (NSAIDs), selective serotonin reuptake inhibitors (SSRIs), phenothiazines, and diuretics may cause drug interactions.

Infectious Disease Pharmacology

ANTIBIOTICS

Antibiotics, produced from microorganisms (such as fungi), are used to combat bacterial infections. Bacteria are critical for human survival and most are benign, but some are **pathogenic**, leading to infection. Bacteria are ubiquitous, with about 10 times as many bacteria in the human body as there are human cells. Bacteria have simple prokaryote structures, with no membrane-encased nucleus or organelles but a tangle of looped DNA called a nucleoid. Bacteria also have plasmids, which are double strands of DNA outside of the nucleoid that allow for transmission from cell to cell or by attaching to viruses. Essentially, bacteria are able to trade genes, making them very adaptable. The cell membrane of most bacteria, except the Mollicutes (mycoplasmas), is surrounded by a cell wall, the composition of which varies. It is the composition of this cell wall that determines the Gram-staining, either negative or positive. Common side effects include nausea, vomiting, diarrhea, rash, and vaginal yeast infections. Severe reactions include anaphylaxis, super-infection with Clostridium difficile, and bone marrow, liver, and renal impairment.

CLASSIFICATION

Antibiotics may be **classified** according to their chemical nature, origin, action, or range of effectiveness. There are hundreds of antibiotics. Broad-spectrum antibiotics are useful against both Gram-positive and Gram-negative bacteria. Medium spectrum antibiotics are usually effective against Gram-positive bacteria although some may be effective against Gram-negative as well. Narrow spectrum antibiotics are effective against a small range of bacteria. Antibiotics function by killing the bacteria by interfering with its biological functions (bacteriocidal) or by preventing reproduction (bacteriostatic). The main classes of antibiotics include:

- **Macrolides**: Medium spectrum antibiotics. They prevent protein production by bacteria and are primarily bacteriostatic but may be bactericidal at high doses. They may be irritating to the gastric mucosa, but are less likely to cause allergic responses than penicillins or cephalosporins. Macrolides include erythromycin (E-Mycin®), clarithromycin (Biaxin®), and azithromycin (Zithromax®).
- **Fluoroquinolones**: Broad-spectrum antibiotics that inhibit bacterial reproduction and repair of genetic material in the bacterial DNA. Drugs include ciprofloxacin (Cipro®), levofloxacin (Levaquin®), and ofloxacin (Floxin®).
- **Sulfonamides**: Sulfonamides are medium spectrum with action against Gram-positive and many Gram-negative organisms as well as Plasmodium and Toxoplasma. Some people are sensitive and may develop an allergic response. Resistance to sulfa drugs is widespread. Sulfa drugs interfere with folate synthesis and prevent cell division, so they are bacteriostatic. Sulfonamides include co-trimoxazole (Bactrim®) and trimethoprim (Proloprim®).
- **Tetracyclines**: Broad-spectrum antibiotics. They are also used for Rickettsias and Psittacosis-producing agents. Tetracyclines include tetracycline, doxycycline (Vibramycin®), and minocycline.
- **Aminoglycosides**: Effective against Gram-negative bacteria. They interfere with protein production in the bacteria and are bacteriocidal. Aminoglycosides cannot be taken orally. They are often given in conjunction with other classes of antibiotics, such as penicillin. Aminoglycosides include gentamicin (Garamycin®) and tobramycin (Tobrex®), neomycin, and streptomycin.
- **Penicillins**: Medium spectrum antibiotics may be combined with β-lactamase inhibitors. They are bacteriocidal and cause breakdown of the bacterial cell wall. They may cause severe allergic reactions in sensitive individuals. Penicillins include penicillin, ampicillin, and amoxicillin.
- **Cephalosporins**: Medium spectrum antibiotics effective against Gram-negative organisms. They are bacteriocidal and inhibit cell wall synthesis. They are divided into different "generations" according to antimicrobial properties with succeeding generations having more powerful effect against resistant strains. First generation includes cephazolin (Kefzol®), cephalexin (Keflex®), and cephradine (Velosef®). Second generation includes cefaclor (Ceclor®), cefuroxime (Zinacef®), and loracarbef (Lorabid®). Third generation includes cefotaxime (Claforan®), cefixime (Suprax®), cefpodoxime (Vantin®), ceftazidime (Fortaz®), and cefdinir (Omnicef®). Fourth generation includes cefepime (Maxipime®).
- **Polymyxins**: Narrow spectrum antibiotics effective against Gram-negative organisms. Interferes with cell membrane of bacteria and are bactericidal. Polymyxins have both neurotoxic and nephrotoxic properties and are not used unless other antibiotics are ineffective. They must be given intravenously. Polymyxins include Polymyxin B Sulfate®.

ANTIFUNGAL AGENTS

Even though **antifungal agents** are available, systemic fungal infections are difficult to treat. Fungi were originally classified as plants, but they do not produce their own food through photosynthesis and must, like animals, get the food from another source. Fungi vary widely, from one-celled microorganisms to multi-celled chains that are miles long. Fungi are used to make antibiotics, but they can also cause infection and disease. Two common classifications of fungi are **molds** (including mushrooms) and **yeast**. Fungi are not motile, but some produce spores, which can be inhaled. Some, such as the yeast Candida albicans, are part of the normal flora of the skin but can overgrow in an opportunistic infection. As microorganisms, fungal infections can invade the sinuses, the mouth, the respiratory system, and the vagina. Antibiotics may affect the balance between bacteria and yeast, causing infection. Fungal infections include histoplasmosis, blastomycosis, and coccidioidomycosis. Fungal infections, such as Pneumocystis jiroveci (formerly carinii), pose a serious problem for the immunocompromised.

Fungal infections are common on the skin and mucous membranes, but the use of vascular access devices and other invasive devices has increased the incidence of fungemia in patients. Additionally, powerful antibiotics contribute to fungal infections by altering the balance of organisms. Fungal cells are more difficult to eradicate than bacterial cells because they are more similar to human cells, so treating a fungus can damage other cells and result in serious side effects, such as nausea, diarrhea, anorexia, rash, itching, especially amphotericin B, which can be lethal and cause fever and chills, headache, hypotension, dyspnea, and multiple organ damage. There are a number of different classes of antifungal agents:

- **Allylamine antifungals** inhibit an enzyme necessary for fungal cell wall synthesis. Terbinafine HCl (Lamisil®) is a synthetic antifungal that is used primarily against fungal infections of the skin. Amorolfine and butenafine are also synthetic antifungals with similar action.
- **Triazole antifungals** have similar action to imidazole but are newer and less toxic. Fluconazole (Diflucan®) may be used for both superficial (skin, mucous membranes) and systemic fungal infections. It is used for both treatment and prophylaxis against candidiasis. It is effective for coccidioidomycosis, cryptococcosis, and histoplasmosis.
- **Polyene antifungals** attack the fungal cell membrane, leading to death of the organism. These antifungals are derived from Streptomyces sp. Natamycin is frequently used to treat corneal infections related to Aspergillus and Fusarium. Nystatin is especially effective against Candida and may be used as a prophylaxis to prevent fungal infections in those vulnerable, such as AIDS patients. Amphotericin B may be used orally for treatment of thrush, but it is more commonly used intravenously for systemic fungal infections, including aspergillosis and candidiasis.
- **Echinocandin antifungals** also inhibit cell wall synthesis. Anidulafungin (Eraxis®) is primarily used for the treatment of systemic candidiasis. It degrades chemically in the presence of normal body pH and is safe to use with liver or kidney impairment. Caspofungin (Cancidas®) is used intravenously for treatment of aspergillosis and candidiasis and is often effective when patients have shown resistance to other drugs. Micafungin (Mycamine®) is used intravenously to treat a wide variety of candidal infections, including candidiasis, candida peritonitis, and esophageal candidiasis. It is also used as a prophylaxis for those having hematopoietic stem cell transplantation.

- **Imidazole antifungals** inhibit an enzyme necessary for fungal cell membrane synthesis. Miconazole has antifungal as well as antiparasitic and some antibacterial action and is used primarily as a topical preparation for athlete's foot, ringworm, and jock itch and an internal preparation for oral or vaginal yeast infections. Clotrimazole (Lotrimin®) has similar uses. Imidazoles also interfere with steroid synthesis.

ANTIPARASITIC AGENTS
PROTOZOAN DISEASES

Antiparasitic agents are used for protozoan diseases. **Protozoa** are one-celled organisms from a number of different phyla. Protozoa consume bacteria, so they have a critical role in the cycle of life, but about 10,000 species are parasites that can infect vertebrates. Protozoan infections, especially of the gastrointestinal tract, have become more prevalent in those who are immunocompromised:

- **Giardia intestinalis** has become the most common cause of water-borne disease and non-bacterial diarrhea in the United States. Antiparasitic agents include metronidazole (Flagyl®), nitazoxanide, and tinidazole.
- **Dientamoeba fragilis** occurs worldwide, especially in children, and those who live or travel to areas with poor sanitation. Antiparasitics include iodoquinol, paromomycin, tetracycline, and metronidazole.
- **Entamoeba histolytica** is more prevalent in developing countries, but increasing rates of infection have been found in Hispanics (33%), Asian and Pacific Islanders (17%), recent immigrants, travelers, institutionalized populations, and men having sex with men. Antiparasitics for asymptomatic infections include iodoquinol, paromomycin, and diloxanide furoate. For mild-severe disease, metronidazole and tinidazole.
- **Balantidium coli** occur most commonly in the tropics among those in contact with pigs, but outbreaks have occurred in psychiatric hospitals in the United States. Antiparasitics include metronidazole, tetracycline, and iodoquinol.
- **Cryptosporidium parvum and Cryptosporidium hominis** have caused a number of outbreaks since first identified in 1976, sometimes related to swimming in pools contaminated with feces or handling of dirty diapers. The antiparasitic agent used for treatment is nitazoxanide, which is effective only in those without HIV. Antiretroviral treatment received for HIV infection is, however, affective against cryptosporidia.
- **Isospora belli** occurs worldwide, primarily in tropical areas, but can occur in travelers and those with HIV. The only effective antiparasitic agent is trimethoprim-sulfamethoxazole. There is no alternative for those allergic to sulfa.
- **Cyclospora cayetanensis** occurs worldwide and has been implicated in a number of foodborne outbreaks in the United States since 1996. The antiparasitic agent is trimethoprim-sulfamethoxazole. Those sensitive to sulfa may be treated with nitazoxanide

PARASITIC WORMS

Antiparasitic agents include antihelmintic agents for treatment of parasitic worms:

- **Nematodes** are unsegmented roundworms, including pin worms, hookworms, whipworms, and roundworms. There are over 80,000 varieties. Those that infest humans range from 0.3 mm to 1 m in length. People usually become infected by ingestion of contaminated food or touching contaminated hands to the mouth. Antiparasitic drugs useful against nematodes include Albendazole (Albenza®), Mebendazole (Vermox®), pyrantel pamoate (Pin-Rid®), and Ivermectin.

- **Cestodes** are segmented flatworms, also called tapeworms, which live in the intestinal tracts of some animals and fish and infect humans who eat raw or undercooked meat/fish. Antiparasitic drugs include praziquantel (Biltricide®), nitazoxanide, and niclosamide.
- **Trematodes** are a type of flatworm called flukes, which can cause diseases in the intestines, blood, liver, and lungs. Fluke infections are caused by ingestion of uncooked meat, plants, or fish from contaminated waters. Antiparasitic drugs include praziquantel and albendazole.

MICROSPORIDIA

Microsporidia are now commonly believed to be basic fungi, closer to fungi than other protozoa, and increasingly recognized worldwide as opportunistic infectious agents, especially in immuno-compromised individuals, such as those with HIV/AIDS, causing microsporidiosis. Fourteen species have been identified as **pathogenic** to humans, some affecting the eyes and muscles. Enterocytozoon bieneusi and Encephalitozoon intestinalis cause most cases of microsporidiosis with gastrointestinal manifestations and are common in HIV/AIDS patients, but there are increasing infections in non-HIV infected travelers and those living in tropical areas. Antiparasitic agents include thalidomide, used for chronic diarrhea unresponsive to other medications. Metronidazole is also useful for the treatment of diarrhea. On-going treatment may be needed to prevent recurrence of symptoms. Drugs of choice include:

- **E. Intestinalis**: Albendazole 400 mg twice daily for 14 days.
- **E. Bieneusi**: Fumagillin 60 mg daily for 14 days.

ANTIRETROVIRAL AGENTS FOR (HIV)/AIDS

There are 4 primary classes of **antiretroviral agents** used for the treatment of HIV/AIDS:

- **Non-nucleoside reverse transcriptase inhibitors** (NNRTIs), such as delavirdine (Rescriptor®), efavirenz (Sustiva®), and Nevirapine (Viramune®), bind to reverse transcriptase and disable it. Reverse transcriptase is a protein required for HIV replication.
- **Nucleoside reverse transcriptase inhibitors** (NRTIs), such as abacavir (Ziagen®), abacavir (Epzicom®), zidovudine (AZT®), and lamivudine (Epivir®), are defective versions of building blocks necessary for replication. When HIV binds to the defective version, it is unable to complete replication.
- **Protease inhibitors** (PIs) disable the protein protease, which HIV requires in order to replicate. PIs include amprenavir (Agenerase®), indinavir (Crixivan®), and nelfinavir (Viracept®).
- **Fusion inhibitors**, such as enfuvirtide (Fuzeon®), are entry blockers.

Sedatives

GHB

Gamma hydroxybutyrate (GHB) is commonly known as "fantasy" or "blue nitro" (when blue dye is added) and is used as a hallucinogen and date rape drug as it causes deep sedation and loss of memory. Similar drugs include butanediol (BD) and gamma butyrolactone (GBL). GHB may produce states of euphoria and hallucinations and is often taken with steroids to increase growth hormones affecting muscles. *Symptoms* of ingestion are dose-dependent:

- <1 g: relaxation, reduced inhibitions.
- 1-2 g: ↑ relaxation, bradycardia, bradypnea, hypotension, and impairment of motor ability.
- 2-4 g: Severe lethargy, motor impairment, and coma.

204

- Other symptoms include nausea, vomiting, amnesia, delusions, seizures, and depression. Diagnosis is by history and clinical examination. Treatment includes:
  - Assessment for rape and rape kit if indicated and tests for sexually transmitted diseases (STDs).
  - Gastric emptying (<1 hour).
  - Charcoal administration.
  - Careful monitoring for central nervous system/respiratory depression.
  - Supportive care.
  - Referral for counseling in instances of rape.

Reproductive Pharmacology

ORAL CONTRACEPTIVES

There are many methods of **birth control**, including the use of condoms, intrauterine devices, spermicides, and barriers, such as diaphragms, sponges, and cervical caps, but **hormonal contraceptives** are commonly used. There are 2 types of oral contraceptives, but there are many different brands with differing amounts of hormones:

- **Combined** (estrogen [ethinyl estradiol] and progestin): These may be monophasic (constant doses), biphasic (constant estrogen but increase of progestin on day 10), or triphasic (varying doses of both).
- **Progestin only**: These have fewer side effects than combined forms, but can increase estrogen levels and incidence of thrombosis.

Oral contraceptives are contraindicated for those who smoke or have evidence or history of breast cancer, coronary artery disease, or elevated cholesterol because they are associated with increased risk of thrombosis.

Common side effects (depending upon the particular drug) include an increase in acne and facial hair growth, weight increase, rash or itching, amenorrhea, decrease in libido, headache, nausea, and breakthrough bleeding. Changing to a different contraceptive may alleviate symptoms.

INJECTABLE, RING, AND PATCH CONTRACEPTIVES

Newer methods of **contraception** include injectable, ring, and patch contraceptives. One primary advantage is that the woman does not need to remember to take pills, but risks are similar to oral contraceptives:

- **NuvaRing®** is a vaginal ring that in inserted vaginally and left in place about the cervix for 3 weeks. It is removed for the 4th week, during which there may be withdrawal bleeding. It is as effective as oral contraceptives.
- **Ortho Evra®** is a small adhesive patch that is applied to the torso, chest (excluding the breasts), arms, or thighs every week for 3 weeks and then the 4th week is patch free. It is as effective as oral contraceptives.
- **Depo-Provera®** is injectable medroxyprogesterone acetate that is given every 13 weeks. It may be used with a history of deep vein thrombosis or smoking. It may relieve symptoms of endometriosis.

HERBAL REMEDIES AND DIETARY SUPPLEMENTS

There are literally thousands of **herbal remedies** and **dietary supplements** and myriad claims of success in treating or preventing disease despite there being very little scientific evidence to support most claims. Many doctors recommend 1 daily multivitamin to ensure adequate vitamin intake and fish oil concentrate to reduce cholesterol, but patients often take high doses of herbal remedies and dietary supplements. This poses a number of problems. High doses of some vitamins can cause **toxicity**:

- **Vitamin A**: Headaches, loss of hair, liver damage, bone disorders, and birth defects.
- **Vitamin C**: Diarrhea and gastrointestinal upset.
- **Vitamin D**: Kidney stones, muscle weakness, and bleeding.
- **Vitamin E**: Inhibits action of vitamin K.
- **Niacin**: Liver damage, gastric ulcers, and increased serum glucose.
- **Vitamin B6**: Neurological damage.

Herbal remedies often contain small amounts of agents found in drugs, so they can cause drug reactions and interactions. Also, patients often fail to inform their physicians when they are using alternative treatments.

Disease-Specific Pharmacology

MEDICAL MANAGEMENT OF LYMPHEDEMA

Medical management of **lymphedema** is intended to reduce the protein accumulation in the tissues and restore lymphatic circulation, but treatment needs to begin before extensive fibrosis occurs. Diuretics do not help and the treatments must be carried out throughout lifetime in order to be successful:

- **Hygiene**: Skin must be kept clean and dry and inspected for open areas or signs of infection. Mild emollients may improve skin barrier.
- **Antimicrobial or antifungal topical agents** are used for infections. About 15-25% require long-term antibiotic prophylaxis.
- **Limb elevation** when possible and at night.
- **Complex decongestive therapy** with massage to improve lymphatic drainage.
- **Static compression bandaging** during the day, providing 40-60 mmHg pressure. May be removed at night if limb elevated.
- **Dynamic compression** (intermittent dynamic compression) may be used but can displace fluid or further damage lymphatics if not monitored carefully.
- **Weight loss** may be advised because obesity further compromises lymphatic circulation.

TREATMENT SELECTION FOR PEDIATRIC HIV PATIENTS

Pediatric HIV treatment involves combination therapy with at least 3 anti-retroviral drugs: nucleoside reverse transcriptase inhibitors (NRTIs), non-nucleoside reverse transcriptase inhibitors (NNRTIs), protease inhibitors (PIs), and fusion inhibitors. Factors to be considered:

- Severity of disease, comorbid conditions.
- Short and long-term effects of treatment.
- Initial treatment's effect on later treatment.
- Compliance of child/parent with regimen.
- Age of child and whether HIV acquired perinatally or through other means.
- Stage of puberty:
  - Those in early puberty typically receive the pediatric regimen.
  - Those in late puberty typically receive the adult regimen.

o   Puberty is often delayed in pediatric HIV patients.
- Antiviral drug resistance testing to ensure proper treatment.

CATEGORIZATION OF PEDIATRIC HIV PATIENTS

The category of treatment selected for pediatric HIV patients is based on CD4 counts, according to age, indicating the amount of immunosuppression.

- **Category 1** (No detectable CD4 suppression):
  o   <1 yr: ≥1500
  o   1-5 yrs: ≥1000
  o   6-12 yrs: ≥500
- **Category 2** (Moderate CD4 suppression):
  o   <1 yr: 750-1499
  o   1-5 yrs: 500-999
  o   6-12 yrs: 200-499
- **Category 3** (Severe CD4 suppression):
  o   <1 yr: <750
  o   1-5 yrs: <500
  o   6-12 yrs: <200

MEDICAL TREATMENTS FOR URINARY INCONTINENCE

The following are medications for urinary incontinence:

- **Antispasmodics** (Detrol®, Ditropan®, and Levsin®): for overactive bladders. These drugs may cause thirst, so longer-acting preparations of these drugs, which have fewer side effects, may be better for some people.
- **Antidepressants** (Tofranil): to relax the bladder and contract the muscles at the bladder neck.
- **Hormone replacement therapy**: Administered as a vaginal cream, ring, or patch to protect bladder and urethral mucosa. Oral estrogen may not be as effective as topical for incontinence.
- **Antibiotics**: To treat infections that may be causing or worsening incontinence.

Some medications, such as sedatives, may increase or cause incontinence, so all medications should be **assessed**.

Medical devices include:

- **Catheters**: Clean intermittent catheterization to empty bladder.
- **Penile clamps**: Apply pressure around the penis to clamp the urethra.
- **Pessaries**: A stiff ring inserted vaginally to treat bladder prolapse.
- **Urethral inserts**: Urethral inserts may be inserted temporarily during times of activity that may prompt incontinence.

CALCULATING FLUID REQUIREMENTS FOR PEDIATRIC PATIENTS

Because children are smaller than adults, and thus have a smaller blood volume, it is necessary to **modify** the amount of intravenous fluids that the child receives. Calculation of the amount of fluids required is based on the **weight** of the child in kilograms and the child's **daily caloric requirements**. For the first 10 kg of weight, 100 calories are required per kg; thus, a 10 kg child requires 1,000 calories (10 kg x 100 calories). 50 cal/kg/day are required for the next 10 kg, and 20 cal/kg/day are required for each kg above 20. Once the child's daily caloric needs are calculated, the fluid needs can be calculated. For a child with acute illness, intravenous fluids must provide a minimum of 20% of the overall daily caloric needs. Knowing that D5 saline provides 200 calories per 1,000 mL, an equation can be used to calculate the child's daily minimum fluid requirements.

Drug Interactions and Complications

DRUG INTERACTIONS

Drug interactions occur when 1 drug interferes with the activity of another in either the pharmacodynamics or pharmacokinetics:

- With **pharmacodynamic interaction**, both drugs may interact at receptor sites causing a change that results in an adverse effect or that interferes with a positive effect.
- With **pharmacokinetic interaction**, the ability of the drug to be absorbed and cleared is altered, so there may be delayed effects, changes in effects, or toxicity. Interactions may include problems in a number of areas. Absorption may be increased or (more commonly) decreased, usually related to the effects within the gastrointestinal system. Distribution of drugs may be affected, often because of changes in protein binding. Metabolism may be altered, often causing changes in drug concentration. Biotransformation of the drug must take place, usually in the liver and gastrointestinal system, but drug interactions can impair this process. Clearance interactions may interfere with the body's ability to eliminate a drug, usually resulting in increased concentration of the drug.

PLACENTAL TRANSFER OF DRUGS

The placenta acts as a barrier to protect the fetus, but its main function is to provide oxygen and nutrients for the fetus by linking the maternal and fetal circulation. Virtually all drugs cross the barrier to some degree, some by active transport. Some drugs are readily diffused across the **placental barrier** and can affect the fetus. Drugs that are non-ionized, fat-soluble and have low molecular weight diffuse easily as does glucose. Once a substance crosses the barrier, the lower pH of the fetal blood allows weakly basic drugs, such as local anesthetics and opioids, to cross into fetal circulation where they become ionized and accumulate because they cannot pass back into maternal circulation (ion trapping). Giving an intravenous injection during a contraction, when uterine blood flow decreases, reduces the amount of the drug that crosses the placental barrier. A few drugs with large molecules (heparin, insulin) have minimal transfer, and lipid-soluble drugs transfer more readily than water-soluble.

DIGITALIS

Digitalis drugs, most commonly administered in the form of **digoxin** (Lanoxin®), are derived from the foxglove plant and are used to increase myocardial contractility, left ventricular output, and slow conduction through the atrioventricular node, decreasing rapid heart rates and promoting diuresis. Digoxin does not affect mortality, but increases tolerance to activity and reduces hospitalizations for heart failure. Therapeutic levels (0.5-2.0 ng/mL) should be maintained to avoid digitalis toxicity, which can occur even if digoxin levels are within therapeutic range, so observation of symptoms is critical. Potassium imbalance may cause toxicity. Evidence of toxicity includes:

- Early signs: Increasing fatigue, lethargy, depression, and nausea and vomiting.
- Sudden change in heart rhythm, such as regular or irregular rhythm.
- Sinoatrial (SA) or AV block, new ventricular dysrhythmias, and tachycardia (atrial, junctional, and/or ventricular).

Treatment of digitalis toxicity involves discontinuing medication and monitoring serum levels and symptoms. **Digoxin-immune Fab** (Digibind®) may be used to bind to digoxin and inactivate it if necessary.

OVERDOSE OF TRICYCLIC ANTIDEPRESSANTS

Tricyclic antidepressants (TCA), such as Elavil® and Tofranil®, cause the most **prescription-related deaths**. They are prescribed for depression and other psychiatric and medical conditions. **Toxicity** may result from intentional overdose, excessive therapeutic dose, poly-drug combinations, serotonin syndrome ($\uparrow$ serotonin in central nervous system [CNS]) and medical conditions.

Symptoms of toxicity vary widely and can include:

- Alterations of consciousness, slurred speech, seizures, coma.
- Dilated or constricted pupils, blurred vision
- Pulmonary edema. Ataxia, tremor, myoclonus, hyperreflexia.
- Tachycardia, hypertension or hypotension, heart block, depressed cardiac contractility.
- Electrocardiogram (ECG): sinus tachycardia with right axis deviation (terminal 40 ms) prolonged PR, QRS, and QT (develop in <6 hours).
- Urinary retention and overflow incontinence.

Diagnosis includes positive serum TCA and clinical findings, urine drug screening, ECG, serum electrolyte, creatinine, glucose levels, admission blood glucose levels. Treatment may include IV access, cardiac monitoring, urinary catheter if necessary, gastric decontamination with gastric lavage (<1 hour) and charcoal, sodium bicarbonate (dysrhythmias, hypotension), IV dextrose, thiamine, naloxone, barbiturates (seizures), isotonic crystalloid fluids and/or vasopressor, such as norepinephrine (hypotension).

SALICYLATE TOXICITY

Salicylate toxicity may be acute or chronic and is caused by ingestion of over-the-counter drugs containing salicylates, such as acetylsalicylic acid (ASA), Pepto-Bismol®, and products used in hot inhalers. *Symptoms* vary according to age and amount of ingestion. Co-ingestion of sedatives may alter symptoms:

- <150 mg/kg: nausea and vomiting. •150-300 mg/kg: Vomiting, hyperpnea, diaphoresis, tinnitus, alterations in acid-base balance.
- >300 mg/kg.

Pediatrics: Metabolic acidosis in children <4 but respiratory alkalosis and metabolic acidosis with alkalemia (pH >7.5) in older children. Chronic toxicity is more serious and includes hyperventilation, volume depletion, acidosis, hypokalemia, and central nervous system (CNS) abnormalities.

Adults (usually intentional): Nausea, vomiting, diaphoresis, tinnitus, hyperventilation, respiratory alkalosis and metabolic acidosis. Chronic toxicity results in hyperventilation, tremor, papilledema, alterations in mental status, pulmonary edema, seizures, and coma.

Diagnosis is by ferrous chloride or Ames Phenistix tests.

Treatment includes:

- Gastric decontamination with lavage (<1 hour) and charcoal.
- Volume replacement (D5W).
- Sodium bicarbonate 1-2 mEq/kg.
- Monitoring of salicylate concentration, acid-base, and electrolytes every hour.
- Whole-bowel irrigation (sustained release tablets).

BENZODIAZEPINE TOXICITY

Benzodiazepine toxicity may result from accidental or intentional overdose with such drugs as Xanax®, Librium®, Valium®, Ativan®, Serax®, Versed®, and Restoril®. Mortality is usually the result of co-ingestion of other drugs. Symptoms are often non-specific neurological changes: lethargy, dizziness, alterations in consciousness, ataxia. Respiratory depression and hypotension are rare complications. Coma and severe central nervous depression are usually caused by co-ingestions. Diagnosis is based on history and clinical exam, as benzodiazepine level does not correlate well with toxicity. *Treatment* includes:

- Gastric emptying (<1 hour).
- Charcoal.
- Concentrated dextrose, thiamine and naloxone if co-ingestions suspected, especially with altered mental status.
- Monitoring for CNS/respiratory depression.
- Supportive care.
- Flumazenil (antagonist) 0.2 mg each minute to total 3 mg may be used in some cases but not routinely advised because of complications related to benzodiazepine dependency or co-ingestion of cyclic antidepressants. Flumazenil is contraindicated in the presence of increased intracranial pressure.

UNFAVORABLE SIDE EFFECTS OF CARDIAC DRUGS

Unfavorable side effects of cardiac medications are as follows:

- **ACE inhibitors** – Coughing (1%-30%), head pain, dizzy feeling.
- **Calcium channel blockers** – Peripheral swelling and fluid, dizzy feeling, head pain, queasiness, tachycardia.
- **Thiazide diuretics** – Queasiness, vomiting, loose bowels, dizzy feeling, head pain.
- **Beta-blockers** – Weakness, impotence, moodiness, and difficulty breathing.
- **Digoxin** – Vision problems, loose bowels, anorexia, queasiness, and vomiting. In an elderly patient, the most frequently seen side effect is an inability to think clearly.

IMPORTANCE OF PATIENT WILLINGNESS TO ADHERE TO MEDICATION REGIMENS

A **patient's willingness to adhere to medication regimens** is often critical to the medications' effectiveness. Noncompliance may result in inadequate relief of symptoms, disease complications, super infections, adverse drug effects, and even death. A patient's willingness to adhere to medication regimens depends on a number of variables:

- **Knowledge base**: The patient must be knowledgeable about the administration (time, dosage) of medications and should be aware of uses and adverse effects in order to understand the importance of adhering to a regimen.
- **Relief of symptoms**: Patients who do not see relief of symptoms immediately may believe medications are ineffective.

- **Financial status**: Patients may not be able to afford medications.
- **Ease of administration**: Patients are more likely to comply with medications that are administered orally.
- **Trust**: Patients must trust healthcare providers to provide appropriate treatment.
- **Cultural values/beliefs**: A patient's cultural attitudes may influence compliance.

PATIENT MOTIVATIONS IN SEEKING PRESCRIPTIONS

Patients **seek prescriptions** for a number of reasons:

- **Alleviation of symptoms**: This is especially true for symptoms that cause discomfort or impair functioning, such as pain, stiffness, diarrhea, nausea, indigestions or dizziness.
- **Friend/Family recommendation**: People often share information about drugs, encouraging others to ask their own doctors about medical treatments the friends or family members have found helpful.
- **Response to advertising**: The drug companies inundate the public with advertisements and commercials about drugs, such as those for erectile dysfunction, indigestion, and depression, creating a market for certain prescriptions by convincing consumers that they need specific drugs.
- **Drug-seeking behavior**: Some who are addicted to medications seek prescriptions, usually for controlled substances, from one or multiple physicians.
- **Hypochondria**: Some people seek prescriptions for conditions that they believe they have even though testing does not substantiate these beliefs. Others seek prescriptions as a means to gain attention through supposed illness.

Non-Pharmacologic Interventions

REMOVING FOREIGN BODIES FROM GENITOURINARY OR GYNECOLOGICAL ORIFICES

Foreign bodies may be intentionally inserted into body orifices. Males, most often children, may insert items, such as paint brushes or ballpoint pens, into the urethra during sexual exploration. This may cause infection and hematuria with difficulty urinating. Diagnosis is by x-ray. Treatment may involve milking the urethra from proximal to distal end or removal by endoscope. In some cases, cystotomy may be necessary. Females, especially children and adolescents, may insert items, such as toilet paper, toys, or other items into the vagina during sexual exploration. More commonly, females may forget that a tampon or contraceptive sponge or cap is in place until they develop signs of infection or discharge. Treatment is a vaginal exam to remove the item, identification of any secondary infection, and then treatment of secondary infections as necessary. Items left in place for more than 48 hours pose a danger of infection with Escherichia coli or other anaerobic bacteria.

REMOVING FOREIGN BODIES FROM THE EYE

Foreign bodies in the eye should be assessed carefully with slit lamp with corneal examination using optical sectioning before attempting removal of the foreign body. Foreign bodies that penetrate the cornea full-thickness should not be removed but should be referred to an ophthalmologist, but superficial foreign bodies can safely be removed. Procedure:

1. Apply **topical anesthetic** to both eyes (to suppress blinking in the unaffected eye).
2. Eye held open by hand or with wire eyelid **speculum**.
3. Foreign body is carefully removed with small gauge **needle** or moistened **cotton swab**.
4. **Rust ring** from metallic objects should be removed with ophthalmic burr (if not over pupil), and patient referred to ophthalmologist for further rust ring removal within 24 hours.

211

5. Eyelid **everted** and examined carefully for further foreign bodies.
6. **Abrasions** treated as indicated.

MANAGEMENT OF RECURRENT EPISTAXIS

Recurrent epistaxis is common in young children (2-10), especially boys, and is often related to nose picking, dry climate, or central heating in the winter. Incidence also increases between 50-80 years and may be caused by NSAIDs and anticoagulants. **Kiesselbach's plexus** in the anterior nares has plentiful vessels and bleeds easily. Bleeding in the posterior nares is more dangerous and can result in considerable blood loss. Bleeding from the anterior nares is usually confined to 1 nostril, but from the posterior nares, blood may flow through both nostrils or backward into the throat and the person may be observed swallowing. People abusing cocaine may suffer nosebleeds because of damage to the mucosa. Hematocrit and hemoglobin should be done to determine if blood loss is significant. Bleeding should stop within 20 minutes. *Treatment* includes:

- **Upright position**, leaning forward so blood doesn't flow down throat.
- **Applying pressure** below the nares or by pinching the nostrils firmly for 10 minutes.
- Packing and/or topical vasoconstrictors for severe bleeding.
- **Humidifiers** to decrease irritation.

MANAGEMENT OF VENOUS DERMATITIS

Venous dermatitis appears on the ankles and lower legs and can cause severe itching and pain, and without treatment to control the dermatitis, it may deteriorate, causing ulcers to form, so *treatment* is needed to alleviate the symptoms:

- **Topical antihistamines** to decrease itching and prevent excoriation from scratching. Low dose topical steroids should be used only for short periods (2 weeks) to reduce inflammation and itching only because of danger of increasing ulceration.
- **Compression therapy**, usually with compression stockings, to affected legs to improve overall venous return.
- **Leg elevation** when sitting to avoid dependency.
- **Topical antibiotics**, such as bacitracin, as indicated to reduce danger of infection. Oral antibiotics as indicated for systemic infection.
- **Hypoallergenic emollients** (without perfume), such as petrolatum jelly, to improve the skin's barrier function is a preventive measure that should be used when the acute inflammation has subsided.

MANAGEMENT OF CHRONIC VENOUS INSUFFICIENCY

Chronic venous insufficiency results in edema of the lower extremities, causing both discomfort and increased risk of ulcers. *Treatment* includes:

- **Leg elevation** when sitting to avoid dependency. Therapy may include lying down and elevating affected limb above the heart for 1-2 hours 2 times daily and during the night. This is important for all patients with CVI, but especially for those unable to comply with compression therapy.
- **Compression therapy**, the type dependent upon the degree of edema.
- **Surgical intervention** is indicated if more conservative treatments are unsuccessful in managing insufficiency:

- o *Ligation and stripping* removes a vein or section of a vein that is damaged or has damaged valves. An incision below the vein allows an endoscope to be threaded into the vein to grasp and remove (strip) it. The vein is tied (ligated). Sometimes only ligation of a faulty valve is done and the vein is left in place.
- o *Deep vein reconstruction* may be considered if other approaches fail.

MANAGEMENT OF EDEMA

Management of **edema** is discussed below:

- **Physical therapy** is important because effective calf muscle pumping requires ankle mobility with dorsiflexion over 90°. Some patients may benefit from gait training and exercises to improve the range of motion and strength of the ankle. Calf muscle exercises may include isotonic exercises. Patients need to alternate sitting and standing with walking on a regular schedule throughout the day.
- **Control of weight** often improves circulation and reduces edema, as obesity may be the primary cause of the circulatory impairment. Patients may need education and referral to a bariatric treatment center.
- **Medications** can't correct venous insufficiency but some can help to control symptoms:
  - o *Pentoxifylline* (Trental®) enhances blood flow in capillaries.
  - o *Horse chestnut seed extract* (HCSE) results in reduced pain and edema. It is widely used in Europe and has been studied in the United States. One problem is that it can cause low blood glucose levels in children and those with diabetes.

MANAGEMENT OF DIARRHEA

Management of **diarrhea** includes the following:

- Institute **dietary modification** includes limiting alcohol and caffeine, which can cause loose stools. Artificial sugar substitutes, such as sorbitol and mannitol, should be avoided. People with lactose intolerance should use Lactaid® with dairy products. Yogurt helps control diarrhea from antibiotic use. Increase foods that thicken stool, such as bananas, and soluble fiber.
- Rule-out bacterial, viral, and parasitic infections and treat as needed.
- Avoid **foods or additives** that trigger diarrhea.
- Stop **medications** that are causing diarrhea. Antibiotics frequently cause diarrhea.
- Restore **fluid and electrolyte imbalance** through diet, adequate fluids, or supplements, Gatorade® (electrolyte beverage).
- Use **antidiarrheals** including antimotilities, such as Lomotil® (diphenoxylate/atropine) and Imodium® (loperamide); bismuth compounds, such as Pepto-Bismol® (bismuth subsalicylate); and absorbents, such as Donnagel® (attapulgite) may be used to get diarrhea under control.
- Treat **underlying disease process**, such as inflammatory bowel disease or Crohn's disease.
- Treat **laxative abuse** that results in cycle of constipation and diarrhea.

213

PROGRESSION IN STRENGTHENING EXERCISES

Strengthening exercise usually progresses as follows:

1. **Isometric exercises** are done with the muscle and limb in static position with no movement of the joint or lengthening of the muscle. The muscle is contracted against resistance.
2. **Isotonic exercises** include movement of the joint during exercise (such as running, weight lifting) and both shortening and lengthening of the muscles through eccentric or concentric contractions. Isotonic refers to tension, so the tension is constant during shortening and lengthening of the muscle.
3. **Isokinetic exercises** utilize machines (such as stationary bicycles that can be set with various parameters) to control the rate and extent of contraction as well as the range of motion. Both speed and resistance can be set so the athlete is limited by the settings of the machine.
4. **Plyometrics** is a particular type of exercise program that uses activities to allow a muscle to achieve maximal force as quickly as possible, and the sequence is a fast eccentric movement (to stretch) followed quickly by a strong concentric (to contract) movement.

SAID PRINCIPLE OF REHABILITATION AND RECONDITIONING

The **Specific Adaptation to Imposed Demands (SAID) principle** suggests that when a person is injured or stressed, that person attempts to overcome the problem by **adapting** to the demands of the situation. This is based on **Wolff's law** (systems adapt to demands). So, if 1 hand is not usable, the person adapts and uses the other hand. Unfortunately, this adaptation can lead to increasing disability, so when the SAID principle is applied to rehabilitation, it means that the person must do exercises that specifically aim to correct the problem. Thus, the functional needs of the person should always be considered when designing a specific exercise program for that individual (such as treadmill running for soccer players). The exercise activities should as closely mirror the functional activities as possible. For example, if the goal is increased strength rather than endurance, then the exercise program should rely more heavily on strengthening exercises.

MASSAGE FOR REHABILITATION AND RECONDITIONING

Massage therapy is commonly used in sports and may be employed before activities, at breaks during activities, and after the activity is completed. Many types of massage are used in sports, and some massage therapists specialize in sports massage, but all FNPs who work with athletes of any age should know the basic techniques of **sports massage** as it is used to both treat and prevent injuries. Sports massage is based primarily on Swedish massage although the massage may be deeper and targeted toward a particular injury and other types of massage may be incorporated into a sports massage program. Massage of an injured area is delayed for the first **48-72 hours** to prevent further injury to tissues. Different techniques include:

- **Compression**: Deep rhythmical compressions of the muscles are done to increase circulation and temperature and make muscles more pliable. It may be used prior to deeper massage techniques.
- **Effleurage**: This is usually the beginning massage and begins softly and increases in intensity with the hands gliding over the tissue, so it is done with some type of oil or emollient. Massage is done in rhythmical broad strokes with the palms of the hands. This massage helps to relax the athlete and identify areas of tightness or pain that may require additional attention.

214

- **Friction**: These are massages either in line with muscle fibers or across the muscle fibers to create stretching and to reduce adhesions and scarring during healing. The tissue is pressed firmly against the underlying tissue and then pressure moves the underlying tissue until resistance is felt. Friction massage may be done deeply, and this can be uncomfortable. Usually the thumb or fingers are used for this type of massage.
- **Pétrissage**: This is kneading massage and is usually used on large muscle areas, such as the calf or thigh. It increases circulation, so it is useful to relax and to improve circulation and drainage as well as to stretch muscles. The full hand is used for this massage with the heel and thumb stabilizing the tissue while the fingers squeeze the tissue.
- **Tapotement**: This type of massage uses quick rhythmic tapping, usually with the edge of the palm and little finger or the heel of the hand with the fingers elevated. It is done to increase circulation or relieve cramped muscles.
- **Vibration**: Vibratory massage is used for deep muscle relaxation and reduction of pain. Usually the entire hand is placed against the skin, compressing the muscle and then vibrating the hand to cause movement.
- **Trigger point**: Pressure is applied with a finger or thumb to areas of point tenderness to reduce spasticity and pain.

PELVIC FLOOR (KEGEL) EXERCISES

The **pelvic floor muscles** cross the floor of the pelvis and attach to the pubic bone and coccyx. The urethra, rectum and vagina all open through the pelvic floor muscles, which support the pelvic organs:

- **Caution**: Avoid holding the breath or tightening the abdominal or buttocks muscles during pelvic floor exercises.
- **Procedure**: Tighten and squeeze the muscles about the rectum, vagina, and urethra and try to "lift" them inside as though trying to stop from passing gas and urine. Hold. Relax. Rest a few seconds. Repeat.
- Schedule:
  - Exercises should be done at least *3 times daily*. They may be done while lying down in the morning and evening and while sitting midday.
  - *1-2 weeks*: Tighten 1 second, relax 5. Repeat 10 times.
  - Then tighten 5 seconds and relax 10. Repeat 10 times.
  - *3-4 weeks*: Tighten 5-10 seconds and relax 10. Repeat 20 times.
  - *5-6 weeks*: Tighten 8-10 seconds and relax 10. Repeat 20 times.

MICROWAVE DIATHERMY

Microwave diathermy is used similarly to shortwave diathermy but has a lower rate of heat increase and penetrance so it is used for muscles and joints near the surface rather than deep muscles, such as the hip. Heat is created by **electromagnetic radiation** (9.15-14.50 MHz) and raises temperature in fatty tissues by about 10-12°C and in muscular tissue by 3-4°C. *Treatment* is usually given for 15-30 minutes per session and is followed by range of motion exercises (passive and active) to increase flexibility. Contraindications are similar to those of shortwave diathermy in that this treatment should not be used where increase in temperature may be detrimental, such as over organs containing fluid, areas of inflammation, and epiphyses of children. Additionally, it should not be used over prostheses or pacemakers and should be avoided in those with cardiac disease.

SHORTWAVE DIATHERMY

Shortwave diathermy uses radio waves (27.12 megahertz) to **increase the temperature in subcutaneous tissue** and is used along with passive and active range of motion exercises to **improve range** in painful conditions such as inflammation of the muscles, tendons, and bursae. The radio waves (eddy currents) are transmitted through a capacitor or inductor in a continuous or pulse waveform. Temperatures increase about 15°C in fatty tissue and 4-6°C in muscular tissue. Shortwave diathermy should not be used over any organs containing fluid, including the eyes, heart, head, or over pacemakers as the diathermy may disrupt the settings. Because this treatment may increase cardiac demand, it should be avoided in those with preexisting cardiac conditions and should not be used over malignancies. Additionally, it is contraindicated in areas of inflammation because heating the tissue increases inflammation. It cannot be used over prostheses as the metal may heat and damage tissue. Shortwave diathermy should avoid the epiphyses in children, as it may stimulate abnormal growth.

SUPERFICIAL HEAT

Superficial heat with externally applied heat sources penetrates only the superficial layers of the skin (1-2 cm after about 30 minutes), but it is believed to relax deeper muscles by reflex, decrease pain, and increase metabolisms (2-3 times for every 10°C increase in skin temperature). Therapeutic temperature range is 40-45°C. Superficial heat modalities include:

- **Moist heat packs** placed on the skin and secured by several layers of towels to provide insulation, applied for 15-30 minutes.
- **Paraffin baths** (52-54° C) with the hand, foot, or elbow dipped 7 times, cooling between dippings, and then wrapping with plastic and towels for 20 minutes.
- **Fluidotherapy** uses hot-air warmed (38.8-47.8°C) cellulose particles into which a hand or foot is submerged for 20-30 minutes.

Passive and active range of motion exercises are done after superficial heat treatment. Contraindications include cardiac disease, peripheral vascular disease, malignant tumor, bleeding, and acute inflammation.

Deep heat differs from superficial heat in that the heat is generated internally using ultrasound, short wave, and microwave diathermy rather than applied to the surface of the skin. Deep heating has penetrance to 3-5 cm.

CRYOTHERAPY

Cryotherapy uses therapeutic cold treatment to cool the surface of the skin and underlying subcutaneous tissues in order to decrease blood flow, pain, and metabolism. Initially response to cold therapy causes **vasoconstriction** to occur within the first 15 minutes but if the tissues are cooled to -10°C, then the body responds with **vasodilation**. Cryotherapy affects sensory response so the person will at first feel cold, which progresses to burning, aching, and finally to numbness and tingling. Treatment is usually given for 15-30 minutes. *Treatment* modalities include:

- **Ice packs** such as refrigerated gel packs (-5°C) or plastic bags filled with water and ice chips are applied directly to the skin for 10-15 minutes for superficial cooling and 15-20 minutes for greater penetrance.
- A **towel dipped in ice and water slurry** is wrapped around limb to provide cold therapy, but this is best used only for emergency situations when ice packs are unavailable, as the towel must be changed frequently as the skin warms the towel rapidly.

- **Ice massage** is applied directly to the affected area for 5-10 minutes, usually rubbing the ice in circular motions on the skin surface. An ice massager is easily made by filled a paper cup with water and freezing it with a tongue depressor or Popsicle stick (to use as a handle) inserted into the center as the water starts to freeze. Then, the paper can be torn away from the bottom and sides when the ice is solid. Ice massage is often followed by friction massage.
- **Ice baths** (13-18°C) are used for limbs, such as the lower leg and/or foot or the hand. The body part is immersed for 20 minutes.

Cryotherapy is usually followed by **active and passive exercises**. Contraindications include impaired circulation or sensation, cardiac disease, Raynaud's disease, and nerve trauma.

THERAPEUTIC ULTRASOUND

Ultrasound treats soft-tissue injuries (such as myositis, bursitis, and tendinitis) with sound waves (frequency 0.8-3 megahertz). Ultrasound utilizes a **piezoelectric crystal** that vibrates, producing sound waveforms, which are transmitted from the transducer through a gel substance into the tissue. The sound waves bounce off of the bone in an irregular pattern that causes an increase in temperature in the connective tissue, such as collagen fibers. Temperatures of the tissue may increase up to 43.5°C, increasing metabolism in the area, neural conduction, as well as blood flow. Ultrasound is used to **decrease both contractures and scarring**. During treatment, the transducer passes in a circular motion about the skin surface, staying in contact with the gel medium. If a distal limb is submerged in water, the treatment is given with the head of the transducer 0.5-1 inch from the skin surface. Treatment is followed by range of motion exercises, passive and active. Contraindications are similar to other heat-producing modalities and include peripheral vascular disease, but ultrasound may be used over metal prostheses.

WHIRLPOOL BATHS

Whirlpool baths are used to increase **circulation** and promote **healing**. They are tubs with a turbine that mixes air with water, which is pressurized and flows into the tub water to create turbulence. Tubs are usually large enough to accommodate the full body although smaller limb-sized whirlpool tubs are available. Water temperature is 95°-104° (adjusted for the individual) and should be deep enough to completely submerge the affected part. The body part should be cleaned with soap and water before immersion or a shower taken. If the full body is treated, then the patient should wear a swimming suit. During the whirlpool treatment, the muscles relax from the heat and **range of motion exercises** can be done while in the water. Typically, treatments last about 20 minutes, but the patient should be monitored, especially for the first 5 minutes, as some people become lightheaded and can lose consciousness.

METHODS OF HEATING AND COOLING

There are a number of different ways to **heat** (thermotherapy) or **cool** (cryotherapy) for **healing**:

- **Conduction**: Conveyance of heat, cold, or electricity through direct contact with the skin, such as with hot baths, ice packs, and electrical stimulation.
- **Convection**: Indirect transmission of heat in a liquid or gas by circulation of heated particles, such as with whirlpools and paraffin soaks.
- **Conversion**: Heating that results from converting a form of energy into heat, such as with diathermy and ultrasound.

217

- **Evaporation**: Cooling caused by liquids that evaporate into gases on the skin with a resultant cooling effect, such as with perspiration or vapocoolant sprays.
- **Radiation**: Heating that results from transfer of heat through light waves or rays, such as with infrared or ultraviolet light.

TENS

Transcutaneous electrical nerve stimulation (TENS) uses electrical stimulation to stimulate **peripheral sensory nerve fibers** to reduce acute or recurrent pain. TENS machines may be 2-lead or 4-lead and have adjustments for both frequency (1-20 Hz) and pulse width (50-300 microseconds, 10-50 mA). Stimulation can be intermittent or continuous. TENS units are small and battery-powered with wires and adhesive electrodes attached so that they can be worn while the person goes about usual activities. The positioning of the electrodes and the settings depend upon the site and type of injury, following guidelines provided by the manufacturer. The TENS machine can be used for a number of hours, but if used for days at a time, it will be less effective. TENS treatment is contraindicated with demand pacemakers and should not be used on the head or neck or over irritated skin.

CONTRAST BATHS

Contrast baths (alternating hot and cold) are used in the sub-acute phase of healing (after edema begins to subside) for **strains and sprains**. It is believed that contrast baths increase the circulation and help to further decrease edema by a pumping action as the **vasoconstriction and vasodilation** alternate. Two containers are filled with water, one with hot and the other with cold. The hot water should be maintained at about 100°-110° F and the cold at 55°-65° F. The cycle begins and ends with immersion in cold water. Cold water immersions usually last about 1 minute and hot water immersions 4 minutes. Typically, the affected limb is immersed in the cold water for 1 minute, removed, and immediately immersed in hot water for 4 minutes. This cycle is repeated about 3-4 times.

VISUALIZATION

There are a number of methods used for **visualization** to reduce anxiety and promote healing. Some include audiotapes with guided imagery, such as self-hypnosis tapes, but the patient can be taught basic **techniques** that include:

- Sit or lie comfortably in a **quiet place** away from distractions.
- Concentrate on **breathing** while taking long slow breaths.
- **Close the eyes** to shut out distractions and create an image in the mind of the place or situation desired.
- Concentrate on that **image**, engaging as many senses as possible and imaging details.
- If the mind wanders, breathe deeply and **bring consciousness back** to the image or concentrate on breathing for a few moments and then return to the imagery.
- End with positive imagery.

Sometimes, patients are resistive at first or have a hard time maintaining focus, so **guiding** them through visualization for the first few times can be helpful.

PROMPTED VOIDING TO PROMOTE CONTINENCE

Prompted voiding is a communication protocol for people with mild to moderate **cognitive impairment**. It uses positive reinforcement for recognizing being wet or dry, staying dry, urinating, and drinking liquids.

- Ask people **every 2 hours** (8 AM to 4-8 PM) whether they are wet or dry.
- Verify if they are correct and give **feedback**, "You are right, Mrs. Brown, you are dry."
- **Prompt** people, whether wet or dry, to use the toilet or urinal. If yes, assist them, record results, and give positive reinforcement by praising and visiting for a short time. If no, repeat the request again once or twice. If they are wet, and decline toileting, change and tell them you will return in 2 hours and ask them to try to wait to urinate until then.
- Offer **liquids** and record amount.
- **Record** results of each attempt to urinate or wet check.

BLADDER TRAINING

Bladder training usually requires the person to keep a toileting diary for at least 3 days so patterns can be assessed. There are a number of different approaches:

- **Scheduled toileting** is toileting or a regular schedule, usually every 2 to 4 hours during the daytime.
- **Habit training** involves an attempt to match the scheduled toileting to a person's individual voiding habits, based on the toileting diary. This is useful for people who have a natural and fairly consistent voiding pattern. Toileting is done every 2-4 hours.
- **Prompted voiding** is often used in nursing homes and attempts to teach people to assess their own incontinence status and prompts them to ask for toileting.
- **Bladder retraining** is a behavioral modification program that teaches people to inhibit the urge to urinate and to urinate according to an established schedule, restoring normal bladder function as much as possible. Bladder training can improve incontinence in 80% of cases.

BLADDER RETRAINING TO PROMOTE CONTINENCE

Bladder retraining teaches people to control the urge to urinate. It usually takes about 3 months to rehabilitate a bladder muscle weakened from frequent urination, causing a decreased urinary capacity. A short urination interval is gradually lengthened to every 2-4 hours during the daytime as the person suppresses bladder urges and stays dry.

- The person keeps **urination diary** for a week.
- An individual program is established with **scheduled voiding times and goals**. For example, if a person is urinating every hour, the goal might be every 80 minutes with increased output.
- The person is taught **techniques** to withhold urination: sitting on a hard seat or on a tightly rolled towel to put pressure on pelvic floor muscles, doing 5 squeezes of pelvic floor muscles, deep breathing, counting backward from 50.
- When the person consistently meets the goal, a **new goal** is established.
- The person keeps a **urination diary**.

THE "KNACK" TO CONTROL URINARY INCONTINENCE

The **knack** is the use of precisely timed muscle contractions to prevent **stress incontinence**. It is "the knack" of squeezing up before bearing down. The knack is a preventive use of **Kegel exercises**.

Women are taught to contract the pelvic floor muscles right before and during events that usually cause stress incontinence. For example, if a woman feels a cough or sneeze coming, she immediately contracts the pelvic floor muscles and holds until the stress event is over. This contraction augments support of the proximal urethra, reducing the amount of displacement that usually takes place with compromised muscle support, thereby preventing incontinence. It is particularly useful if used before and during stress events, such as coughing, sneezing, lifting, standing, swinging a golf club, or laughing. Studies have shown that women who are taught this technique for mild to moderate urinary incontinence and use it consistently are able to decrease incontinence by 73-98%.

MANAGEMENT STRATEGIES FOR CONSTIPATION AND FECAL IMPACTION

Management strategies for **constipation** and **impaction** include:

- **Enemas** and **manual removal of impaction** may be necessary initially.
- Add **fiber** with bran, fresh/dried fruits, and whole grains, to 20-35 grams per day.
- Increase **fluids** to 64 ounces each day.
- **Exercise** program should include walking if possible, and exercises on a daily basis.
- Change in **medications** causing constipation can relieve constipation. Additionally, use of stool softeners, such as Colace® (docusate), or bulk formers, such as Metamucil® (psyllium), may decrease fluid absorption and move stool through the colon more quickly. Overuse of laxatives can cause constipation.
- Careful **monitoring** of diet, fluids, and medical treatment, especially for irritable bowel syndrome.
- **Pregnancy-related constipation** may be controlled through dietary and fluid modifications and regular exercise.
- **Delayed toileting** should be avoided and bowel training regimen done to promote evacuation at the same time each day. During travel, stool softeners, increased fluid, and exercise may alleviate constipation.

BOWEL TRAINING

Bowel training for defecation includes keeping a bowel diary to chart progress:

- **Scheduled defecation** is usually daily, but for some people 3-4 times weekly, depending on individual bowel habits. Defecation should be at the same time so work hours or activities must be considered. Defecation is scheduled for 20-30 minutes after a meal when there is increased motility.
- **Stimulation** is necessary. Drinking a cup of hot liquid may work, but initially many require rectal stimulation, inserting a gloved, lubricated finger into the anus and running it around the rim of the sphincters. Some people require rectal suppositories, such as glycerine. Stimulus suppositories, such as Dulcolax® (bisacodyl), or even Fleet® enemas are sometimes used, but the goal is to reduce use of medical or chemical stimulants.
- **Position** should be sitting upright with knees elevated slightly if possible and leaning forward during defecation.
- **Straining** includes attempting to tighten abdominal muscles and relax sphincters while defecating.

ADDITIONAL BOWEL TRAINING AND EXERCISES

Additional bowel training and exercises include:

- **Exercise** increases the motility of the bowel by stimulating muscle contractions. **Walking** is one of the best exercises for this purpose, and the person should try to walk 1 or 2 miles a day. If the person is unable to walk, then other activities, such as chair exercises that involve the arms and legs and bending can be very effective. Those who are bed bound need to turn from side to side frequently and change position.
- **Kegel exercises** increase strength of the pelvic floor muscles. Kegel exercises for urinary incontinence and fecal incontinence are essentially the same, but the person tries to pull in the muscles around the anus, as though trying to prevent the release of stool or flatus. The person should feel the muscles tightening while holding for 2 seconds and then relaxing for 2, gradually building the time holding time to 10 seconds or more. Exercises should be done 4 times a day.

FIBER IN THE DIET

Most constipation is caused by insufficient **fiber** in the diet, especially if people eat a lot of processed foods. An adequate amount of fiber is 20-30 grams daily. There are both soluble and insoluble forms of fiber, and both add bulk to the stool and are not absorbed into the body. Some foods have both types:

- **Soluble fiber** dissolves in liquids to form a gel-like substance, 1 reason why liquids are so important in conjunction with fiber in the diet. Soluble fiber slows the movement of stool through the gastrointestinal system. Food sources include bananas, starches (potatoes, bread), cheese, dried beans, nuts, apples, oranges, and oatmeal.
- **Insoluble fiber** changes little with the digestive process and increases the speed of stool through the colon, so too much can result in diarrhea. Food sources of insoluble fiber include oat bran, seeds, skins of fruits, vegetables, and nuts.

Therapeutic Communication

Expressing implied messages:

- Patient: "This treatment is too much trouble."
- Nurse: "You think the treatment isn't helping you?"

Exploring a topic but **allowing the patient to terminate the discussion** without further probing:

- "I'd like to hear how you feel about that."

Indicating reality:

- Patient: "Someone is screaming."
- Nurse: "That sound was an ambulance siren."

Commenting on distortions **without directly agreeing or disagreeing**:

- Patient: "That nurse promised I didn't have to have any shot!"
- Nurse: "Really? That's surprising because this medicine can only be given as an injection."

Working together:

- "Maybe if we talk about this, we can figure out a way to make the treatment easier for you."

Seeking validation:

- "Do you feel better now?" "Did the medication help you breathe better?"

PROMOTING THERAPEUTIC COMMUNICATION

Therapeutic communication begins with respect for the patient/family and the assumption that all communication, verbal and non-verbal, has meaning. Listening must be done empathetically. Techniques that facilitate communication include:

- Making a **personal introduction**, using the patient's name and listening intently.
- Using an **open-ended opening statement**: "Is there anything you'd like to discuss."
- **Acknowledging comments**: "Yes," "I understand."
- Reflecting statements back (used sparingly):
  - Patient: "I hate it here!"
  - Nurse: "You hate it here?"
- **Making observations**: "You are shaking" or "You seem worried."
- Recognizing feelings:
  - Patient: "I want to go home."
  - Nurse: "It must be hard to be away from your family and friends."
- **Allowing silence** and **observing non-verbal behavior** rather than trying to force conversation.
- **Providing information** as honestly and completely as possible about condition, treatment, and procedures.
- **Asking for clarification** if statements are unclear.

NON-VERBAL THERAPEUTIC COMMUNICATION

Nonverbal communication is involved in most communication, and is usually automatic and is not a conscious process. Non-verbal communication is good for connecting with patients and communicating feelings or mood, but is not useful for communicating specific information. Nonverbal communication can include body language, facial expressions, vocalizations, and eye contact.

- Facial expressions: The face can show numerous emotions, and the words being used should usually match the facial expression. If the voice and face do not match, miscommunication can take place, as the listener may perceive the speaker as ingenuine or lying. Facial expressions should be used to reinforce the intended message and tone.
- Vocal signals: Nonverbal vocal signals refer to sounds made, other than words, such as sighing, saying "mmm-hmm" to communicate tone or mood. The method of delivery of speech, such as pace, pitch, and volume are considered part of verbal communication, but can also indicate and reinforce emotions in conversation.
- Eye contact: Eye contact varies with cultures, and one should follow cultural cues, but for most Americans, there is a line between maintaining eye contact and staring. A good balance includes enough eye contact to communicate attention, but not so much eye contact that it makes someone uncomfortable by communicating intimidation or overconfidence.

222

- <u>Body language:</u> People may present their bodies with different tones by changing how they stand. An open position, arms to the side or outstretched, and leaning forward suggest trust and care. A closed position, with arms folded, legs crossed, and leaning backwards can serve as a barrier to conversation. Body language is helpful, but unreliable by itself. A closed position can indicate pain, feeling cold, unwillingness, or mistrust. An open position can be used to help connect and build trust between a professional and their client. Leaning toward a person when speaking shows interest and helps to put the other person at ease.
- <u>Gestures:</u> Hand gestures can be used to signify understanding or confusion, to accentuate a point, to indicate directions, or pantomime an activity. People often nod their heads in agreement or disagreement.
- <u>Personal Space:</u> The personal space and distance between people at which people feel comfortable varies by culture, and the laboratory professional should observe and match the distance established by their patients and family. For communication in a professional space, a healthy distance of four to seven feet is generally preferred.

COMMUNICATION AND ENVIRONMENT WHEN DEVELOPING A RELATIONSHIP WITH AN ELDERLY PATIENT

Do not talk fast. Use a low tone of voice so that the patient can hear better. Aid the patient in illuminating what he or she might be feeling, and get them to verify this. Express kindness and connection by paying attention and the use of suitable physical contact. Watch for indications of stress, tiredness, or uneasiness. Try to comprehend social backgrounds, ethnic differences, language issues, or individual partialities. Make sure the conversation is in a soothing environment, where no one can overhear. Put a restriction on how long the interview goes because an aged patient gets tired faster. Talk facing each other to be able to meet the patient's eyes. Be calm but concerned. Make sure there is good lighting and air, and make sure the light does not come from behind (to avoid shadowing or shining in the eyes).

INTERPRETERS

Interpreters have a vital and often overlooked role and function in healthcare management and delivery. Interpreters enable the patient to **communicate effectively** with healthcare providers and also enable the patient to have a **clear understanding of the medical system**. Interpreters also serve to assist the healthcare team in providing the patient with information about the medical condition and treatment options. There are no licensing requirements for interpreters or accreditation requirements. Some interpreters may obtain training in medical terminology to facilitate interpretation in the healthcare setting. Many interpreters are informal native speakers and often function on a volunteer basis.

AVOIDING NON-THERAPEUTIC COMMUNICATION

While using therapeutic communication is important, it is equally important to **avoid interjecting non-therapeutic communication**, which can effectively block effective communication. Avoid the following:

- **Meaningless clichés**: "Don't worry. Everything will be fine." "Isn't it a nice day?"
- **Providing advice**: "You should…" or "The best thing to do is…." It's better when patients ask for advice to provide facts and encourage the patient to reach a decision.
- **Inappropriate approval** that prevents the patient from expressing true feeling or concerns:
  - Patient: "I shouldn't cry when Mommy goes home."
  - Nurse: "That's right! You're a big boy!"

223

- Asking for explanations of **behavior that is not directly related to patient care** and requires analysis and explanation of feelings: "Why are you crying?"
- **Agreeing with rather than accepting and responding to patient's statements** can make it difficult for the patient to change his/her statement or opinion later: "I agree with you," or "You are right."
- **Negative judgments**: "You should stop arguing with the nurses."
- **Devaluing patient's feelings**: "Everyone gets upset at times."
- **Disagreeing directly**: "That can't be true," or "I think you are wrong."
- **Defending against criticism**: "The doctor is not being rude; he's just very busy today."
- **Subject change** to avoid dealing with uncomfortable topics:
  o Patient: "I'm never going to get well."
  o Nurse: "Your parents will be here in just a few minutes."
- **Inappropriate literal responses**, even as a joke, especially if the patient is at all confused or having difficulty expressing ideas:
  o Patient: "There are bugs crawling under my skin."
  o Nurse: "I'll get some buy spray,"
- **Challenge to establish reality** often just increases confusion and frustration:
  o "If you were dying, you wouldn't be able to yell and kick!"

LANGUAGE BARRIERS TO COMMUNICATION

Language barriers often compromise patient's access to care and compliance with treatment, especially if the family members are non-English speaking or have poor English skills. If the nurse practitioner's practice draws from a minority population, then the nurse should consider proactive steps to resolving the issue of language barriers, such as hiring bilingual staff, taking language classes, providing translated materials (i.e., treatment guidelines and pamphlets), or symbol-based signs. Many practices depend on family members, often children, to translate, but this is not a good solution as children often lack the maturity to assume this responsibility and may also lack the vocabulary or understanding to translate effectively, leading to serious misunderstandings. Interpreters should have training in **medical vocabulary**. In some cases, volunteer translators can be trained. Another solution is to pool translation resources among a number of practices so that costs are manageable.

Culturally Congruent Practice

CULTURALLY COMPETENT HEALTH CARE

Cultural sensitivity is an important attribute for APRNs and other clinicians to possess; ignorance of other cultural beliefs can lead to alienation of the patient, which will obviously compromise the therapeutic relationship and the overall healing process. An APRN who is culturally sensitive, moreover, does not make **assumptions** about cultures based on broad generalizations and stereotypes. Although there may be characteristics that seem to apply to a specific culture as a whole, it is important for the APRN to remember that each person has his or her own beliefs and attitudes, regardless of cultural differences. An APRN who practices culturally competent health care is attentive and intuitive, and is able to recognize how the patient is feeling based on the patient's behavior, even if the behavior is unexpected.

CULTURAL COMPETENCE

Different **cultures** view health and illness from very different perspectives, and patients often come from a mix of many cultures, so the FNP must be not only accepting of cultural differences but must be sensitive and aware. There are a number of characteristics that are important for an FNP to have cultural competence:

- **Appreciating diversity**: This must be grounded in information about other cultures and understanding of their value system.
- **Assessing own cultural perspectives**: Self-awareness is essential to understanding potential biases.
- **Understanding intercultural dynamics**: This must include understanding ways in which cultures cooperate, differ, communicate, and reach understanding.
- **Recognizing institutional culture**: Each institutional unit (hospital, clinic, office) has an inherent set of values that may be unwritten but is accepted by the staff.
- **Adapting patient service to diversity**: This is the culmination of cultural competence as it is the point of contact between cultures.

CULTURAL DIFFERENCES/ISSUES

Often healthcare providers who strive to be **culturally competent** are unaware that patients have very different perspectives about issues central to their health. According to the National Center for Cultural Competence there are a number of specific cultural differences/issues that healthcare providers should understand:

- Attitudes about illness and the cause of illness may be very different from one culture to another.
- Understanding of general health, mechanisms of healing, and issues of wellness may be very diverse.
- Attitudes about healthcare providers may range from very positive to very negative.
- The manner of help seeking for medical problems may vary, and healthcare providers may not recognize help-seeking behavior when it is not direct.
- Attitudes about traditional and non-traditional treatment influence the individual's medical choices.
- Attitudes of healthcare workers may project biases to which the patients are subjected.
- The current health system is often not culturally or linguistically diverse, so patient needs may be overlooked.

CULTURAL COMPETENCE WHEN COMMUNICATING WITH CHILDREN/FAMILY

There are a number of issues related to **cultural and spiritual competence** in communicating with children/family:

- **Eye contact**: Many cultures use eye contact differently than is common in the United States. They may avoid direct eye contact, considering it rude, or may look away to signal disapproval, or may look down to signal respect. Careful observation of the way family members use eye contact can help to determine what will be most comfortable for the child//family.
- **Distance**: Some cultures stand close to others (<4 feet) when speaking (Middle Easterners, Hispanics) and others stand at a further distance (>4 feet) (Northern Europeans, many Americans). There is considerable difference relating to concepts of personal space among cultures. Allowing the family to approach or observing whether they tend to move closer, lean forward, or move back can help to determine a comfortable distance for communication.
- **Time**: Americans tend to be time-oriented, and expect people to be on time, but time is more flexible in many cultures, so scheduling may require flexibility.

225

TAILORING DELIVERY OF CARE TO MEET THE DIVERSE NEEDS OF PATIENTS

Studies indicate that those who are **diverse**, that is ethnical, cultural, or life-style minorities, are often treated differently by healthcare providers in the sense that they may receive less than optimal care. It is incumbent upon nurse practitioners to ensure that all patients/families receive equal quality care but with delivery of care **tailored** to meet the **individual needs** of the patients. This begins with asking other staff to assess their own attitudes and open discussion about differences to help people to gain self-awareness and determine if their ideas are stereotypical and/or based on lack of knowledge. The care plan should be formatted to specifically address diversity issues so that discussions of diversity and preferences are part of the care plan development and not an addendum. The original assessment should include questions about family, country of birth, educational level, religious preferences, and native language, with explanations as to why the questions are asked, establishing a relationship of trust and respect that encourages the patient/family to express individual differences.

INTEGRATING CONCERNS AND VALUE SYSTEMS INTO PATIENT'S PLAN OF CARE

Integrating concerns and value systems of patient/family, nursing staff, other healthcare team members, administrators, and payors into every patient's plan of care requires a determination and understanding of what is important to each participant. Planning for this type of integration is an ongoing effort as it's not practical to call a participant meeting to discuss each care plan, but general concerns and values can be identified for the institution or the unit and these can then be individualized for each patient. Participants may have widely divergent concerns. For example:

- A child may want her parents to be with her at all times.
- A parent may want religious/ cultural concerns about medical care to be respected.
- A payor may want appropriate and cost-effective treatments.
- A nurse may want treatments to be clearly outlined and carried out competently.
- A nutritionist may want the patient to have adequate nutrition.
- An adequate care plan should allow for all of these concerns to be addressed.

PROVIDING SPIRITUALLY AND CULTURALLY COMPETENT CARE

The ability to **communicate** among **different cultures** is an important skill, built on respect for others and knowledge. The nurse practitioner should learn the **basic cultural values** of specific groups that will be seen in practice so that these can be integrated into the care plans. It's especially important to understand what each patient believes about illness or health matters. Many cultures use complementary medicine, and the nurse practitioner should respect traditional healing and methods as long as the safety of the patient/child is not compromised. Such things as healers, massage, aromatherapy may provide emotional support to both children and parents and should be accommodated. If complementary treatment poses a health risk, such as Greta (a lead-based drink), then the reasons why it should not be used should be clearly stated. Families can be advised that herbs often contain the same chemical compounds found in medications and the patient might have an overdose to an ingredient or a reaction to prescribed medications to encourage them to describe herbal treatments.

IDENTIFICATION OF ISSUES OF CULTURAL DIVERSITY AND FACILITATION OF AWARENESS

Issues of **cultural diversity** must be an integral part of the plan of care so that they are always addressed. Individuals vary considerably in their attitudes, so assuming that all members of an ethnic or cultural group share the same values is never valid. The individual must be assessed as well as the group. However, basic **cultural guidelines** should be understood, addressing issues such as eye contact, proximity, and gestures. It is important to take time to observe family dynamics

226

and language barriers, arranging for translators if necessary, to ensure that there is adequate communication. In patriarchal cultures, such as the Mexican culture, the eldest man may speak for the patient. In some Muslim cultures, women will resist care by men. The attitudes and beliefs of the patient in relation to care and treatment must be understood, accepted, and treated with respect. In some cases, the use of healers or cultural traditions must be incorporated into a plan of care.

Leadership Concepts

INTRA- AND INTERDISCIPLINARY TEAMS

COLLABORATION

The complexity of patient care requires **collaboration** and among intra- and interdisciplinary teams. Collaboration may begin between the FNP and patient or FNP and doctor, but often the expertise of others in the healthcare community must be included. Often the FNP is in the position to seek collaboration and to recognize when multiple perspectives can be helpful in solving conflicts or making decisions about healthcare. Collaboration requires open sharing of ideas and respect for the expertise of the individual. Collaboration requires more than just talking, however. In many cases it may be more formalized, with specialized committees formed in order to solve specific problems. Studies have indicated that patients benefit from collaborative efforts between nurse and physician, and this benefit extends to others as well. In a collaborative environment, all of the participants benefit from sharing ideas and discussion that can lead to **innovative problem-solving**.

COORDINATION

There are a number of skills that the FNP needs to lead and facilitate **coordination of intra- and interdisciplinary teams**:

- **Communicating openly** is essential with all members encouraged to participate as valued members of a cooperative team.
- **Avoiding interrupting** or interpreting the point another is trying to make allows free flow of ideas.
- **Avoiding jumping to conclusions**, as that can effectively shut off communication.
- **Active listening** requires paying attentions and asking questions for clarification rather than to challenge other's ideas.
- **Respecting others' opinions and ideas**, even when opposed to one's own, is absolutely essential.
- **Reacting and responding to facts** rather than feelings allows one to avoid angry confrontations or diffuse anger.
- **Clarifying information or opinions** stated can help avoid misunderstandings.
- **Keeping unsolicited advice out of the conversation** shows respect for others and allows them to solicit advice without feeling pressured.

BENEFITS OF INTERDISCIPLINARY TEAM APPROACH

The **interdisciplinary team approach** to care coordination is beneficial to the patient in several ways. First, the quality of patient care is improved because several different medical services are involved in the care of the patient, and each service is familiar with the patient's situation as a result of increased communication with other health care workers. The interdisciplinary team approach also allows the patient to have a more active role in his or her care because of the emphasis on communication between the patient and all the team members. When the clinicians work together, they also make better use of time spent with the patient, so that the patient is not subjected to lengthy history-taking sessions and redundant testing by unaware clinicians.

TEAM BUILDING

Leading, facilitating, and participating in performance improvement teams requires a thorough understanding of the dynamics of **team building**:

- **Initial interactions:** This is the time when members begin to define their roles and develop relationships, determining if they are comfortable in the group.
- **Power issues:** The members observe the leader and determine who controls the meeting and how control is exercised, beginning to form alliances.
- **Organizing:** Methods to achieve work are clarified and team members begin to work together, gaining respect for each other's contributions and working toward a common goal.
- **Team identification:** Interactions often become less formal as members develop rapport, and members are more willing to help and support each other to achieve goals.
- **Excellence:** This develops through a combination of good leadership, committed team members, clear goals, high standards, external recognition, spirit of collaboration, and a shared commitment to the process.

LEADERSHIP STYLES

Leadership styles often influence the perception of leadership values and commitment to collaboration. There are a number of different leadership styles:

- **Charismatic** - Depends upon personal charisma to influence people, and may be very persuasive, but this type leader may engage "followers" and relate to one group rather than the organization at large, limiting effectiveness.
- **Bureaucratic** - Follows organization rules exactly and expects everyone else to do so. This is most effective in handling cash flow or managing work in dangerous work environments. This type of leadership may engender respect but may not be conducive to change.
- **Autocratic** - Makes decisions independently and strictly enforces rules, but team members often feel left out of the process and may not be supportive. This type of leadership is most effective in crisis situations, but may have difficulty gaining commitment of staff.
- **Consultative** - Presents a decision and welcomes input and questions although decisions rarely change. This type of leadership is most effective when gaining the support of staff is critical to the success of proposed changes.
- **Participatory** - Presents a potential decision and then makes final decision based on input from staff or teams. This type of leadership is time-consuming and may result in compromises that are not wholly satisfactory to management or staff, but this process is motivating to staff who feel their expertise is valued.
- **Democratic** - Presents a problem and asks staff or teams to arrive at a solution although the leader usually makes the final decision. This type of leadership may delay decision-making, but staff and teams are often more committed to the solutions because of their input.
- **Laissez-faire (free rein)** - Exerts little direct control but allows employees/ teams to make decisions with little interference. This may be effective leadership if teams are highly skilled and motivated, but in many cases, this type of leadership is the product of poor management skills and little is accomplished because of this lack of leadership.

Managing Care Across Systems

COLLABORATION WITH EXTERNAL AGENCIES

The nurse practitioner must initiate and facilitate collaboration with **external agencies** because many have direct impacts on patient care and needs:

- **Industry** can include other facilities sharing interests in patient care or pharmaceutical companies. It's important for nursing to have a dialog with drug companies about their products and how they are used in specific populations because many medications are prescribed to women, children, or the aged without validating studies for dose or efficacy.
- **Payors** have a vested interest in containing health care costs, so providing information and representing the interests of the patient is important.
- **Community groups** may provide resources for patients and families, both in terms of information and financial or other assistance.
- **Political agencies** are increasingly important as new laws are considered about nurse-patient ratios and infection control in many states.
- **Public health agencies** are partners in health care with other facilities and must be included, especially in issues related to communicable disease.

MEDICAL HOME MODEL

The **medical home model** is a healthcare approach to providing care (primary and comprehensive) to patients. This healthcare model serves to **coordinate and improve relationships** between patients, their families, and their personal physicians. In March 2007, the American Academy of Family Physicians, American Academy of Pediatrics, American College of Physicians, and American Osteopathic Association developed joint principles for the medical home model. The characteristics of these principles are a personal physician, physician-directed medical practice, focus on the whole person, coordinated care, focus on quality and safety of medical care, enhanced patient access, and payment.

ASSISTED LIVING FACILITIES

Assisted living facilities are considered as alternative care facilities. Assisted living is designed to aid community residents with the activities of daily living. Some state regulations will allow an assisted living facility to provide assistance or reminders for medications. Assisted living facilities are different from nursing homes in that such facilities do not provide **complex medical services**. Assisted living communities vary from a stand-alone facility to being one tier of care in a continuing care retirement facility. Usually, the assisted living environment is more like a personal home or apartment. The cost for an assisted living facility is usually paid via private funds; however, some exceptions exist. Some long-term-care insurance policies provide for such fees; Medicaid and waivers may also be available.

GROUP HOMES

Group homes are considered another type of alternative care facility. Typically, a group home is small, residential, and it functions to care for patients with **chronic disabilities**. These group homes are usually small and have six or fewer residents. Group homes are staffed around the clock by trained personnel. The typical group home is a single-family residence that is paid for by the group home administrators. It is usually adapted to meet the special needs of its patients. Group home residents may have chronic mental or physical disabilities that require assistance or supervision or aid with the activities of daily living.

RESIDENTIAL TREATMENT FACILITIES

Another alternative care facility is a **residential treatment facility**. Resident treatment facilities may also be referred to as rehab facilities. Residential treatment facilities serve as a live-in situation in which **therapies** for substance abuse, behavioral issues, and mental illness are provided. Residential treatment facilities may be either locked or unlocked. Locked facilities are quite restrictive and may confine the patient to a single room or cell. Unlocked residential treatment facilities generally afford the patient much more freedom in the facility, but there are certain conditions/supervision required in order to leave the facility. In general, most residential treatment facilities are of a clinical focus and often utilize behavior modification techniques.

CONTINUUM OF CARE

The **continuum of care** refers to a series of services provided for patients or adults needing assistance across a span of time or through stages of change. The continuum of care may involve care practices used from the home, in the community, in a residential care facility, or another institution that provides care. This continuum meets the needs of the adult through **stages of health or disability**. By having a continuum of care, providers can better identify the needs of patients to provide and coordinate services as needed. For example, if a person needs to move from his home to a long-term care facility for residential treatment because of declining health, the continuum of care can give providers resources for helping the patient to make the transition. The care continuum ensures that all of the client's needs are met while making the transition. The process is tracked and evaluated to ensure competency and that services are complete.

SERVICE ACROSS THE CONTINUUM OF CARE

The continuum of care is a **series of care levels** that meet patients where they are in terms of health. By identifying the level of the patient's needs, the continuum can guide clinicians for services. On one end is home care and intervention. This provides care for the patient in his home and identifies any additional needs. The next level might be outpatient services, in which the patient receives services at a healthcare center, but remains living at home. Beyond this level, the patient may need hospitalization or short-term care. This is more of an acute stage, but the patient does not need services for long. Following this, the patient might need inpatient care or assisted living services, this includes being monitored on a regular basis and no longer living at home. Finally, the end of the continuum involves high-need care, in which the patient requires intensive treatments because of a fragile state of health.

Advocacy

PATIENT ADVOCACY AND ANA'S DEFINITION OF NURSING

Patient advocacy is defined as the process of speaking on behalf of a patient to ensure that his or her rights are protected, and that he or she is provided with necessary information and services. The nurse practitioner frequently serves as patient advocate, although physicians, social workers, and other individuals in the health care industry may act on behalf of the patient as well.

The ANA defines **nursing** as "the protection, promotion, and optimization of health and abilities, prevention of illness and injury, alleviation of suffering through the diagnosis and treatment of human response, and advocacy in the care of individuals, families, communities, and populations."

EMPOWERING PATIENTS/FAMILIES TO ACT AS THEIR OWN ADVOCATES

Patients and families are empowered to act as their own advocates when they have a clear understanding of their **rights and responsibilities.** These should be given (in print form) and/or presented (audio/video) to patients and families on admission or as soon as possible:

- **Rights** should include **competent, non-discriminatory medical care** that respects privacy and allows participation in decisions about care and the right to refuse care. They should have clear understandable explanations of treatments, options, and conditions, including outcomes. They should be apprised of transfers, changes in care plan, and advance directives. They should have access to medical records information about charges.
- **Responsibilities** should include providing **honest and thorough information** about health issues and medical history. They should ask for clarification if they don't understand information that is provided to them, and they should follow the plan of care that is outlined or explain why that is not possible. They should treat staff and other patients with respect.

FACILITATORS OF PATIENT ADVOCACY

Perhaps the greatest facilitator of patient advocacy is the **nurse practitioner-patient relationship**; if a strong relationship exists between the nurse practitioner and the patient, the nurse practitioner will be motivated to perform the duties of advocate. If the patient and nurse practitioner have a strained or limited relationship, advocacy can be difficult. **Recognizing the patient's needs** is another facilitator, one that goes hand in hand with a good nurse practitioner-patient relationship. If the nurse practitioner feels a sense of responsibility and accountability on behalf of the patient, he or she is more likely to serve as a good patient advocate; conscience is a strong motivator. Another facilitator is if the **physician acts as a colleague**, instead of a superior; this strengthens the nurse practitioner-physician relationship, and the nurse practitioner feels that he or she can question the physician's judgment instead of constantly deferring. That being said, the greater the knowledge base and skill level of the nurse practitioner, the greater he or she will be as an advocate.

FACILITATING SAFE PASSAGE

Facilitating **safe passage** is part of caring practice that ensures patient safety, in a broad sense, from a variety of perspectives:

- **Giving appropriate medications and treatment** without errors that endanger the patient's health is essential.
- **Providing information** to the patient/family about treatments, changes, conditions, and other aspects related to care helps them to cope with the situations as they arise.
- **Preventing infection** is central to patient safety and includes staff using proper infection control methods, such as handwashing.
- **Knowing the person** requires the nurse to take the time and effort to understand the needs and wishes of the patient/family.
- **Assisting with transitions** involves not only helping the patient/family cope with moving from one form of treatment, or one unit to another but also with transitions in health, such as from illness to health or from illness to death.

ANALYSIS OF PATIENT/CUSTOMER SATISFACTION

Patient/customer satisfaction is usually measured with **surveys** given to patients upon discharge from an institution or on completion of treatment. One problem with analyzing surveys is that establishing benchmarks can be difficult because so many different survey and data collection methods are used that comparison data may be meaningless. Internal benchmarking may be more

231

effective, but the sample rate for surveys may not be sufficient to provide validity. As patients become more knowledgeable and demand for accountability increases, patient satisfaction is being used as a guide for performance improvement although patient perceptions of clinical care do not always correlate with outcomes. The results of surveys can provide feedback that makes healthcare providers more aware of customer expectations. Currently, surveys are most often used to evaluate service elements of care rather than clinical elements. Analysis includes:

- Determining the patient/customer's **degree of trust**.
- Determining the **degree of satisfaction** with care/treatment.
- Identifying **needs** that may be unmet.
- Identifying patient/customer **priorities**.

PROBLEM SOLVING TO ANTICIPATE AND PREVENT RECURRENCES OF PATIENT/FAMILY DISSATISFACTION

Problem solving in any nursing context involves arriving at a hypothesis and then testing and assessing data to determine if the hypothesis holds true. If a problem has arisen, taking steps to resolve the immediate problem is only the first step if recurrence is to be avoided:

- **Define the issue**: Talk with the patient or family and staff to determine if the problem related to a failure of communication or other issues, such as culture or religion.
- **Collect data**: This may mean interviewing additional staff or reviewing documentation, gaining a variety of perspectives.
- **Identify important concepts**: Determine if there are issues related to values or beliefs.
- **Consider reasons for actions**: Distinguish between motivation and intention on the part of all parties to determine the reason for the problem.
- **Make a decision**: A decision on how to prevent a recurrence of a problem should be based on advocacy and moral agency, reaching the best solution possible for the patient and family.

IMPORTANCE OF INTERPRETING AND COMMUNICATING NEEDS IN THE COORDINATION OF CARE

The nursing environment is increasingly complex and must include meeting the needs of various members of the healthcare community and administration as well as those of the patient/family. The nurse often stands at a central point between the patient/family on one side and other care providers and/or interested parties on the other. Especially in situations of severe illness, the patient/family often feel as though they are at the mercy of the healthcare community and are powerless. Because of this, the nurse practitioner must always represent the best interests of the patients/families and must interpret and communicate on their behalf so that there is **consistency of care** and **consideration and understanding of their needs**. It's important for the nurse practitioner to recognize that the patients/families are in a vulnerable position and need **advocacy** and care to ensure that other caregivers respect their needs and preferences.

PATIENT ADVOCACY AND MEDICAL ERROR

Patient advocacy must include a review of medical errors, unintentional but preventable mistakes in providing care. Errors are classified as failures to carry out a planned action or using the wrong plan while an adverse event is the negative result of that error, such as an injury:

- Errors may result from **commission** (doing something) or **omission** (failing to do something).
- Errors can be **active** (resulting from contact between the patient and an aspect of the medical system, such as a nurse or piece of equipment).
- Errors can be **latent**, resulting from a failure of design in the system.
- **Error chains** are the series of events that lead to a negative outcome, usually identified through root cause analysis.

Medical errors are most often identified after an adverse event occurs, but some may not be identified and are found on medical record reviews. Typical errors include incorrect diagnosis, mistakes in medications (such as wrong medication or dose), delays in reporting of results, failure of communication, improper or inadequate care, and mistaken identity.

BARRIERS TO PATIENT ADVOCACY

Patient advocacy is often seen as a moral obligation that the nurse practitioner must fulfill, and is a rewarding part of the nurse practitioner's job; however, patient advocacy can be difficult in certain situations. One barrier to advocacy is a feeling of **powerlessness** on the part of the nurse practitioner; sometimes it may feel as if it is the nurse practitioner against the world, especially if the nurse practitioner has no support; lack of support in general is another barrier. A **lack of knowledge of the law** is another barrier; certain laws may exist, though the nurse practitioner may not be aware of them. If the nurse practitioner and his or her peers are lacking in time, communication, or motivation, advocacy will also prove difficult. Another problem that nurse practitioners frequently encounter is the **risk** associated with advocacy; included are disagreeing with other nurse practitioners and physicians, and lack of legal support for the advocate.

ICD-10, CPT, AND HCPC

ICD-10 – International Classification of Diseases, 10th Edition; this has diagnostic codes that tell what medical problem, sickness, or harm the medical attention is for; utilized with billing insurance companies.

CPT – Current Procedural Terminology; these codes tell what procedure or medical attention was done; there are more than 7000. Both Medicare and state Medicaid carriers have to utilize these codes under the law.

HCPC – Health Care Financing Administration Common Procedure Coding System; this is utilized to make an account of supplies and medical tools.

Conflict Resolution

Conflict is an almost inevitable product of teamwork, and the leader must assume responsibility for **conflict resolution.** While conflicts can be disruptive, they can produce positive outcomes by forcing team members to listen to different perspectives and opening dialogue. The team should make a plan for dealing with conflict resolution. The best time for conflict resolution is when differences emerge but before open conflict and hardening of positions occur. The leader must pay close attention to the people and problems involved, listen carefully, and reassure those involved that their points of view are understood. Steps to conflict resolution include:

- Allow **both sides** to present their side of conflict without bias, maintaining a focus on opinions rather than individuals.
- Encourage **cooperation** through negotiation and compromise.
- Maintain the **focus**, providing guidance to keep the discussions on track and avoid arguments.
- Evaluate the need for **renegotiation**, formal resolution process, or third party.
- Utilize **humor and empathy** to diffuse escalating tensions.
- **Summarize** the issues, outlining key arguments.
- Avoid forcing resolution if possible

STRATEGIES

There are many ways to attempt conflict resolution, some of them beneficial, some of them not.

- **Avoidance** is a strategy that is not typically considered to be beneficial to conflict resolution; when the clinician is not committed to the relationship with the patient, or if the situation is nonemergent, the clinician may ignore or deny the conflict in an effort to avoid facing it.
- **Coercion** is another strategy that does not usually end in a favorable outcome, at least for one of the parties involved. This strategy is used when the clinician feels that he or she is right, does not have time to devote to proper resolution, and has not invested time into a relationship with the patient.
- **Accommodation** is a somewhat similar strategy, albeit with less resistance, where one party concedes that the other's position is right.
- **Compromise and collaboration** are usually the best methods of resolution, and allow both sides to be heard.

Quality Improvement

INTEGRATION OF KEY QUALITY CONCEPTS WITHIN THE ORGANIZATION

There are a number of **key concepts** related to quality that must be communicated to all members of an organization through inservice, workshops, newsletters, fact sheets, and team meetings. Quality care/performance should be:

- **Appropriate** to needs and in keeping with best practices.
- **Accessible** to the individual despite financial, cultural, or other barriers.
- **Competent**, with practitioners well-trained and adhering to standards.
- **Coordinated** among all healthcare providers.
- **Effective** in achieving outcomes based on the current state of knowledge.
- **Efficient** in methods of achieving the desired outcomes.
- **Preventive**, allowing for early detection and prevention of problems.
- **Respectful** and caring with consideration of the individual needs given primary importance.
- **Safe** so that the organization is free of hazards or dangers that may put patients or others at risk.

OPTIMIZING OUTCOMES FOR PATIENTS, FAMILIES, OR PAYORS

Optimal outcomes can be achieved when the characteristics of the patient and the nurse competencies match within the framework of an inter-related system in which the patient/family is an equal partner. Outcomes are derived from different components:

- **Patient**: Trust in the healthcare provider based on perceived caring and competency is an essential outcome and links with the functional ability of the patient and the quality of life. Patients and their families must feel satisfied with care.
- **Nurse**: Measurable outcomes are associated with nursing and include physiological changes, occurrence or prevention of infection, and effectiveness of nursing care and treatments. The nurse serves to coordinate many aspects of care relating to outcomes.
- **System**: Outcomes relate to the delivery of care that is consistently both high quality and cost-effective. This includes data regarding rates of rehospitalization, length of hospitalization, and optimal utilization of resources linked to cost data.

CQI RELATED TO IMPROVEMENT EXERCISES FOR CLINICAL PRACTICE

Continuous Quality Improvement (CQI) emphasizes the organization, systems, and processes within that organization rather than individuals. It recognizes internal customers (staff) and external customers (patients) and utilizes data to **improve processes**. CQI represents the concept that most processes can be improved. CQI uses the scientific method of experimentation to meet needs and improve services and utilizes various tools, such as brainstorming, multivoting, various charts and diagrams, storyboarding, and meetings. Core concepts include:

- Quality and success are meeting or exceeding internal and external customer's needs and expectations.
- Problems relate to processes, and variations in process lead to variations in results.
- Change can be in small steps.
- Steps to CQI include:
  - Forming a knowledgeable team.
  - Identifying and defining measures used to determine success.
  - Brainstorming strategies for change.
  - Plan, collect, and utilize data as part of making decisions.
  - Test changes and revise or refine as needed.

INTEGRATION OF CONTINUOUS PROCESS IMPROVEMENT INTO NURSE PRACTITIONER PRACTICE

The primary principle of **continuous process improvement** is that improvement can be accomplished by small incremental steps. In larger organizations, with multiple staff, CQI can be instituted and a formal process carried out, but in small practices, while the basic procedures are the same, the staff may be much smaller, often only the nurse practitioner, so procedures are modified accordingly. Continuous process improvement begins by identifying **one process that needs improvement**, and it might be something as small as improving telephone service, but once a problem is identified, and then first steps to solving the problem are initiated. Once the first step is accomplished (contacting various telephone services), then the next step is accomplished (picking a new service). When the steps to improving one process are completed, another project is picked for improvement. In some cases, multiple continuous improvement projects may be in process at the same time.

EVALUATION OF PERFORMANCE IMPROVEMENT MODELS

A number of different **performance improvement models** have been developed over the year. Evaluating and applying these models are part of strategic management and quality healthcare. In some offices/organizations, one approach may be used, but often models are **combined** in various ways in order to meet specific needs. Planning and understanding how these models can facilitate change are important for those in leadership roles because, in order for these models to be effective, there must be cooperation and consensus across the organization. The various models share some like elements:

- The models focus on continuous improvement and are planned, systematic, collaborative and apply to the entire organization.
- They share common focus on identifying problems, collecting data, assessing current performance, instituting actions for change, assessing changes, team development, and use of data.

A model or models should be chosen that seem appropriate to the needs of the organization and to those who will work with the model.

JURAN'S QIP

Joseph Juran's quality improvement process (QIP) is a 4-step method, focusing on **quality control**, which is based on a trilogy of concepts that includes quality planning, control, and improvement. The steps to the QIP process include:

1. **Defining** the project and organizing includes listing and prioritizing problems and identifying a team.
2. **Diagnosing** includes analyzing problems and then formulating theories related to cause by root cause analysis and test theories.
3. **Remediating** includes considering various alternative solutions and then designing and implementing specific solutions and controls while addressing institutional resistance to change. As causes of problems are identified and remediation instituted to remove the problems, the processes should improve.
4. **Holding** involves evaluating performance and monitoring the control system in order to maintain gains.

SHEWHART CYCLE (PLAN-DO-CHECK-ACT)

The Shewhart cycle (Plan-Do-Check-Act) is a method of continuous improvement that is part of quality management and is used to solve problems:

1. **Plan** involves identifying and analyzing the problem, clearly defining the problem, setting goals, and establishing a process that coordinates with coordinates with leadership. Extensive brainstorming, including fishbone diagrams, identifies problematic processes and lists current process steps. Data is collected and analyzed and root cause analysis completed.
2. **Do** involves generating solutions from which to select 1 or more and then implementing the solution on a trial basis.
3. **Check** involves gathering and analyzing data to determine the effectiveness of the solution. If effective, then continue to Act; if not, return to Plan and pick a different solution.
4. **Act** involves identifying changes that need to be done to fully implement the solution, adopting the solution, and continuing to monitor results while picking another improvement project.

Healthcare Economics, Policy, and Organizational Practices

USE OF HEALTH POLICY

Health policy – Movement in the direction of primary medical attention and getting prevention earlier encourages utilization of APRNs. The main elements that control healthcare delivery are payors, insurance companies, providers, and suppliers. Legislation regarding ways to do things and politics is included in this topic.

MEDICAL ATTENTION

Medical attention – May be primary health care or managed care. Managed care includes Health Maintenance Organizations (HMO), Preferred Provider Organizations (PPO) and Point of Service (POS) plans.

HIPAA

HIPAA is the Health Insurance Portability and Accountability Act of 1996, under Public Law 104-191. This has a goal of better organization and helpfulness in the medical system, which is to be done by regulating the way that electronic communications for administrative and economic information is done. The requirements include particular transaction regulations (including code sets), security and electronic signatures, privacy and particular identifiers that also have utilization permissions for bosses, health plans and people who give medical attention.

IMPACT OF SOCIAL, POLITICAL, REGULATORY, AND ECONOMIC FORCES ON THE DELIVERY OF CARE

The **delivery of care** is impacted by numerous forces:

- **Social forces** are increasing demand for access to treatment and medical services, both traditional and complementary. As society views equitable medical care as a right, then delivery of care must be available to all.
- **Political forces** affect medical care as the Federal and state governments increasingly become purchasers of medical care, imposing their guidelines and limitations on the medical system.
- **Regulatory forces** may be local, state, or Federal and can have a profound effect of delivery of care and services, differing from one state or region to another.
- **Economic forces**, such as managed care or cost-containment committees, try to contain costs to insurers and facilities by controlling access to and duration of treatment, and limiting products. Economic pressure is working to prevent duplication of services in a geographical area, and providers are creating networks to purchase supplies and equipment directly.

SYSTEMS THINKING

The promotion of organizational values and commitment requires that the organization embody systems thinking and the associated concepts. **Systems thinking** focuses on how systems interrelate, with each part affecting the entire system: Concepts include:

- **Individual responsibility**: Individuals are encouraged to establish their own goals within the organization and to work toward a purpose.
- **Learning process:** The internalized beliefs of the staff are respected while building upon these beliefs to establish a mindset based on continuous learning and improvement.
- **Vision**: A sharing of organizational vision helps staff to understand the purpose of change and builds commitment.

237

- **Team process:** Teams are assisted to develop good listening and collaborative skills so that there is an increase in dialogue and an ability to reach consensus.
- **Systems thinking:** Staff members are encouraged to understand the interrelationship of all members of the organization and to appreciate how any change affects the whole.

STEPS

An approach to systems thinking is especially valuable in organizations in which there is lack of consensus, effective change is stalemated, and standards are inconsistent. Systems thinking is a critical thinking approach to problem solving that takes an organization-wide perspective. **Steps** include:

1. **Define the issue:** Describe the problem in detail without judgment or solutions.
2. **Describe behavior patterns:** This includes listing factors related to the problem, using graphs to outline possible trends.
3. **Establish cause-effect relationships:** This may include using the Five Whys or other root cause analysis or feedback loops.
4. **Define patterns of performance/behavior:** Determine how variables affect outcomes and the types of patterns of behavior currently taking place.
5. **Find solutions:** Discuss possible solutions and outcomes.
6. **Institute performance improvement activities:** Make changes and then monitor for changes in behavior.

COST CONTAINMENT PRINCIPLES

The rapidly rising costs of health care need to be curtailed; the system is now focusing on attaining better outcomes while controlling costs. Over- and underutilization of services in health care is one principle in **cost containment**. Improved coordination and cooperation over the entire quality of care continuum is another principle. Another principle is placing greater emphasis upon prevention by awarding incentives for wellness behaviors in patients as well as stressing early detection of disease. Increased usage of evidence-based guidelines in the treatment of various diseases helps to contain costs. Electronic medical records and improved information regarding the costs of products and services used by providers and patients allow informed decisions about the comparative effectiveness of treatments.

INTERNATIONAL PATIENT SAFETY GOALS

FNPs may work in institutions under accreditation of the Joint Commission, but even those in private practice can incorporate the **International Patient Safety Goals** as a management strategy that includes adhering to goals, educating support staff, and monitoring for compliance:

- **Identify patients correctly**: 2 identifiers for medicines, blood, or blood products.
- **Checklist before beginning surgery**: Ensure correct patient, procedure, and body part.
- **Improve effective communication**: Establish process for taking orders/report and read back for verbal/telephone orders.
- Remove concentrated electrolytes from patient care units: Including potassium.
- **Surgical checklist**: Ensure proper documentation and necessary equipment in working order.
- **Mark surgical site**: Clear identifiable marking.
- **Comply with handwashing standards**: Centers for Disease Control (CDC) guidelines.
- Assess risk of falls: Eliminate risks.

MEDICARE AND MEDICAID

An American is **eligible for Medicare** if he/she is age 65 or older and either receiving or is eligible to receive Social Security benefits. Patients younger than 65 are also eligible if they receive Social Security disability benefits or have end-stage renal disease (ESRD).

- **Part A** of Medicare is free and covers inpatient costs, nursing facilities, home healthcare and hospice care.
- **Part B** requires a premium payment and covers outpatient care, x-rays and lab work.
- **Part C** (Medicare Advantage) covers enrollment in HMOs or PPOs if they are approved.
- **Part D** is the Medicare prescription drug benefit.

Persons eligible for Medicaid include pregnant women and children under the age of six whose family income is <133% of the poverty level. All children under 18 are eligible if their family income is <100% of the poverty level. Elderly and disabled individuals who are below the poverty level are also eligible. There are no premiums associated with Medicare and most medical services are covered.

> **Review Video: Medicare & Medicaid**
> Visit mometrix.com/academy and enter code: 507454

MEDIGAP AND MEDICARE SELECT

Patients are responsible for Medicare's coinsurance, deductible fees and many medical services not covered, e.g., prescriptions. **Medigap** is private insurance that helps pay these "gaps." Medigap's open enrollment period is 6 months from the date of enrollment in Medicare Part B and age 65 or older. Open enrollment means the patient cannot be turned down or charged higher premiums due to poor health, factors that limit Medigap options after the open enrollment period. Another type of supplemental health insurance is **Medicare Select**. Medicare Select is a health maintenance organization-type policy that specifies the hospitals and in some cases the providers a patient must use, unless there is an emergency. Due to the provider restrictions, Medicare Select usually offers more reasonable premiums than Medigap policies.

EXAMPLES OF WHEN INSURANCE OTHER THAN MEDICARE PAYS PROVIDERS FIRST

Many people have **both** Medicare and private health insurance coverage. The private policy will pay first when:

1. The patient is 65 or older, and the patient or spouse works for a company (20 or more employees) that provides a group health plan.
2. The patient is disabled, and the patient or family member works for a company (100 or more employees) that provides a large group health plan.
3. The patient has End-Stage Renal Disease and either group plan coverage or COBRA, and is within his or her first 30 months of Medicare eligibility.
4. The patient is covered for the illness or injury under worker's compensation, the federal black lung program, or no-fault or liability insurance.

ITEMS COVERED BY MEDICARE UNDER THE BALANCED BUDGET ACT OF 1997

The Balanced Budget Act of 1997 provided **coverage of preventive care** recognizing it as cost-effective. Procedures covered include:

- One influenza vaccination per year and one pneumococcal vaccine per lifetime.
- One mammogram for women over 40 with no Part B deductible.

239

- One PAP smear and one pelvic exam every 3 years, unless the woman is at high risk and the Part B deductible waived and one colorectal cancer screening each year for people over 50.
- Diabetic education and glucose test strips to achieve outpatient self-management.
- Osteoporosis bone mass tests for people who are clinically at risk for osteoporosis.
- Yearly prostate cancer screening for men over 50.

MEDICAID

Medicaid is a national insurance program, created by Title XIX of the Social Security Act, for the poor and "needy" in all states and territories. There are no "out of pocket" medical expenses for persons covered by Medicaid. Medicaid is funded by federal and state governments and usually administered by state welfare or health departments. Although coverage varies from state to state/territory, it must always cover inpatient hospital care and outpatient services, physicians' services, skilled nursing homes for adults, laboratory and x-ray services, family planning services, and preventative and periodic screening, diagnosis and treatment for children under age 21.

CATEGORICALLY NEEDY AND NEEDY ELIGIBILITY GROUPS

Title XIX of the Social Security Act established Medicaid as a national insurance program for the poor and categorically or medically needy. States set the eligibility requirements using the minimum standards set by CMS. **Categorically needy** are families and certain children who qualify for public assistance, e.g., Aid to Families with Dependent Children (AFDC) or Supplemental Security Income (SSI), and include the aged, blind and physically disabled adults and children. **Medically needy** are eligible individuals or families with sufficient earnings to meet their basic needs but do not have the resources to pay healthcare bills. Low income is not the only criteria for Medicaid eligibility; assets and other resources are considered. Medically needy often qualify for coverage due to excessive medical expenses and the benefits may be confined to that specific illness only, e.g., tuberculosis (TB).

SCHIP PROGRAM AND OASDI

SCHIP is the State Children's Health Insurance Program. It was established in 1997 by the federal government to provide matching funds to states for health insurance coverage for children. States set their eligibility following federal guidelines. Recipients must have low income, not be eligible for Medicaid and have no health insurance coverage. SCHIP covers, at a minimum, inpatient and outpatient hospital services; doctors' surgical and medical services; laboratory and x-ray services; and well-baby and child care, including immunizations. **OASDI** is the Old-Age, Survivors and Disability Insurance program which is the centerpiece of the Social Security Act. It provides hospital insurance to the elderly and supplementary medical insurance for other medical costs.

TYPES OF HEALTH INSURANCE COVERAGE

Indemnity health insurance plan is a legal entity, licensed by the state insurance department, providing reimbursement for healthcare claims. Managed indemnity companies are those who have adopted cost-saving approaches to healthcare coverage. **Self-insured** is an alternative option adopted by many companies where all or part of the coverage risk, up to a threshold amount, is assumed by the employer rather than an insurance company. For costs incurred over the individual employee's threshold amount, the employer purchases a re-insurance or stop-loss policy, which then pays the remainder of a claim. **Automobile insurance** provides coverage for medical expenses and lost wages when the car owner/policy holder has an accident. They must also be aware that when auto insurance maximums are reached, the healthcare plan may be used to complete treatment. Many auto accidents go to court and the Case Manager records may be subpoenaed. **Managed Care** is a cost-containment healthcare system overseen by an organization other than the physician or patient. Managed care encompasses HMOs (health maintenance

240

organizations), PPOs (preferred provider organizations), EPOs (exclusive provider organizations), and POS (point of service) plans.

HEALTH CARE REFORM

Health care reform initiatives are spurring the switch from paper to electronic health records and sharing of health care information among health care providers, increasing the demand for **health information technology** and people with expertise in **informatics**. New programs have been developed to focus on wellness with an increased emphasis on cost-effective measures because of increases in health costs. Internal data analysis and research are becoming important means by which to identify waste, institute best practices, and reduce costs. Increasing numbers of people are covered by health plans, even those with preexisting conditions, placing more demand on health care providers for services. There is an increased need for health literacy so that people are better informed about the services available, especially those newly insured. Medicaid costs have increased, resulting in some cutbacks in care. Early transfer from acute care facilities to extended care or home health care is also increasing.

HEALTH IMPACT ASSESSMENT

Health impact assessment is a method of assessing the potential effects of a health policy or health program on the overall health of the population targeted by the policy or program. The purpose of health impact assessment is to maximize the benefits of health programs (in addition, of course, to minimizing the negative impact that the program may potentially have). There are typically 5 steps involved in the health impact assessment project; these steps include a screening process to ensure that the program is necessary or beneficial; scoping, which determines which population(s) will be impacted by the program; identification and assessment of all potential health impacts if the program is mandated; decision making and recommendations based on the assessment of potential impact; and evaluation and monitoring, which continues throughout the life of the program.

Creating and Modifying the Plan of Care

MODIFYING A PLAN OF CARE AFTER EVALUATING PATIENT OUTCOMES

After evaluating patient outcomes, the plan of care may be **modified** in a number of ways:

- **Change in nursing diagnosis**: Nursing diagnoses may be deleted if problems are resolved or added if new problems become evident.
- **Change in recommended processes/procedures**: Every process/procedure related to patient outcomes should be evaluated to determine if it needs modification, replacement, or deletion. This is especially true if the nursing diagnoses change.
- **Reconsideration of times/durations**: Patients may require more or less time to achieve outcome goals.
- **Increased collaboration**: Patients' outcomes should be evaluated in relation to the type of collaboration that is present between the patient/family and healthcare providers to determine if patients are collaborating effectively.
- **Examination of the nursing process**: The entire nursing process should be evaluated if patients are not achieving the expected patient outcomes to determine if the fault lies within the process.

241

ADVANCE CARE PLANNING

Advance care planning is the process of planning for potential medical situations or crises that would impact a person's health or disability. It involves considering potential situations that could occur before they actually happen and then making plans for what to do in case those situations were to occur. Advance care planning gives people **security** about health care in the future, in case they are unable to make medical decisions for themselves. An example of advance care planning is to develop an **advance directive**, which guides clinicians as to the types of treatments the patient would like if he/she became unable to make those decisions. Advance care planning may also involve appointing a power of attorney to make legal decisions regarding medical care. Taking steps to plan for potential problems through advance care planning provides peace of mind for people to face the future with possible health problems.

ROLE OF NURSE PRACTITIONER

Advance care planning outlines the **desires of the patient** and has been planned in advance. If the patient is unable to make decisions, the advanced care plan speaks the wishes of the patient. Nurse practitioners can play a crucial role in helping patients with advance care planning by beginning the conversation with a patient about whether or not they have an advance care plan in place, and guiding the patient on steps to create one if the patient does not have one. The nurse practitioner should be available to explain disease processes and expectations regarding symptoms and pain that could occur based on the patient's condition, as well as procedure options and their ability to prolong life. The nurse practitioner can also explain what types of care can be provided in different settings and answer questions about quality at the end of life. It is also the nurse practitioner's responsibility to be aware of what type of advance care planning a patient has in place, especially if the patient has a terminal or chronic disease. If something were to happen, the nurse practitioner's **awareness of the patient's wishes** will guide her decision making for the patient's care. Finally, when applicable, the nurse practitioner can use the patient's advanced care planning to write orders for the patient that hospital personnel can actually follow, such as translating an advanced directive that states the patient does not want CPR into an actual Do Not Resuscitate Order.

STANDARDS OF ADVANCE PRACTICE

The family nurse practitioner (FNP) is guided by the **standards of advance practice**, which provide the framework for practice and describe the FNP's responsibilities related to the values and priorities of the profession:

- **Care process**: In assessing, diagnosing, developing, and implementing a plan of care, and evaluating the patient's response, the FNP must use the scientific method and national standards as the basis for care.
- **Establishing priorities**: Providing education and encouraging the patient/family to take an active role in self-care is of primary concern. The FNP must ensure that the patient can make informed decisions. The FNP must assist the patient through all aspects of health care to ensure patient safety and optimal care.
- **Collaboration**: The FNP is a member of the interdisciplinary health team and consults with others when appropriate and refers the patient to specialists as needed. When collaboration is mandated by law, the FNP complies with all requirements.

Professional Role

Healthcare Informatics and Technology

EHR

The Healthcare Information and Management Systems Society (HIMSS) define the **electronic health record (EHR)** as a "secure, real-time, point-of-care, patient-centric information resource for clinicians."

HIMSS has also published a series of guidelines for EHR known as the HIMSS Electronic Health Record Definitional Model. According to the model, the EHR should record and manage information for both the short- and long-term. The EHR should be the healthcare professional's main resource when taking care of patients. Evidence-based care can be planned using the EHR on both the individual and community level. Another important job of the EHR is its use in continuous quality improvement, performance management, risk management, utilization review, and resource planning. The EHR aids in the billing process as well. Finally, the EHR is a boon to evidence-based research, clinical research, and public health reporting. Since it is computerized, clinicians are assured that the EHR information is up to date and relevant for patients and research protocols.

SAFEGUARD AGAINST HOSPITAL ERRORS

Traditionally, the patient chart consisted of a clipboard with admission notes, progress notes, lab orders and results, and other patient information. There existed the potential for the chart to be lost or misplaced; in addition, serious errors in medication, patient identification, and ordering of tests could be attributed to a clinician's inability to decipher another clinician's handwritten notes. This one set of notes also made it difficult for other clinicians and allied health personnel in other departments to assess the patient. The advent of the electronic medical record helped to eliminate some of the problems associated with paper charts. Since the notes are entered into a computer system, illegible handwriting is no longer a source of error. The computerized system also allows clinicians in other areas of the hospital to access necessary information on patients, which improves the communication between clinicians and departments.

STANDARDS FOR COMPUTERIZED SYSTEMS USED IN HEALTHCARE

The Joint Commission has described the need for **computer system standards** in the following areas:

- Access to **databases** that are located outside the organization and used to compare information, need to be supported and secured.
- **Patient confidentiality** related to personal health information (PHI) and data security must be ensured.
- **Knowledge-based systems** should be developed and promoted to allow resident organizational expertise to be used throughout the organization.
- A means to **link physician information systems** while protecting patient privacy and data security.
- Projects that are designed to **achieve quality improvements** should be supported.
- Data integrity and overall system security must be ensured.
- **Procedural controls** that are currently in place for documentation should be integrated into the new computerized standards.
- A **regular assessment** of needs and system capacity for growth should be supported.

243

IMPORTANT FACTORS IN INFORMATION SYSTEMS IN THE ACCREDITATION PROCESS

The Joint Commission outlined factors it believes are important for **information standards**:

- Measures must be adopted that are designed to **protect an individual's personal health information**. This may be accomplished by limiting access to information based on a user's need to know, having strict policies regarding the removal of records, and making sure data is physically and electronically safeguarded.
- A **national standard for data entry** should be created and followed. All users should be trained both in system use and information management. Educational courses may include lectures on how information that is entered into a computer system is transformed into data that can later be used to perform statistical analysis and support decision-making.
- All information should be available both on the computer and in print form.

CURRENT PROCEDURAL TERMINOLOGY CODES

Current procedural terminology (CPT) codes were developed by the American Medical Association and used to define those **licensed to provide services** as well as **medical and surgical treatments, diagnostics, and procedures**. The CPT 2012 codes cover specific procedures as well as typical times required for treatment. The CPT codes are usually updated each October with revisions (additions, deletions) to coding. The use of CPT codes is mandated by both the Centers for Medicaid and Medicare and the Health Insurance Portability and Accountability Act (HIPAA) to provide a uniform language and to aid research. These codes are used primarily for billing purposes for insurance (public and private). Under HIPAA, Health and Human Services has designed CPT codes as part of the national standard for electronic health care transactions. **Category I codes** are used to identify a procedure or service. **Category II codes** are used to identify performance measures, including diagnostic procedures. **Category III codes** identify temporary codes for technology and data collection.

HIPAA PRIVACY PROVISIONS

The Health Insurance Portability and Accountability Act (HIPAA) addresses the rights of the individual related to privacy of health information. The NP must not release any information or documentation about an individual's **condition or treatment** without consent, as the individual has the right to determine who has access to personal information. Personal information about the individual is considered **protected health information** (PHI), and consists of any identifying or personal information about the individual, such as health history, condition, or treatments in any form, and any documentation, including electronic, oral, or written. Personal information can be shared with spouse, legal guardians, those with durable power of attorney for the individual, and those involved in care of the individual, such as physicians, without a specific release, but the individual should always be consulted if personal information is to be discussed with others present to ensure there is no objection. Failure to comply with HIPAA regulations can result in the NP and their employer being held liable and assessed heavy penalties.

SENSITIVE INFORMATION

Sensitive information is classified under HIPAA as protected health information (PHI) and includes

- Any information about an individual's past, present, or future health or condition (mental or physical).
- Any information describing health care provided to the individual.
- Any information related to payment for healthcare services that can be used to identify the person.

- Any identifying information: name, address, Social Security number, birthdate, and any document or material that contains the identifying information (such as laboratory records).

Information that is to be shared or aggregated for research purposes must first be deidentified. The HIPAA privacy rule provides two methods of deidentification:

- Expert determination (based on applying statistical or scientific principles): The expert must have appropriate knowledge and must document the method and analysis results.
- Safe harbor (removing 18 types of identifiers): includes names, geographic information, zip codes, telephone numbers, license numbers, account numbers, fax numbers, serial numbers of devices, email addresses, URLs, full-face photographs, dates (except year) and biometric identifiers.

INDIVIDUAL RIGHTS REGARDING HIPAA

HIPAA individual rights:

- **Covered entity duties** and contact name, title, or telephone to take delivery of grievances with effectual month, day, and year.
- **Access**, with the right to look at and get a copy of PHI in a designated record set (DRS) in an appropriate time frame.
- **Amendment**, so that each patient has the right for Covered Entity amend PHI, but this can be not approved by Covered Entity even when the account is correct and finished.
- **Accounting**, so that the patient has the right to get a record of what information was given out from PHI for 6 years (or less) before the month, day and year that it was asked for.
- **Asked for restrictions**, so that the patient can ask for limitations of utilization and giving out PHI (although Covered Entity may not allow).
- **Confidential communication**, so that the provider has to allow and accommodate justifiable desires for PHI information that was exchanged by alternative methods and to alternative places.
- Grievances to covered **Entity**.
- Grievances to **Secretary** (HHS/OCR).

FORMATS FOR MEDICAL RECORD DOCUMENTATION

Different methods of documentation used for patient's medical records include:

- **Narrative**: This charting provides a chronological report of the athlete's condition, treatment, and responses. It is an easy method of charting but may be disorganized and repetitive, and if different people are making notes, they may address different issues, making it difficult to get an overall picture of the athlete's progress.
- **SOAP** (subjective data, objective data, assessment, plan of action): This problem-oriented form of charting includes establishing goals, expected outcomes, and needs and then compiling a numbered list of problems. A SOAP note is made for each separate problem.
  - o *Subjective*: Client's statement of problem.
  - o *Objective*: Trainer's observation.
  - o *Assessment*: Determination of possible causes.
  - o *Plan*: Short- and long-range goals and immediate plan of care.

If there are multiple problems (edema, pain, restricted activity, etc.,), this charting can be very time-consuming, as each element of SOAP must be addressed. SOAP notes may be extended to **SOAPIER** (including intervention, evaluation, and revision.)

CHARTING BY EXCEPTION

This form of charting was developed in response to problem-oriented charting in an attempt to simplify charting. It includes extensive use of flow sheets and intermittent charting to document unexpected findings and interventions. However, because this focuses on interventions, those problems that require no particular intervention (such as increased discomfort after a particular exercise) may be overlooked, and charting may not be adequate for legal challenge because lack of charting may be construed as lack of care of evaluation.

COMPUTERIZED CHARTING

All record keeping is done electronically, usually at point of care. Computer terminals must be placed where others cannot read notes being written, and access must be password protected. These systems may include clinical decision support systems (CDSS), which provide diagnosis and treatment options based on symptoms. Computerized charting has some advantages: it is legible, tamper-proof, and tends to reduce errors as many systems signal if a treatment is missed or the wrong treatment given.

PIE

PIE (problem, intervention, evaluation) is a problem-oriented form of charting that is similar to SOAP but less complex. It combines use of flow sheets with progress notes and a list of problems. Each problem is numbered sequentially and a PIE note is made for each problem, at least 1 time daily (or during treatment, depending on the frequency).

DAR

Focus/DAR (data, action, response) is a type of focused charting that includes documentation about health problems, changes in condition, and athlete concerns or events, focusing on data about the injury, the action taken by the trainer, and the response. The written format is usually in 3 columns (D-A-R) rather than traditional narrative linear form. A DAR note is used for each focus item.

FLOW SHEETS

Flow sheets are often a part of other methods of charting and are used to save time. They may be used to indicate completion of exercises or treatments. They usually contain areas for graphing data and may have columns or rows with information requiring checkmarks to indicate an action was done or observation made.

CRITICAL PATHWAYS

Critical pathways are specific multi-disciplinary care plans that outline interventions and outcomes of diseases, conditions, and procedures. Critical pathways are based on data and literature and best practices. The expected outcomes are delineated as well as the sequence of interventions and the timeline needed to achieve the outcomes. There are many different types of forms that appear similar to flow sheets but are more complex and require more documentation. Any variance from the pathway or expected outcomes must be documented. Critical pathways are increasingly used to comply with insurance limitations to ensure cost-effective timely treatment.

GOOD USE OF DOCUMENTATION DURING AND AFTER PATIENT VISITS

Documentation provides invaluable diagnostic and treatment information, but it is also a legal document that outlines the **effectiveness of care** provided by the nurse practitioner:

- Make note of any **complaints** and evaluate them in relation to health history and assessment to determine if there are changes or additional cause for concern.
- Note serious **concerns** about the child on the record and record that the child/parent was advised of the need for any follow-up testing or visits.
- Identify **abnormal findings** of any kind in the documentation as well as when the child/parent was informed and intervention.
- Note **referrals** in the documentation as well as the fact that a request was made for a report.
- **Flag** the documentation (electronically if computerized or with other coding methods if using standard paper documentation) for any type of follow-up to ensure that it is done and recorded.
- Document all **follow-up communications**, such as telephone calls, e-mails, and letters, including the date, time, and communication content.

DOCUMENTATION TO SHOW THAT SERVICES PROVIDED ARE CONSISTENT WITH INSURANCE COVERAGE

The family nurse practitioner should always verify **coverage** provided by the patient's insurance plan and ensure that the type of **billing** (direct or incident-to) is supported by the plan. When billing for services, the correct CPT/HCPCS level II code (or ICD-10 PCS for inpatients) should be provided and should be appropriate for the ICD-10-CM diagnostic code. All codes should be supported in the documentation and should indicate the medical necessity for the services provided. If the diagnosis is not confirmed or is uncertain, then an "unspecified" diagnostic code for the symptoms should be utilized. Each encounter should include the reason for the encounter and any history and test results that are relevant as well as the type of physical exam conducted. Assessment should include the diagnosis, treatment provided, and the plan of care and follow-up. Documentation must meet the requirements of the payer, and this may vary somewhat.

MEDICARE DOCUMENTATION GUIDELINES

HISTORY

Under Medicare documentation guidelines, **history** includes the assessment of 4 elements:

- **Chief complaint** (CC): Reason for patient encounter, including symptoms, problems, patient condition, and diagnosis. Always required.
- **History of present illness** (HPI): Location of symptoms, quality, severity (1-10 scale), duration, timing, context, modifying factors, and associated signs and symptoms. The number required depends on the type of history billed.
- **Review of systems** (ROS): Review of all body systems (minimum of 10) and constitutional symptoms.
- Pertinent past, family, and/or social history (PFSH): Current and previous.

There are 4 types of history, with each type requiring specific elements and a specific billing code:

Type	HPI	ROS	PFSH
Problem-focused	Brief (1-3)	----	----
Expanded problem-focused	Brief	Problem-pertinent	----
Detailed	Extended (≥4)	Extended	Pertinent
Comprehensive	Extended	Complete	Complete

EXAMINATION

Under Medicare documentation guidelines, **examination** requires an inspection of one or more organ systems. Abnormal findings require elaboration, while ordinary findings may be documented by "negative" or "normal." There are 4 types of examinations, with each type requiring specific performance and documentation elements and specific billing code.

Type	Single Organ system	Multi-system
Problem-focused	1 to 5 elements	1 to 5 elements
Expanded problem-focused	Minimum of 6 elements.	Minimum of 6 elements.
Detailed	Minimum of 12 elements OR Minimum of 9 elements for eye and psychiatric examinations.	Minimum of 6 organ systems/body areas with two elements for each OR 12 elements in 2 or more organ systems/body areas.
Comprehensive	All elements.	Minimum of 9 organ systems/body areas with at least 2 elements for each.

MEDICAL DECISION-MAKING

Under Medicare documentation guidelines, **medical decision-making** relates to the complexity of the diagnosis or medical data and associated risks or morbidity/mortality. Complex decision-making includes decisions made without a diagnosis or conditions requiring further consultation. Data is considered complex if old records must be reviewed or test results are contradictory/unexpected. There are 4 types of medical decision-making, with each type requiring specific performance and documentation elements and specific billing codes:

Type	Diagnoses or management options	Amount or complexity of data	Risk of complications, morbidity, mortality
Straight-forward	Minimal	Minimal/None	Minimal (one or minor)
Low complexity	Limited	Limited	Low (Two or more minor, one stable chronic, or one acute uncomplicated)
Moderate complexity	Multiple	Moderate	Moderate (progression, uncertainty, two stable chronic)
High complexity	Extensive	Extensive	High (exacerbations, risks, abrupt changes, complications)

FACTORS NECESSARY FOR INFORMATION QUALITY

Quality information is defined by the following factors:

- **Timeliness:** The necessary data is available (and retrievable) as needed.
- **Precision:** System dictionaries shall describe uniform wording and clear definitions.
- **Accuracy:** The data should be as error-free as possible.
- **Measurability:** The information should be quantifiable so that comparisons can be made.
- **Independently verifiable:** The integrity of the information remains constant regardless of the individual reporting it.
- **Availability:** The information should be accessible where it is needed. In the hospital or clinic environment, the information should usually be available at the patient's location.

CLINICAL DECISION SUPPORT SYSTEMS AND ELECTRONIC PRESCRIBING

Clinical decision support systems are interactive software programs that assist the family nurse practitioner to make clinical decisions. The two basic components of the CDSS are a **knowledge base** and an **inferencing mechanism**. The family nurse practitioner enters data (knowledge) into the system and the program applies logic through the inferencing mechanism to the data to produce an output (the decision). CDSS may assist with diagnoses or may be used for alerts and reminders, clinical guidelines (based on best practices), online information retrieval (such a drug information), and clinical protocols.

Electronic prescribing: E-prescribing allows computerized ordering of medications and treatments from local pharmacies and mail-order pharmacies, such as Express Scripts®. E-prescribing reduces errors resulting from illegible writing, illegal alterations, or miscommunications. E-prescribing saves time and is more convenient for the patient. Computerization increases formulary adherence as well. Most programs send reminders to ordering physicians and/or patients so that prescriptions remain current.

Scope and Standards of Practice

LIFELONG LEARNING WHILE GAINING SKILLS NEEDED IN PRACTICE

Lifelong learning requires commitment on the part of the nurse, the organization/facility, and the profession:

- The nurse must make an **individual commitment to lifelong learning** as a professional and ethical responsibility. This includes not only experiential learning but also formal learning, such as classes, and additional training.
- The organization/facility must give lifelong learning a **priority focus**, requiring that staff acquire ongoing education, both formal and informal. This commitment requires an allocation of resources to increase salaries, provide release time, and reimburse educational costs.
- The profession must continue to lobby legislatures throughout the United States to require that **all licensed nurses complete continuing education courses** to renew their licenses to practice. The profession, through professional organizations and the efforts of all nurses, must continue to set standards for certification and continue to delineate the evolving role of nurses as part of the healthcare team.

SCOPE OF PRACTICE FOR APRN

The scope for the APRN is dependent on each state and what the advanced practice registered nurse (APRN) in this position can do beneath the Nurse Practice Act for that state. The scope gives guidelines instead of particular directives. There is a big range, depending on the state. Many times, the scope is founded on what is allowed legally both in the state and in the nation. The initial Scope of Practice for PNPs occurred in 1983 by the National Association of Pediatric Nurse Practitioners. This has been updated in 1990 and in 2000. Scope is always changing and improving.

NURSING PRACTICE ACTS

See the NCSBN Web site to find the complete list of state practice acts (not for every state, but 31 states are included): http://www.ncsbn.org. An authorizing board of nursing is available in every state to lead statutes with regard to licenses for an RN. They have responsibility for how titles are used, scope of work, and how to handle discipline cases. Nurse practice acts come out of statutory law.

CERTIFICATION FOR APRN

The government has no responsibility for **certification**. An agency or group verifies that the nurse has a license and has finished specific, set-forth standards as must be met in the particular area of expertise. It might be necessary to receive a state license or reimbursement. It is necessary to become an APRN in certain states.

Writing Prescriptions

NPs and Certified Nurse-Midwives (CNM) have had the ability to write certain **prescriptions** since the mid-1970s. Since 1998, every state allows a degree of ability to write prescriptions. It is necessary that pharmacology instruction be included in the master's degree; the APRN has to get continued instruction to keep the authority to write prescriptions. Certain guidelines differ between the states. The range of what prescriptions are allowed is different between the states. Total ability for prescriptions includes the capability to get a federal DEA registration number.

PRESCRIPTION AND DIAGNOSTICS

Both prescribing medications and treatment and ordering diagnostic tests are within the **scope of practice** of nurse practitioners, but as with other aspects of practice, each state establishes how that will be carried out. Additionally, insurance reimbursement varies from one area to another and must be considered:

- **Prescription**: Terminology varies from state to state with nurse practitioners allowed to "furnish" or "prescribe" some types of medications. In some states they may do so independently; in others, they must be "supervised" by a physician under whose auspices they provide care to patients. The nurse practitioner should maintain a list of medications and consider cost-effectiveness when ordering medications.
- **Diagnostics**: Nurse practitioners can order laboratory, electrocardiogram, and radiographic tests for routine screening and health assessment as well as diagnosis based on assessment. There are limitations, depending upon the individual state nursing practice act.

CREDENTIALS FOR APRN

Credentials for APRN are as follows:

- Make sure there is answerability and conscientiousness for proficient work.
- Authenticates that the practitioner has received the correct instruction, has a license, and is certified.
- Compulsory to make sure that the local and national laws are followed. Recognizes the furthered scope for the APRN.
- Allows for needed ways for patients to make a grievance.
- Allows for responsibility for the community by making sure standards of practice are met.
- Debates between the State boards of Nursing and different education accrediting organizations were more heated in the 1990s due to more NP programs coming available.
- National task force with regard to the excellence of NP schools met in 1995. Many organizations were present.
- The government does not have a hand in credentialing.
- Credentials may be obtained through an AACN-acknowledged certifying body.

APRN ACCORDING TO THE NCSBN

According to the National Council of State Boards of Nursing (NCSBN), advanced practice registered nursing (APRN) is acting as a nurse with a **foundation on information and proficiency** that was obtained in basic nursing school. This nurse has a license to be an RN and has completed and received a diploma from graduate school in an APRN program that has been accredited from a nationwide accrediting body. This nurse has up-to-date certification from a nationwide certification board to work in the proper APRN area. Being an APRN defines the nurse as someone that has more responsibility, which may or may not come with more pay or gain for the nurse.

Some **responsibilities** include:

- Give professional education and leadership.
- Handle patient and medical center leadership.
- Support the patient and local area by keeping the ideal concerns for the patient or community.
- Assess reactions of involvement and how well medical routines are working.
- Be in touch with and act together with patients, patient relatives, and colleagues.
- Employ research; get and use new information and equipment.
- Educate others regarding APRN.

Additional advanced practice registered nurse (APRN) **responsibilities** include but are not limited to the following:

- Evaluate the patient, produce and assess information; comprehend higher nursing practice in action at this rank.
- Assess many kinds of information; find differential diagnosis; determine proper medical care.
- Without supervision, determine how to handle difficult patient issues.
- Create a way to identify the condition, create objectives for the patient's medical management, and stipulate the medical routine or plan.
- Identify, set the routine for medical management, oversee, and give out the medical plan. This includes medicine and drugs as appropriate that fall inside of the APRN's area.
- Handle the patient's bodily and mental condition.

- Make sure there is protected and pertinent nursing being done, whether direct or indirect with regard to the patient.
- Keep protected and beneficial surroundings.

FNP's Scope of Practice

Each state has a nurse practice act that outline the **scope of practice** of advanced practice nurses, such as nurse practitioners. Additionally, the American Academy of Nurse Practitioners has established guidelines in relation to activities allowed under scope of practice. Primary responsibilities include activities aimed at health promotion and disease prevention:

- **Assessing** includes history, physical evaluation, screening tests, identifying risks, and ordering routine laboratory/radiographic tests.
- **Diagnosing** includes integrating information from assessment with specific laboratory tests to arrive at a clinical diagnosis.
- **Managing** includes establishing a plan of care, providing interventions and education, referring to other healthcare providers or agencies, and reassessing the care plan based on outcomes.

Nurse practitioners with a specific clinical focus have added responsibilities. For example, pediatric and family nurse practitioners' scope of practice includes:

- **Monitoring** growth and development, assessing risk factors, and differentiating normal from abnormal development in all areas, such as physical, social, and psychological.

Delegation of Tasks to Unlicensed Assistive Personnel

The **scope of nursing practice** includes **delegation** of tasks to unlicensed assistive personnel, providing those personnel have adequate training and knowledge to carry out the tasks. Delegation should be used to manage the workload and to provide adequate and safe care. The nurse who delegates remains accountable for patient outcomes and for supervision of the person to whom the task was delegated, so the nurse must consider the following:

- Whether knowledge, skills, and training of the unlicensed assistive personnel provides the **ability** to perform the delegated task.
- Whether the patient's condition and needs have been properly **evaluated and assessed**.
- Whether the nurse is able to provide **ongoing supervision**.

Delegation should be done in a manner that reduces **liability** by providing adequate **communication**. This includes specific directions about the task, including what needs to be done, when, and for how long. Expectations related to consultation, reporting, and completion of tasks should be clearly defined. The nurse should be available to assist if necessary.

Standards of Advance Practice

The family nurse practitioner must practice within the standards of advance practice and the individual's **scope of practice**, which is directly related to the individual's educational preparation and certification.

A family nurse practitioner (FNP) must have 2 types of licenses/certificates: an RN and an advanced practice certificate. **Advance practice nurses** are those who have completed additional education in an accredited nursing program (usually at a Master's level) and have received certification with a national certifying organization, such as the American Nurse's Credentialing Center or the American Academy of Nurse Practitioners.

The FNP must function legally under the **Nurse Practice Act** of the state in which the person resides. In some cases, an FNP license/certification in 1 state is automatically recognized in other states through the Compact agreement, but advance practice nurses are often excluded from these agreements. Educational experience and scope of practice must relate to patient population in terms of age, disease, diagnosis, and treatment.

PROFESSIONAL ROLE AND POLICY

Advanced nurse practitioners, such as family nurse practitioner are regulated by state rather than federal law, but federal law has some implications. **Laws and regulations** include:

- The **Balanced Budget Act** (1997) provided for reimbursement for care of Medicare patients. FNPs must follow Medicare guidelines for coding. Most regulation of Medicaid is done at the state level, but the Centers for Medicare and Medicaid Services (CMS) of the federal government requires that the states reimburse pediatric and FNPs.
- States must also follow **CMS regulations** in relation to enrolling Medicaid recipients in managed care. This requires a state waiver that must specifically identify the FNP as a primary care provider. If the state has not done this, then the FNP will not be able to care for Medicaid patients in managed care.
- Federal law allows FNPs to supervise care of patients in a **nursing home** but a physician must be available in case of emergency.
- All laboratories, including those in hospitals, clinics, and offices, are under oversight of the **Clinical Laboratory Improvement Amendments** (CLIA), which has regional and state offices. Labs must meet state and federal requirements and may be subject to both state and federal inspection. If an FNP limits office laboratory studies to urine pregnancy, urinalysis (dip stick), blood glucose, fecal occult blood, and office microscopic examination, the FNP may apply to CLIA for an exemption from inspection.
- **National Provider Identifier (NPI) numbers** may be applied for at the CMS website by healthcare providers, including FNPs. This unique identifier number is intended to eliminate the need for multiple identifier numbers.

FAMILY NURSE PRACTITIONER PRIVILEGES

Depending upon the state's nurse practice act, **FNP privileges** vary:

- FNPs may be able to practice independently or in **collaboration/agreement** with a physician, podiatrist, or chiropractor. The type of physician oversight and collaboration required varies considerably. Only 12 states have no collaboration requirement.
- Nurse practitioners can be **reimbursed** by Medicare, Medicaid, the Civilian Health and Medical Program of the Uniformed Services (CHAMPUS), and private insurance. Currently, governmental reimbursement for nurse practitioners is at the rate of 85% of the customary physician reimbursement. However, a billing rate of 100% is allowed with "incident to" billing that allows the physician to charge for services that are incident to practice as though he/she performed the service.
- **Prescriptive authority** varies from state to state. Many states require physician oversight for all or some prescriptions. There are often limits to the types of treatments/drugs that can be prescribed. Only 11 states and Washington, D.C. allow FNPs to be completely independent in prescribing.

DETERMINING WHAT IS WITHIN SCOPE OF PRACTICE

APRNs must consider a number of different factors in determining what is within their scope of practice:

- **State nurse practice acts/legislation**: The APRN must always be in compliance with state regulations, which vary from state to state (especially in relation to issues such as supervision and prescriptive authority). The APRN may be responsible to different agencies in different states. CMS outlines what APRN services will be covered by Medicare/Medicaid, and this affects practice.
- **Professional organizations**: Organizations such as the American Academy of Nurse Practitioners often publish standards related to scope or practice. Certifying agencies provide certification that a nurse has adequate knowledge to function as an APRN.
- **Institutional policies**: Institutions may outline specific limits to practice.
- **Liability issues**: APRNs often must consider risk management and the liability associated with aspects of the scope of practice.
- **Personal choice**: The APRN may limit practice in some way as a matter of self-determination.

CONSULTATION, REFERRAL, AND COORDINATION SERVICES

As part of the scope of practice, the nurse practitioner is able to provide and augment **primary care to children and families** through a number of different services:

- **Consultation services** may include a variety of services, such as assessment of growth and development and risk factors, providing interventions, such as diet and exercise programs, and educating children and parents.
- **Referral services** include referring children to physicians, such as orthopedic specialists, and to organizations or agencies, such as drug rehabilitation programs.
- **Coordination services**, with the nurse maintaining contact and receiving reports from referrals in order to provide an integrated plan of care, serves as a valuable service to children and parents, who often must deal with many different healthcare providers who have little or no contact with each other. This type of service can prevent unnecessary duplications of service but also ensure that findings are not overlooked.

TRANSLATIONAL SCIENCE AND TWO AREAS OF TRANSLATION RELATED TO THE NURSE PRACTITIONER

Translational science is a multi-disciplinary approach to science that attempts to bridge the gap between laboratory or research findings and clinical applications and outcomes by analyzing and understanding the processes involved in each stage of translation in order to develop new approaches. Translation involves researchers taking the research findings and developing **interventions** to improve patients' health. The different **phases of translation** include basic research, pre-clinical research, clinical research, clinical implementation, and public health. While some family nurse practitioners may be involved in clinical research, the family nurse practitioner is most often involved in the last two phases of translation:

- **Clinical implementation**: Utilizing new interventions as part of the clinical care of patients, identifying any remaining problems associated with the interventions, and developing new questions.
- **Public health**: Evaluating the effect of the interventions on the larger population to determine if the interventions have improved health outcomes and/or provided prevention.

CLINICAL SCHOLARSHIP

Clinical scholarship is a constant process in which the family nurse practitioner examines practice, questions interventions, makes observations, tests ideas, synthesizes information, and disseminates results through presentations, journal articles, or other means in order to **improve application**. The methods utilized and resultant findings should be peer-reviewed, replicable, and documented. The family nurse practitioner develops, utilizes, and shares new knowledge through 4 processes involved in clinical scholarship:

- **Discovery**: Studying and observing. May include empirical research, historical research, and philosophical inquiry.
- **Integration**: Creating new ideas from multidisciplinary studies in order to advance knowledge and producing writings or other products that show this integration.
- **Application**: Developing clinical knowledge and skills in order to improve the delivery of health care.
- **Teaching**: Transferring of knowledge from the expert nurse to the novice through a learning environment that recognizes differences in learning styles and approaches to teaching and includes development of innovative approaches and new course material as well as mentoring.

Regulatory Guidelines

CONFIDENTIALITY AND CHILDREN

Children, especially adolescents, may have areas of concern in relation to their health or activities that they do not want divulged to their parents. Young people may be uncomfortable addressing concerns verbally and may be more forthcoming if given a questionnaire to fill out as a beginning point for discussion. The nurse practitioner is often faced with ethical concerns about dealing with **confidentiality**, but the best course is to deal with the issue directly by informing adolescents that what they say will be held in confidence within certain limitations:

- **Mandatory reporting requirements** must be upheld, including reports of child abuse, sexual abuse, and communicable diseases.
- **Health endangerment**, such as through the abuse of drugs or alcohol, eating disorders, or suicidal thoughts, must be reported to the parents, while assuring the child that the nurse practitioner will be there to support and help them to discuss these matters with parents.

MALPRACTICE

Family nurse practitioners, as all advance practice nurses, are usually insured for **malpractice** at a higher rate than for registered nurses because their scope of practice is much wider. An FNP may be sued individually or as part of a medical group to which the FNP is associated. Because a suit is a civil matter, loss of judgment may not be reported to the state board of nursing. If a charge of **negligence** is brought to the attention of the board, the board may initiate an investigation and disciplinary action. Negligence may involve a number of failures, such as not referring a patient when needed, incorrect diagnosis, incorrect treatment, and not providing the patient/family with adequate or essential information. Once an FNP has established a duty to a patient—by direct examination or even casual or telephone conversation that involves professional advice—the FNP may be liable for malpractice if he/she does not follow up with adequate care.

NEGLIGENCE

Risk management must attempt to determine the burden of proof for acts of **negligence**, including compliance with duty, breaches in procedures, degree of harm, and cause. Negligence indicates that proper care has not been provided, based on established standards. Reasonable care uses rationale for decision-making in relation to providing care. State regulations regarding negligence may vary but all have some statutes of limitation. There are a number of different types of negligence:

- **Negligent conduct** indicates that an individual failed to provide reasonable care or to protect and assist another, based on standards and expertise.
- **Gross negligence** is willfully providing inadequate care while disregarding the safety and security of another.
- **Contributory negligence** involves the injured party contributing to his/her own harm.
- **Comparative negligence** attempts to determine what percentage amount of negligence is attributed to each individual involved.

PROFESSIONAL LIABILITY

Defining professional **liability** is a function of risk management and ensures that related risks are minimized. Direct providers of care, such as FNPs, must obtain consents for medical care, provide adequate care, and obey drug laws. FNPs may have liability for a wide range of issues, including misdiagnosing, lack of supervision of other staff, providing incorrect or substandard treatment, treating patients outside area of expertise, failure to provide follow-up care, failure to seek necessary consultation, infections resulting from procedures, premature discharge, and lack of proper documentation. Nursing staff may also be liable for improper administration of drugs, failing to follow standard medical procedures, failure to follow orders or take correct oral or verbal orders, failure to report changes in patient's conditions or defective equipment, miscounting sponges and instrument surgical equipment, and avoidable injuries to patients from falls or burns as well as mishandling of patient's personal belongings.

RISK AVOIDANCE AND PREVENTION

Risk management aligns with quality management in determining measures for risk avoidance and prevention. In the analysis process, adverse events may be shown to relate to dysfunction in the organization, increasing risk exposure, so risk management may need to take steps to decrease this exposure:

- **Financial management** includes determining both risk retention and risk transfer.
  - *Risk retention* occurs when the organization assumes financial responsibility for risks.
  - *Risk transfer* occurs when the financial responsibility for risks is transferred, as with insurance policies.
- **Risk event control** involves development of specific programs/processes to limit risk exposure:
  - *Avoidance* is eliminating that which causes risk, such as a particular high-risk program.
  - *Shifting* is changing from internal responsibility for risk to external through contract services or referrals.
  - *Prevention* is making changes in processes to reduce adverse events, such as using disposable equipment to reduce infection rates.

LOSS AND RISK EXPOSURE

Risk management includes **loss prevention**, taking proactive measures to prevent, eliminate loss, and loss reduction, taking reactive measures to decrease potential loss. Risk management must identify risk exposure through continuous data collection of occurrences or events, including external review, patient complaints, financial audits, referrals, observations, and contracts, current litigation, and risky practices. Continuous **analysis** must also be conducted in a number of areas:

- **Liability**, including malpractice and defamation actions.
- **Employer-related issues**, including Worker compensation issues, hiring, terminating, intellectual property losses, and death or disability of employees.
- **Property and environment issues**, including injuries related to equipment or physical plant, chemical or nuclear wastes, and transportation vehicles.
- **Financial or contract issues**, including embezzlement, theft, anti-trust actions related to peer review, contracts, fraud and abuse, and securities violations.

FNP's RESPONSIBILITY IN REPORTABLE DISEASES

The Centers for Disease Control (CDC) issues a list of **reportable diseases**, and each state also has a list, which may include additional diseases, such as cancer or hospital-acquired infections. The nurse practitioner is required to report those diseases in which mandatory reporting is required and should also report diseases of interest that do not require reporting but are a public health concern. Reporting to the CDC is not name-based, so no personal information is maintained at the federal level; however, some state reporting, such as for human immunodeficiency virus (HIV), is name-based, so the nurse practitioner must be familiar with reporting statutes for the state of practice. In some cases (chickenpox) just the total number of cases is reported. Different types of reports are required, depending upon the disease:

- **Written reports** are required for those diseases that require follow-up to identify source of disease or contacts, such as syphilis and salmonella infection.
- **Telephone reports** are required for those diseases in which statistics are maintained, such as measles and pertussis.

STANDARD OF CARE

The **standard of care** is the criteria or guideline provided to nurses and health care providers that defines the quality of care that should be given. High-quality care should be given everywhere, but the standard of care can vary between specific types of care areas, and the related tasks and decisions depend on the area. For example, tasks associated with standards of care for cardiac patients in a critical care unit will vary from task standards for residents of long-term care facilities. Although the standards will be high in quality in both areas, the tasks associated with each are different. Standards of care can be broken down into several steps, including assessment of the patient, nursing diagnosis, identifying patient outcomes, planning for nursing interventions, implementing the interventions, and finally, evaluating the results. Following these steps through the nursing process will help to fully implement the standard of care.

STANDARDS OF CARE AND CLINICAL GUIDELINES FOR OLDER ADULTS

Standards of care and clinical guidelines vary between populations and levels of acuity of care provided. Common standards of care and clinical guidelines among older adults include such measures as patient safety, pharmacologic intervention, and quality of life. Older adults may be at higher risk of falls, impaired skin integrity, the development of certain illnesses or disabilities, and impaired mobility. Common clinical guidelines for nurses working with this population center on improving patient safety and mobility to avoid the risk of falls, improving nutrition to avoid malnutrition and maintain skin integrity, and assist with health screenings and medication administration. Older adults may take many different types of medications to manage their health conditions. Clinical guidelines are in place to assist patients with medication administration as well as knowledge of side effects. Additionally, common clinical guidelines and care standards exist that can help to maintain quality of life among older adults, such as addressing depression and mental health issues.

CLINICAL PRACTICE GUIDING PRINCIPLES AND PRACTICE

Clinical practice guiding principles and practice are needed so that the NP and the patient will know what is suitable with regard to medical treatment. It is different from state to state because of the different nurse practice acts for the states. **Publications and notable references** may be used to determine protocol needs. For instance, in pediatric care, with regard to guidelines for prevention of medical conditions, guidelines include Bright Futures (MCHB), Guidelines for Adolescent Preventative Services (AMA) and Guide to Preventative Services. As examples for pediatric care guidelines for sicknesses, there are asthma (NIH, AAP), hearing screening (NIH, AAP), HIV (AHRQ), otitis media including effusion (AHRQ), pain (AHRQ), and sickle cell disease (AHRQ).

PEDIATRIC ADVANCE LIFE SUPPORT (PALS) GUIDELINES REGARDING LENGTH-BASED RESUSCITATION TAPE

Length-based resuscitation tape is used to estimate weight according to length in infants and small children. The measurement is taken from head to heel with the child in supine position. The results are used to determine **dosages of drugs and sizes of equipment**. Dosages of common emergency drugs are printed on the tape for different lengths although some calculations for volume and concentration may be required. The marked tape is usually extended alongside the child. A straight edge should be used when possible to increase accuracy at both ends. The **Broselow® tape** is commonly used by emergency departments and first responders. Lengths are divided by colors into different "zones," related to length/estimated weight. In some emergency departments, pediatric carts are color coded to correspond to the zones on the tape. It is important to use the tape properly, with the top at the head of the child, colored red (for head) on the Broselow® tape.

CDC ISOLATION GUIDELINES

Through the years, the Centers for Disease Control (CDC) has issued a number of different guidelines for isolation precautions. The 1996 **CDC isolation guidelines** were an update from the "Universal precautions" guidelines that dealt with blood and some body fluids but did not directly address other types of transmission. There are now 2 tiers of isolation precautions. **Tier I** deals with standard precautions that should be in place for all patients:

- Standard precautions include **protection** from all blood and body fluids and include the use of gloves, face barriers, and gowns as needed to avoid being splashed with fluids. **Hand washing** remains central to infection control and should be with plain (not antimicrobial) soap or instant antiseptic. **Private rooms** are used for those who contaminate the environment (uncontrolled diarrhea, cough, etc.) or are unhygienic. If no private room is available, patients with the same type of infection, same colonizing organism, may share a room.

Tier II of the **CDC isolation guidelines** protects from 3 types of transmission:

- The first type provides protection from diseases spread by **small airborne droplets** (<5 mm), including measles, tuberculosis, and Varicella. Airborne precautions include placing the patient in a private room with monitored negative airflow and the door closed. People who are susceptible to the disease, such as those not immune against measles, should not enter the room. Respiratory precautions (a mask) should be worn if the patient has suspected or confirmed tuberculosis. The patient should wear a mask outside of his or her room.
- The second type provides protection from diseases spread by **large airborne droplets** (>5 mm), easily spread by talking, coughing, or sneezing, but do not travel more than 3 feet. Diseases include viral influenza, pertussis, streptococcal pharyngitis or pneumonia, Neisseria meningitides, and mumps. Droplet precautions include private room. Staff and visitors who are within 3 feet of the patient must wear masks, and the patient must wear a mask outside of room.

Tier II of the **CDC Isolation guidelines** includes the third type, contact, which provides protection from diseases spread by direct **hand-to-hand or skin-to-skin contact**, such as those with significant infection or colonization and those who have suspected or confirmed multi-drug resistance, which may include vancomycin-resistant Enterococci and Staphylococcus aureus.

Contact precautions include placing the patient in a **private room** or in a room with someone with the same infection. **Gloves** should be used as for standard precautions but should immediately be removed and hands sanitized after contact with infective material. A clean protective **gown** should be worn inside the room for close contact with patient, including caring for a patient who is incontinent or has uncontained drainage. The patient should not leave the room if possible and equipment should be dedicated for patient use or disinfected before use by other patients.

Some diseases may require some combination of airborne, droplet, and contact precautions: Lassa fever, Marburg virus, and smallpox.

DIAGNOSIS OF DIABETES MELLITUS

The American Diabetes Association Clinical Practice Recommendations outline the 4 **diagnostic categories of diabetes mellitus:**

- **Type 1** with insulin deficiency caused by destruction of β cells.
- **Type 2** with insulin resistance and progressive defect in insulin secretion.
- **Gestational** occurring during pregnancy.
- **Other types**, such as genetic defect, pancreatic disease, or drug induced.

Criteria for diagnosis of diabetes include ONE of the following:

- **Fasting blood sugar ≥126 mg/dL** after 8 hours of fasting. (The hemoglobin A1C and 75-g oral glucose tolerance test [OGTT] are not recommended for initial diagnosis, although A1C should be done on diagnosis and every 3 months to monitor average glucose level.)
- **Hyperglycemic symptoms** (polyuria, polydipsia, weight loss, blurred vision) with non-fasting plasma glucose ≥200 mg/dL. If symptoms are not equivocal, the test should be repeated on another day.
- **Two-hour plasma glucose** ≥200 mg/dL during a 75-g OGTT.

Criteria for pre-diabetes include:

- Impaired fasting glucose: 100-125 mg/dL.
- **Impaired glucose tolerance**: 2-hour plasma glucose of 140-199 mg/dL.

DIAGNOSIS OF GESTATIONAL DIABETES

Assessment of risk should be done at initial visit and further testing for those at high risk: obese, previous GDM or delivery of infant >9 pounds, glycosuria, PCOS, or family history of type 2 diabetes. All women except those at very low risk should be tested at 14-28 weeks of gestation with 1 of 2 methods.

Plasma/serum glucose 1 hour after 50-g glucose load with >140 mg/dL (threshold) diagnosing 80% of those with GDM. Those who exceed this threshold level should have a 100-g OGTT on another day.

100-g OGTT in the AM after 8-hour fast with 2 of the following fasting glucose levels diagnostic of GMS:

- Fasting ≥95 mg/dL
- 1 hour ≥180 mg/dL
- 2 hours ≥155 mg/dL
- 3 hours >140 mg /dL

Very low risk women are <25 years with normal weight, no family or abnormal glucose history, no poor obstetrical outcomes or membership in high-risk ethnic group.

TARGET PLASMA GLUCOSE AND A1C LEVELS FOR TYPE 1 DIABETES IN INFANTS AND YOUTH

American Diabetes Association Clinical Practice Recommendations for **target plasma glucose and A1C levels** for **type 1 diabetes** in infants and youths varies according to age:

Age (yrs)	Plasma glucose before meals	Plasma glucose HS (night)	A1C	Discussion
0-6	100-180 mg/dL	110-200	>7.5% and <8.5%	Increased risk for hypoglycemia.
6-12	90-180	100-180	<8%	Risks for hypoglycemia remain high and complications are usually low pre-puberty.
13-19	90-130	90-150	<7.5%	Individualized goals may be lower, based on benefits and risks.

Hypoglycemia can result in **permanent cognitive impairment** in children <5, so management must recognize that normal plasma glucose levels are usually not attainable. Adolescents often have A1C about 1% higher than adults although the increased use of insulin pumps has helped patients maintain proper levels.

DIABETES MANAGEMENT

The American Diabetes Association Clinical Practice Recommendations for **management of diabetes** include:

- **Complete evaluation**: Appropriate laboratory testing and history.
- **Management plan**: Development of plan and educational goals and strategies.
- **Glycemic control**: Self-monitoring of blood glucose (3-4 times daily if on multiple insulin injections or insulin pump) and hemoglobin A1C (<7%) twice yearly for patients meeting treatment goals and quarterly for those not meeting goals or with change in therapy.
- **Medications**: Intensive insulin (≥3 insulin injections daily or continuous subcutaneous infusion) or insulin analogs for type 1, and oral medications for type 2 if needed (after initial insulin if hyperglycemic).
- **Diabetes self-management education (DSME)**: Education should be provided according to national standards (covering 9 areas of diabetes management) and should include self-management and psychosocial issues in a skill-based approach.
- **Intercurrent illness**: Increased monitoring of blood glucose or blood ketones and intervention may be needed to prevent hyperglycemia or hypoglycemia.
- **Hypoglycemia**: Immediate treatment with 15-20 g glucose for conscious patients, repeated in 15 minutes if self-monitored blood glucose indicates continued hypoglycemia. Snack should be eaten when normal glucose level reached. Those at risk should carry glucagon.
- **Immunizations**: Adults should receive 1 lifetime pneumococcal vaccine and one-time revaccination for those >65 who had original injection >5 years ago or who have nephrotic syndrome, chronic renal disease or immunocompromised. All those ≥6 months of age should have annual influenza vaccine.
- **Medical nutrition therapy** (MNT): Diet modifications should be individualized and may include low fat, low carbohydrate. Saturated fats should be restricted to <7% of total calories and carbohydrates monitored through use of carbohydrate counting or exchanges. Sugar alcohols and non-nutritive sweeteners (aspartame, Splenda® [sucralose]) may be used. Alcohol intake should be limited to 1 drink per day for women and 2 drinks per day for men.
- **Physical activity**: Aerobic activity ≥150 min/week (ideally 30 minutes daily) to 50-70% of maximum heart rate and (unless contraindicated) those with type 2 should do resistance training 3 times weekly.
- **Psychosocial assessment and care**: Screening should be done for such issues as depression, eating disorders, financial resources, psychiatric history, and cognitive impairment.
- **Failure to meet treatment goals**: Assessment of barriers to compliance or changes in treatment may be indicated.

PREVENTION OF DIABETES

RENAL COMPLICATIONS

The American Diabetes Association Clinical Practice Recommendations for **preventing renal complications** of diabetes include:

- **Screening and diagnosis:** Annual test of urine albumin for those with type 1 diabetes for ≥5 years and all type 2 diabetics (from diagnosis). Serum creatinine should be done annually to estimate glomerular filtration rate (GFR) and determine degree of chronic kidney disease.

- **Treatment**: Angiotensin-converting enzyme (ACE) inhibitors or angiotensin receptor blockers (ARBs; with monitoring serum creatinine and potassium) and reduction of protein intake to 0.8-1.0 g/kg body weight per day in early stages of chronic kidney disease and 0.8 g/kg/body weight per day with advanced chronic kidney disease.
- **Glucose monitoring**: Maintaining normal steady glucose levels is critical to avoid renal disease. Between 20-40% of patients with diabetes develop diabetic nephropathy with persistent albuminuria, a marker for both type 1 and type 2.

CARDIOVASCULAR COMPLICATIONS

The American Diabetes Association Clinical Practice Recommendations for **preventing cardiovascular complications** (*the most common cause of morbidity and mortality*) include:

- **Control of hypertension**: Screening, diagnosis, and treatment to lower blood pressure to <140/80 (preferably <130/80).
- **Lipid management**: Lifestyle modifications include diet and exercise. Statin therapy is indicated for overt CVD or those >40 without cardiovascular disease (CVD) but with other risk factors. Lower risk patients should have statin therapy if low-density lipoprotein (LDL) >100 mg/dL or with multiple risk factors. Statin is optional with CVD if LDL is <70 mg/dL.
- **Antiplatelet agents**: Acetylsalicylic acid (ASA) 75-162 mg daily (not recommended <30 years). Combination therapy with clopidogrel if CVD is severe.
- **Smoking cessation**: No patient should smoke. Counseling and intervention should be provided.
- **Coronary heart disease screening**: Combination of ASA, statin, and angiotensin-converting enzyme (ACE) inhibitor may be used to reduce risk of acute cardiovascular events. Metformin and thiazolidinedione should not be used for those treated for congestive heart failure.

NEUROPATHIC COMPLICATIONS

The ADA Clinical Practice Recommendations for **preventing neuropathic complications** of diabetes include:

- **Screening**: Type 1 and type 2 diabetics should be screened for distal symmetric polyneuropathy at initial diagnosis and every year with pinprick, vibration sensation, and 10-g monofilament testing. Type 1 diabetics >5 years and type 2 diabetics at diagnosis should be screened for autonomic neuropathy. Cardiovascular autonomic neuropathy is characterized by tachycardia (>100 at rest), and orthostatic hypotension. Gastrointestinal (GI) neuropathies, such as gastroparesis and esophageal enteropathy, may present as constipation alternating with diarrhea. Genitourinary neuropathy may cause erectile dysfunction. Comprehensive foot exam should include screening for PAD with ankle-brachial index.
- **Education**: All patients must be taught about foot care, including examination of feet and wearing of protective shoes.
- **Treatment**: Maintaining stable glucose levels and smoking cessation is critical. Drug treatments include tricyclic antidepressants (amitriptyline, nortriptyline, and imipramine), anticonvulsants (gabapentin, carbamazepine, and pregabalin), 5-hydroxytryptamine and norepinephrine uptake inhibitors (duloxetine), and substance P inhibitor (capsaicin cream) and other treatments specific to the neuropathy (such as penile implants).

RETINAL COMPLICATIONS

The American Diabetes Association (ADA) Clinical Practice Recommendations for **preventing retinal complications** of diabetes include:

- **Screening**: Type 1 diabetics should be screened for diabetic retinopathy within 5 years of diagnosis and type 2 after initial diagnosis with subsequent yearly exam or 2-3 years if 1 or more yearly exam is normal.
- **Pregnancy**: Women planning pregnancy or already pregnant should be examined during the first trimester with monitoring throughout pregnancy and 1 year after delivery.
- **Treatment**: Prompt referral to ophthalmologist for laser photocoagulation therapy to prevent vision loss.
- **Diabetic retinopathy**, a vascular complication, is the most common cause of new cases of blindness in adults 20-74. Other eye disorders, such as cataracts, are also more common in those with diabetes.

COMPLICATIONS IN CHILDREN AND ADOLESCENTS WITH TYPE 1 DIABETES

About 75% of those diagnosed with **type 1 diabetes** are <18 years. These children, according to the American Diabetes Association Clinical Practice Recommendations, have increased risk for a number of **complications**:

- **Nephropathy**: Screening for microalbuminuria should be done yearly >10 years of age or 5 years of diabetes. Angiotensin-converting enzyme (ACE) inhibitors are indicated for persistent increased microalbuminuria.
- **Hypertension**: Increased blood pressure (BP) should be treated initially with diet and exercise, and if it remains elevated (>95% for age, gender, and height or >130/80 mm Hg) after 3-6 months, ACE inhibitors may be used.
- **Dyslipidemia**: With family history, initial screening >2 years of age on diagnosis. Without family history, initial screening ≥10 years. Annual monitoring is required if lipid findings are abnormal; otherwise, monitoring is done every 5 years. Medical nutrition therapy (MNT) with Step 2 American Heart Association diet is initial treatment with statin for those >10 with persistent elevation and other risk factors with goal of low-density lipoprotein (LDL) <100 mg/dL.
- **Retinopathy**: Screening should be done after 3-5 years of diabetes if the child is ≥10 years. It is most common after puberty and after 5-10 years of diabetes.
- **Celiac disease**: 1-16% of children with type 1 diabetes also have celiac disease, so those with symptoms (weight loss, diarrhea, fatigue, malnutrition, abdominal pain) should be tested for tissue transglutaminase or anti-endomysial antibodies and referred to a gastroenterologist if results are positive and should be seen by a dietitian for education regarding a gluten-free diet.
- **Hypo- or hyperthyroidism**: 17-30% of children with type 1 diabetes also have autoimmune thyroid disease (usually hypothyroidism), so thyroid peroxidase and thyroglobulin antibodies should be checked at diagnosis and thyroid-stimulating hormone (TSH) after diabetes is controlled. TSH should be rechecked every 2 years if normal.

AMERICAN DIABETES ASSOCIATION CLINICAL PRACTICE RECOMMENDATIONS FOR TESTING CHILDREN

The American Diabetes Association Clinical Practice Recommendations advise **routine testing** of asymptomatic **children** who are overweight (BMI >85% for age and sex, weight for height >85%, or weight >120% of ideal) at age 10 or onset of puberty and have at least 2 additional risk factors, which can include:

- **Family history type 2 diabetes** (1st or 2nd degree family member) or maternal history of diabetes or gestational diabetes.
- **High-risk ethnicity**: African American, Native American, Asian, Latino, and Pacific Islander.
- **Indications of insulin resistance** or associated conditions, such as elevated blood pressure, elevated cholesterol levels, or polycystic ovarian syndrome.

The **fasting plasma glucose test** is recommended for diagnosis of children with tests repeated every 2 years. At present, 8-45% of children are presenting with diabetes Type 2 (insulin deficient) although it may be difficult to determine the type with initial diagnosis. Most cases of diabetes are diagnosed during puberty when hormone changes affect insulin, but children as young as 4 have been identified.

AMERICAN DIABETES ASSOCIATION CLINICAL PRACTICE RECOMMENDATIONS FOR TESTING ADULTS

The American Diabetes Association Clinical Practice Recommendations advise **routine testing** of asymptomatic **adults** who are overweight (BMI ≥25 kg/m2) although may be lower in some ethnic groups) with additional factors that put them at risk:

- Lack of physical activity.
- Family history (first-degree relative with diabetes).
- High-risk ethnicity: African American, Native American, Asian, Latino, and Pacific Islander.
- Gestational diabetes mellitus and delivery of infant >9 pounds.
- Hypertension (treatment for hypertension).
- Polycystic ovarian syndrome (PCOS).
- Pre-diabetes indicated by impaired fasting glucose (IFG) or impaired glucose tolerance (IGT) on earlier testing.
- HDL cholesterol level <35 mg/dL and/or triglycerides >250 mg/dL.
- Cardiovascular disease.
- Insulin-resistant conditions, such as severe obesity and acanthosis nigricans.

HIGH BLOOD PRESSURE

The 7th and 8th Reports of the Joint National Committee on Prevention, Detection, Evaluation, and Treatment of High Blood Pressure provide evidence-based approaches to the treatment and prevention of **hypertension,** but the reports differ. The 8th report has been interpreted by some experts as not being extensive enough in defining hypertension. The 7th Report makes important conclusions that experts continue to rely on, specifically that systolic blood pressure (BP) >140 mm Hg poses a greater risk for those age 50 or older than increased diastolic BP. Increased diastolic pressure is more common under age 50 and is a cardiovascular risk factor until age 50, after which increased systolic blood pressure is a risk factor as diastolic pressure tends to level off or decrease after age 50:

- **Normal BP**: <120/80.
- **Prehypertension**: 120-139/80-89 mm Hg.
- **Stage 1 hypertension**: 140-159/90-99 mm Hg.
- Stage 2 hypertension: ≥160/100.

BP should be checked with properly sized, inspected, and validated equipment using the auscultation method. Patients should be seated with feet on the floor for 5 minutes before check with avoidance of caffeine, exercise, and smoking for 30 minutes. At least 2 measurements should be made to arrive at an average reading.

GUIDELINES FOR TREATMENT

The 8th Report of the Joint National Committee on Prevention, Detection, Evaluation, and **Treatment of High Blood Pressure** has developed an **algorithm** that incorporates guidelines for treatment:

Lifestyle modifications ↓ BP		
Initial medication treatment (if goal blood pressure [BP] not reached)↓		
Age > 60 (goal BP < 150/90) OR Age < 60 (goal < 140/90)	Compelling indications* with Diabetes (no CKD)	Compelling indications* with CKD
Nonblack: Thiazide diuretic, ACEI, ARB, or CCB, alone or in combo Black: Thiazide or CCB alone or in combo	Nonblack: Thiazide diuretic, ACEI, ARB, or CCB, alone or in combo Black: Thiazide or CCB alone or in combo	Initiated ACEI or ARB, alone or in combo with another class
Goal BP not achieved↓		
Reinforce lifestyle changes. Increase dosage or add additional medications. Consider referral to hypertension specialist.		

*Heart failure, post-myocardial infarction, coronary disease risk, diabetes, chronic kidney disease, prevention of recurrent stroke, and pregnancy.

EVALUATION GUIDELINES

The 8th Report of the Joint National Committee on Prevention, Detection, Evaluation, and Treatment of High Blood Pressure does not make specific recommendations regarding **reevaluation of hypertension**, but the 7th Report provides important information for the family nurse practitioner to consider that are still relevant:

- **Follow-up**: Recheck in 2 years for normal, 1 year for prehypertension, 2 months for stage 1, and 1 month for stage 2. Immediate treatment for blood pressure (BP) >180/110 mm Hg.
- **Ambulatory BP**: Done for suspected white-coat (reactive) hypertension if no target damage to organs (heart, brain, chronic kidney disease, peripheral artery disease, or retinopathy), drug resistance, hypotension related to antihypertensives, episodic hypertension, and autonomic dysfunction.
- **Diagnostic tests**: 12-lead electrocardiogram, urinalysis, blood glucose, hematocrit, potassium, creatinine (with estimated glomerular filtration rate), calcium, lipoprotein profile.

DASH

The National Institutes of Health and National Heart, Lung, and Blood institute have developed **Dietary Approaches to Stop Hypertension (DASH)**. Nutrient goals (based on a 2100 calorie diet) include:

- Total fat: 27%
- Saturated fat: 6%
- Protein: 18%

- Carbohydrates: 55%
- Cholesterol: 150 mg
- Na: 1500-2300 mg
- K: 4700 mg
- Ca: 1250 mg
- Mg: 500 mg
- Fiber: 30 g

Food group	Daily servings
Grains (whole grains preferred)	6-8
Vegetables and fruits	4-5 each
Fat-free or low-fat milk/milk products	2-3
Lean meat, poultry, fish	<6 (serving=1 ounce)
Nuts, seeds, legumes	4-5 per week
Fats and oils	2-3
Sweets and added sugars	<5 per week

Note: Serving sizes vary considerably, depending on the food, so nutritional label or food guides should always be checked.

DIAGNOSIS AND TREATMENT OF ASTHMA

ASSESSMENT AND MONITORING

The NIH and NHBLI have developed guidelines for diagnosis and treatment of asthma. There are 4 primary components. The first is **Component 1—Assessment and monitoring**. The severity of the disease (including degree of impairment and risks), the degree of control, and the responsiveness to therapy must be assessed. Assessment is emphasized for initial diagnosis and monitoring for continued care. *Diagnosis* is based on:

- **History**: Cough, wheeze, triggers (precipitating factors or comorbid conditions), time of day variations.
- **Physical examination**: Hyperexpansion of thorax, wheezing, increased nasal secretions, polyps, swelling, and allergic skin conditions.
- **Spirometry (for those age 5 and older)**: Episodic symptoms of airflow obstruction that are at least partially reversible and not caused by other conditions. Responsiveness to therapy is demonstrated by forced expiratory volume in 1 second (FEV_1) increase $\geq12\%$ from baseline or $\geq10\%$ of predicted FEV_1 after inhalation of short-acting bronchodilator. Additional pulmonary function studies, bronchoprovocation, chest x-ray, allergy testing, and biomarkers for inflammation may be assessed.

EDUCATION

The NIH and NHBLI have developed guidelines for diagnosis and treatment of asthma. There are 4 primary components. The second is **Component 2—Education**:

- **Education** should begin with diagnosis, should be at multiple points of care (office, hospital, emergency department, school, and home), should involve periodic clinical review, and should include a written asthma action plan for daily management and recognition of exacerbation.
- Patients (adult and pediatric) and family should be aware of **system-based interventions** and should be educated about asthma management through self-monitoring of symptoms and/or peak flow.

- Adult patients should take an **active role** in decision-making through a partnership with the health professional.
- **Allergen-control interventions** should be taught, such as use of impermeable mattress/pillow covers and high-efficiency particulate (HEPA)-filter vacuum cleaners, replacing carpet with vinyl or wooden flooring, and exterminating cockroaches and rodents. Additionally, smoking cessation classes are useful as well as education about preventing exposure to secondhand smoke.

ENVIRONMENTAL FACTORS AND COMORBID CONDITIONS

The NIH and NHBLI have developed guidelines for diagnosis and treatment of asthma. There are 4 primary components. The third is: **Component 3—Environmental factors and comorbid conditions**:

- Patients should be **evaluated** for role of allergens through history and skin testing as well as assessment of occupational exposure. Allergen immunotherapy instituted if indicated and steps taken to reduce exposure.
- Patients should **avoid** allergens, exposure to environmental smoke, and respiratory irritants (such as substances with strong odors). Inhaled allergens tend to precipitate asthma more than food allergens, which are more commonly related to anaphylactic responses.
- Outdoor exertion, nonselective β-blockers, and sulfite-containing foods should be **avoided**.
- Patients with sensitivity to nonsteroidal anti-inflammatory drugs (NSAIDs) and acetylsalicylic acid (ASA) should be counseled about possibility of **exacerbation** with these drugs.
- Those over 6 months old may receive **inactivated influenza vaccination** to avoid complications related to influenza.
- **Air conditioners and dehumidifiers** prevent entry of outdoor allergens (from open windows) and reduce house-dust mite levels.

PHARMACOLOGIC TREATMENT

The NIH and NHBLI have developed guidelines for diagnosis and treatment of asthma. There are 4 primary components. The fourth is: **Component 4—Pharmacologic treatment**: Pharmacologic treatment includes both medications for long-term control and for acute exacerbations. Long-term control includes the use of:

- **Corticosteroids**: Short-term administration is used to reduce symptoms and gain control when initiating long-term therapy and may be used long-term for severe asthma.
- **Cromolyn sodium and nedocromil**: May prevent asthmatic response to exercise or allergens.
- **Immunomodulator (omalizumab)**: Used as adjunctive therapy for those aged 12 or older with allergies and severe asthma.
- Leukotriene modifiers (leukotriene receptor antagonists and 5-lipoxygenase inhibitor): Used for mild persistent asthma.
- Long-acting β2-adrenergic agonists (LABAs) (salmeterol and formoterol): Used for bronchodilation
- **Methylxanthines** (theophylline): Used for bronchodilation.

Medications for relief of acute exacerbations include:

- **Anticholinergics**: Used as adjunct to SABA or alternative bronchodilator.
- Short-acting β agonists (SABAs) (albuterol, levalbuterol, pirbuterol): Used for bronchodilation.
- Systemic corticosteroids: To speed recovery.

LIPID CLASSIFICATIONS

The NIH, NHLBI Report of the National Cholesterol Education Program Expert Panel on Detection, Evaluation, and Treatment of High Blood Cholesterol in Adults classifies total cholesterol, low-density lipoprotein (LDL), and high-density lipoprotein (HDL) to help to determine the need for treatment. **Classification** includes:

- LDL cholesterol:
  - <100: Optimal
  - 100-129: Near optimal
  - 130-159: Borderline high
  - 160-189: High
  - ≥190: Very high
- Total cholesterol:
  - <200: Optimal
  - 200-239: Borderline high
  - ≥240: High
- HDL cholesterol:
  - <40: Low
  - ≥60: High

The optimal LDL goal for those with coronary heart disease (CHD) or equivalent risk is <100 mg/dL; 0-1 risk factors, <160 mg/dL; and more than 2 risk factors, <160 mg/dL. Those with coronary heart disease or equivalent risk factor have a risk of having major coronary events at the rate of >20% per 10 years.

ASSESSMENT OF CHOLESTEROL

The NIH, NHLBI Report of the National **Cholesterol** Education Program Expert Panel on Detection, Evaluation, and Treatment of high Blood Cholesterol in Adults stresses that low-density lipoprotein (LDL) cholesterol is the major cause of coronary heart disease (CHD). Optimal LDL level is <100 mg/dL. **Management** strategies include:

- **Risk assessment**: A fasting lipoprotein profile should be obtained for adults ≥20 every 5 years. Major risk factors that modify LDL goals include smoking, hypertension, high-density lipoprotein (HDL) <40 mg/dL, family history of premature CHD (or risk equivalent, such as diabetes, peripheral arterial disease, abdominal aortic aneurysm, and carotid arterial disease), and age ≥45 for men and ≥55 for women.
- **Determining primary or secondary cause**: If LDL is elevated, causes of secondary dyslipidemia should be assessed prior to treatment. Secondary causes include diabetes, hypothyroidism, obstructive liver disease, chronic kidney failure, and drugs (progestins, anabolic steroids, corticosteroids).

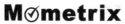

Evidence-Based Practice

Evidence-based practice is the use of current research and individual values in practice to establish a **plan of care** for each individual. Research may be the result of large studies of best practices or individual research from observations in practice about the effectiveness of treatment. Evidence-based practice requires a commitment to **ongoing research and outcomes evaluations**. Many resources are available, such as the *Guide to Clinical Preventive Services* by the Agency for Healthcare Research and Quality of the U. S. Department of Health and Human Services (http://www.ahrq.gov/clinic/cps3dix.htm). Evidence-based practice requires a thorough understanding of research methods to evaluate the results and determine if they can be generalized. Results must also be evaluated in terms of cost-effectiveness. Steps to evidence-based practice include:

- Making a diagnosis.
- Researching and analyzing results.
- Applying research findings to a plan of care.
- Evaluating outcomes.

FUNCTION OF GUIDELINES

Evidence-based clinical guidelines are recommendations for **clinical care practices**. These guidelines are supported by evidence-based practice measures, meaning that the evidence to support the guidelines has been reviewed through a systematic process. Evidence-based practice uses the latest **clinical research results and practices** to define the best methods. It is this evidence that is used to develop the guidelines. Once developed, clinicians should use these guidelines to direct their practices. Evidence-based guidelines may also be used for other measures, such as educational tools for patients and their families. They may back up the practice of clinicians so that if a measure is put into question, such as by insurance companies, the guidelines can be used as a standard of measurement. Evidence-based clinical practice guidelines are also useful for **quality improvement measures**, to determine where upgrades can be made.

DEVELOPING GUIDELINES

Steps to **developing evidence-based practice guidelines** include the following:

1. **Focus on the topic/methodology**: This includes outlining possible interventions/treatments for review, choosing individual populations and settings, and determining significant outcomes. Search boundaries (e.g., journals, studies, dates of studies) should be determined.
2. **Evidence review**: This includes review of literature, critical analysis of studies, and a summary of results, including pooled meta-analysis.
3. **Expert judgment**: Recommendations based on personal experience from a number of experts may be used, especially if there is inadequate evidence based on review, but this subjective evidence should be explicitly acknowledged.
4. **Policy considerations**: This includes cost-effectiveness, access to care, insurance coverage, availability of qualified staff, and legal implications.
5. **Policy**: A written policy must be completed with recommendations. Common practice is to use letter guidelines, with "A" the most highly recommended, usually based on the quality of supporting evidence.
6. **Review**: The completed policy should be submitted to peers for review and comments before instituting the policy.

Support Strategies

Evidence-based practice must be part of the mission and goal of a health care organization, and **strategies** to attain this must be supported at all levels. Information technology tools, such as Internet capability or access to information databases, should be available at the point of care so that health care providers are able to access journal articles and other clinical information. Links may be available through the patient's health risk evaluation as well. All staff should receive **training** in the use of equipment and methods of researching and retrieving information and have an understanding of how to interpret research findings; the inability of health care providers to understand and interpret findings can be a significant barrier to evidence-based practice. Because evidence-based practice often results in change, institutional support for change must be evident and may involve incentives. Continuing education classes should be available on-site to help health care providers gain the research skills they need.

Theory-Practice Gap

The **theory-practice gap** refers to the lack of communication between researchers and clinicians; while researchers are working to develop new treatments and methodologies, clinicians are busy treating patients and may not have the time to educate themselves about what is new in the **research world**. On the other side, the research community is probably not familiar with the **clinical applications** of the current methodologies. It is important for both sides to take an active role in communicating with one another in an effort to bridge the gap; active communication between researchers and clinicians can help disseminate new research ideas and methods into practice, and can educate researchers about what will and will not work in the clinical setting.

The theory-practice gap exists because clinicians and researchers traditionally work in 2 separate worlds; the clinical community is directly involved in patient care on a daily basis, while the research community is removed from the realm of patient care. Both communities, however, have the same **goal**, and that is to **improve patient care and quality of life**. Establishing communication and camaraderie between the 2 communities is incredibly beneficial for both sides. Training sessions in which clinicians are educated about research practices and researchers are trained about clinical practices are a good start. Facilitating research collaborations between researchers and clinicians is another great way to improve communication. Clinician-researchers can function as intermediaries between the 2 communities, and can educate others. The development of standard operating procedures or best practice guidelines for the transfer of knowledge is also important.

Using Evidence-Based Research to Provide Care

Evidence-based research is the use of current research and patient values in practice to establish a **plan of care** for each patient. Research may be the result of large studies of best practices or individual research from observations in practice about the effectiveness of treatment. Evidence-based practice requires a commitment to **ongoing research and outcomes evaluations**. Many resources are available, including:

- Guide to Clinical Preventive Services by the Agency for Healthcare Research and Quality of the US Department of Health and Human Services (http://www.ahrq.gov/clinic/cps3dix.htm).

Evidence-based practice requires a thorough understanding of research methods in order to evaluate the results and determine if they can be generalized. Results must also be evaluated in terms of cost-effectiveness. Steps to evidence-based practice include:

- Making a diagnosis.
- Researching and analyzing results.
- Applying research findings to plan of care.
- Evaluating outcomes.

MODEL OF INTEGRATION FOR APPLYING RESEARCH FINDINGS

Integrating the results of data analysis and research into performance improvement or best practice guidelines varies from one organization to another, depending on the **model of integration** that the organization uses:

- **Organizational:** Processes for improvement are identified, and teams or individuals are selected to participate in different areas or departments, reporting to one individual, who monitors progress.
- **Functional/coordinated:** While staff specialties, such as risk management and quality management, are not integrated, they draw from the same data resources to determine issues related to quality of care and efficiency.
- **Functional/integrated:** While staff specialties remain, there is cross-training among specialties. A case management approach to individual care is used so that one person follows the progress of a patient through the system and coordinates with the various specialties, such as infection control and quality management.

CONSENSUS-BASED PRACTICE

The **nurse practitioner** is assuming an increasingly autonomous role as a health care provider because an emphasis is placed on the nurse practitioner being an "advanced practice" clinician. The nurse practitioner may find him or herself managing a clinic with a high patient volume, or he or she may be considered an equal to resident physicians as far as responsibilities are concerned. Nurse practitioners find that they are given more patient-management responsibilities, and do not have time for teaching, education, and research. This can lead to the nurse practitioner making clinical decisions based on results that he or she observes in the clinical setting (**"consensus-based" practice**) instead of making decisions based on results gained from actual **research-based practice**.

OUTCOMES EVALUATION

Outcomes evaluation is an important component of evidence-based practice, which involves both internal and external research. All treatments are subjected to review to determine if they produce positive outcomes, and policies and protocols for outcomes evaluation should be in place. Outcomes evaluation includes the following:

- **Monitoring** over the course of treatment involves careful observation and record keeping that notes progress, with supporting laboratory and radiographic evidence as indicated by condition and treatment.
- **Evaluating** results includes reviewing records as well as current research to determine if outcomes are within acceptable parameters.
- **Sustaining** involves continuing treatment, but continuing to monitor and evaluate.

- **Improving** means to continue the treatment but with additions or modifications in order to improve outcomes.
- **Replacing** the treatment with a different treatment must be done if outcomes evaluation indicates that current treatment is ineffective.

PROCESS OF CRITICAL ANALYSIS

The nurse practitioner must be taught and understand the **process of critical analysis** and know how to conduct a survey of the literature. Basic concepts related to research include:

- **Survey of valid sources:** Information from a juried journal and an anonymous or personal website are very different sources, and evaluating what constitutes a valid source of data is critical.
- **Evaluation of internal and external validity:** Internal validity shows a cause and effect relationship between 2 variables, with the cause occurring before the effect and no intervening variable. External validity occurs when results hold true in different environments and circumstances with different populations.
- **Sample selection and sample size:** Selection and size can have a huge impact on the results, but a sample that is too small may lack both internal and external validity. Selection may be so narrowly focused that the results can't be generalized to other groups.

Ethical/Legal Principles

RESPECT FOR AUTONOMY

Respect for autonomy is one of the four principles that constitute **principle-based ethics**; it means that people should recognize and respect that each individual has a right to make his or her own choices and formulate his or her own opinions. The individual will make decisions and form opinions based on his or her own **guiding values and principles**. There are exceptions to the principle of autonomy, however, and these occur when the individual is not capable, for whatever reason, of making his or her own decisions. In these cases (which must be evaluated with care), the respect for autonomy may be trumped in the interest of safety for the individual. Typically, the individual will have an appointed family member or caretaker who will be in charge of making decisions in the instance that the individual cannot.

BIOETHICS

Bioethics is a branch of ethics that involves making sure that the medical treatment given is the most **morally correct choice** given the different options that might be available and the differences inherent in the varied levels of treatment. In the acute/critical care unit, if the patients, parents, and the staff are in agreement when it comes to values and decision-making, then no ethical dilemma exists; however, when there is a difference in value beliefs between the patients and parents and the staff, there is a bioethical dilemma that must be resolved. Sometimes, discussion and explanation can resolve differences, but at times the institution's **ethics committee** must be brought in to resolve the conflict. The primary goal of bioethics is to determine the most morally correct action using the set of circumstances given.

COMPLAINTS, GRIEVANCES, AND APPEALS

Healthcare organizations that participate in federal programs, such as Medicare or Medicaid, must have procedures for patient **complaints, grievances, and appeals** as directed by Condition of Participation. Under these regulations, a team of individuals assigned by the governing board of an institution, such as a hospital, must receive any type of complaint rather than an individual. FNPs must have policies in place. Patients must be notified of their right to file complaints, grievances, and appeals. Additionally, state regulations may vary somewhat:

- **Complaint**: A specific oral or written report of lack of satisfaction with the quality of care of processes of care.
- **Grievance**: In some cases, this is the same as a complaint, but sometimes it's differentiated as a formal oral or written complain about quality of care or financial issues.
- **Appeals**: This is a process by which a person can ask for review of previous decisions issued by an organization.

INFORMED CONSENT FOR MINORS

Children <18 (minors), unless legally emancipated, lack the legal right to give **consent** for medical treatments until they reach the **age of majority** except in those areas approved by law, such as for birth control, abortion, and human immunodeficiency virus (HIV) testing, and even these vary from 1 state to another, with some requiring parent notification. However, children must be included in discussions about treatment options in accordance to their age and level of understanding. Because children do not always appreciate cause and effect relationships, the law allows the parents to override decisions of the child and teenager, but forcing a child to have treatment puts the child in a poor emotional state for healing and is cause for ethical concern. Therefore, the nurse practitioner should work with **both the parents and the child**, explaining the benefits and disadvantages of treatment, to try to bring about agreement or assent on the part of the child. This is especially important for adolescents, who are seeking autonomy. Discussions about when to stop treatment and advance directives should include the child whenever possible.

ADVANCE DIRECTIVES
LIVING WILLS, DNR, DURABLE POWER OF ATTORNEY

In accordance to Federal and state laws, individuals have the right to self-determination in health care, including decisions about end of life care through **advance directives** such as living wills and the right to assign a surrogate person to make decisions through a durable power of attorney. Patients should routinely be questioned about an advanced directive as they may present at a healthcare provider without the document. Patients who have indicated they desire a do-not-resuscitate (DNR) order should not receive resuscitative treatments for terminal illness or conditions in which meaningful recovery cannot occur. Patients and families of those with terminal illnesses should be questioned as to whether the patients are Hospice patients. For those with DNR requests or those withdrawing life support, staff should provide the patient **palliative** rather than curative measures, such as pain control and/or oxygen, and **emotional support** to the patient and family. Religious traditions and beliefs about death should be treated with respect.

ISSUE OF ADVANCE DIRECTIVES

An **advance directive** is a way that a patient can communicate to his/her family and physician what kind of **medical intervention** he/she desires. Advance directives are legal documents and the specific laws regarding them vary by state. A patient must be competent in order to make an advance directive. A **living will** is a type of advance directive. It generally describes what type of intervention a patient desires in the face of terminal illness. A "**Do Not Resuscitate**" or DNR order is another type of advance directive. A DNR order must be written in the patient's chart by the attending physician in order to be valid. All discussions with the patient and the family should be clearly documented in the chart. In the absence of a written DNR order, call a full Code Blue and proceed with resuscitation.

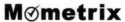

RESOURCES TO FACILITATE RESOLUTION OF ISSUES RELATED TO ADVOCACY AND MORAL AGENCY

Utilization of internal and external sources is an important aspect of **advocacy and moral agency**:

- **Advocacy** is working for the best interests of the patient when an ethical issue arises, despite personal values that might be in conflict.
- **Agency** is openness and recognition of issues and a willingness to act.
- **Moral agency** is the ability to utilize recognition and willingness to take action to influence the outcome of a conflict or decision.

Ethical issues can be difficult to assess because of **personal bias**, and that is one of the reasons that sharing concerns with other resources sources and reaching consensus is so valuable. Issues of concern might include options for care, refusal of care, rights to privacy, adequate relief of suffering, and the right to self-determination. Internal sources might include the ethics committee, whose charge is to make decisions regarding ethical issues. Risk management can provide guidance related to personal and institutional liability. External agencies might include government agencies, such as the public health department.

ETHICAL DECISION-MAKING AND PATIENT ADVOCACY

An environment for **ethical decision-making** and **patient advocacy** does not appear when it's needed; it requires planning and preparation. The expectation for an institution or practice should clearly communicate that nurses are **legally and morally responsible** for assuring competent care and respecting the rights of patients. Decisions regarding ethical issues often must be made quickly with little time for contemplation; therefore, ethical issues that may arise should be identified and discussed. Clearly defined procedures and policies for dealing with conflicts, including an active ethics committee, in-service training, and staff meetings, must be established. Patients and families need to be part of the ethical environment, and that means empowering them by providing patient/family information (print form, video, audio) that outlines patient's rights and procedures for expressing their wishes and dealing with ethical conflicts. Respect for privacy and confidentiality and a non-punitive atmosphere are essential.

ENVIRONMENT

An environment for ethical decision-making and **patient advocacy** does not appear when it is needed; it requires planning and preparation. The expectation for the institution should clearly communicate that nurses are legally and morally responsible for assuring competent care and respecting the rights of patients and other stakeholders. Decisions regarding ethical issues often must be made quickly with little time for contemplation; therefore, ethical issues that may arise should be identified and discussed. Clearly defined procedures and policies for dealing with conflicts, including an active ethics committee, in-service training, and staff meetings, must be established. Patients and families need to be part of the ethical environment, which means empowering them by providing patient and family information (e.g., print form, video, audio) that outlines patient's rights and procedures for expressing their wishes and dealing with ethical conflicts. Respect for privacy and confidentiality and a nonpunitive atmosphere are essential.

VARIABLES IN RESOLVING ETHICAL CONFLICTS

In the health care setting, it is important that ethical conflicts be **resolved** without harming the patient or compromising care. There are several factors that will affect the course and outcome of an ethical conflict. First, the **level of commitment** the clinician has to the patient will determine the amount of effort put forth in resolving an ethical conflict. Second, the **degree of moral certainty** the clinician has will determine the approach to resolution; if the clinician feels that he or she is correct, he or she will most likely not waver in the decision. Third, the **amount of time** available for resolution is important; if the clinician is pressed for time, he or she will most likely come to a decision faster than if there is not a time constraint, in which case avoidance may occur. Fourth is the **cost-benefit ratio**; if the patient refuses to negotiate a certain point, for example, it is not worth the time to the clinician to try to influence the patient's decision.

FACILITATION OF ETHICAL AND CLINICAL CONFLICTS AMONG PATIENT/FAMILY AND OTHER HEALTHCARE PROFESSIONALS

Ethical and clinical conflicts among patients and their families and healthcare professionals are not uncommon. Issues frequently relate to medications and treatment, religion, concepts of truth telling, lack of respect for patient's autonomy, and limitations of managed care or incompetent care. Additionally, healthcare providers are in a position to easily manipulate patients/families by providing incomplete information to influence decisions, and this can give rise to ethical conflicts. **Facilitation** involves questioning and listening, acknowledging each person's perspective while sharing different viewpoints:

- **Open communication** is critical to solving conflicts. Asking what steps could be taken to resolve the conflict or how it could be handled differently often leads to compromise because it allows for exchange of ideas and validates legitimate concerns.
- Sharing **cultural perspectives** can lead to better understanding.
- **Advocacy** for the patients/families must remain at the center of conflict resolution.

ETHICAL ISSUES RELATED TO GENETIC TESTING IN CHILDREN

Genetic testing poses a number of ethical issues because parents can authorize genetic testing without the consent of the minor. The nurse practitioner must serve as an **advocate** for the child in cases where genetic testing is done to determine if the child is a carrier or has an adult-onset genetic disease for which there is no cure or adequate treatment, such as Huntington's disease. In both of these cases, the information derived from testing cannot be used for health promotion or disease prevention, so the parents should be counseled to wait until the child is at least in the teen years and can make an informed decision about whether to have testing. This type of information can be devastating to young people who are not provided adequate support and counseling prior to testing. Some people with adult-onset diseases choose not to be tested, and childhood testing robs them of this choice.

ETHICAL ASSESSMENT

While the terms *ethics* and *morals* are sometimes used interchangeably, ethics is a study of morals and encompasses concepts of right and wrong. When making **ethical assessments,** one must consider not only what people should do but also what they actually do, as these two things are sometimes at odds. Ethical issues can be difficult to assess because of personal bias, and that is one of the reasons that sharing concerns with other internal sources and reaching consensus is so valuable. Issues of concern might include options for care, refusal of care, rights to privacy, adequate relief of suffering, and the right to self-determination. Internal sources might include the ethics committee, whose charge is to make decisions regarding ethical issues. Risk management can provide guidance related to personal and institutional liability. External agencies might include government agencies, such as the public health department.

Research Appraisal

HEALTH BELIEF MODEL

The **Health Belief Model (HBM)** is a model used to predict health behavior with the understanding that people take a health action to avoid negative consequences if the person expects that the negative outcome can be avoided and that he/she is able to do the action. The HBM, as modified, is based on 6 basic **perceptions**:

- **Susceptibility**: Belief that the person may get a negative condition.
- **Severity**: Understanding of how serious a condition is.
- **Benefit**: Belief that the action will reduce risk of getting the condition.
- **Barriers**: Direct and psychological costs involved in taking action.
- **Action cues**: Strategies used to encourage action, such as education.
- **Self-efficacy**: Confidence in the ability to take action and achieve positive results.

This model attempts to encourage people to make changes or take action (such as stopping smoking) in order to avoid negative consequences, so this model—when used for education—focuses on the **negative consequences** (such as quitting smoking to avoid cardiovascular and pulmonary disease).

THEORY OF PLANNED BEHAVIOR

The **Theory of Planned Behavior**, by Icek Ajzen, evolved from the Theory of Reasoned Action in 1985 when studies showed that behavioral intention does not necessarily result in action. The Theory of Planned Behavior is more successful in **predicting behavior**. To the basic concepts of attitudes, subjective norms, and behavioral intentions encompassed by the earlier theory, Ajzen added the concept of perceived behavioral control, which relates to the individual's attitudes about self-efficacy and outcomes. Ajzen's theory shows that **beliefs** are central:

- **Behavioral beliefs** lead to attitudes toward a behavior/action.
- **Normative beliefs** lead to subjective norms.
- **Control beliefs** lead to perceived behavioral control.

All of these beliefs interact to influence intention and action. Basically, this theory relates to the person's **confidence**, based on beliefs and social influence of others, that he/she can actually do an action and that the outcome of this action will be positive. This theory looks at the power of emotions—such as apprehension or fear—when predicting behavior.

THEORY OF REASONED ACTION

The **Theory of Reasoned Action**, developed in 1975 by Fishbein and Ajzen is based on the idea that the actions people take voluntarily can be predicted according to their **personal attitude** toward the action and their **perception** of how others will view their doing the action. There are 3 basic concepts to the theory:

- **Attitudes**: These are all of the attitudes about an action, and they may be weighted (some more important than others).
- **Subjective norms**: People are influenced by those in their social realm—family, friends—and their attitudes toward particular actions. The influence may be weighted. For example, the attitude of a spouse may carry more weight than the attitude of a neighbor.

- **Behavioral intention**: The intention to take action is based on weighing attitudes and subjective norms (opinions of others), resulting in a choice to either take an action or avoid the action.

STRESS APPRAISAL AND COPING THEORY

The **Transactional Stress Appraisal and Coping Theory** is used to evaluate how people cope with stressors by going through a series of appraisals, based on personal ideas and resources (social, cultural) available to the person:

- **Primary appraisal**: The person considers and evaluates the importance of a current or future event that has resulted in stress.
- **Secondary appraisal**: The person considers his/her ability to control the stressor and to cope with it in terms of personal, social resources.
- **Coping**: The person develops strategies based on the primary and secondary appraisal in order to attempt to change the stressor or to think about the stressor in a different way.
- **Meaningful coping**: The person uses coping processes that lead to positive emotions in order to continue coping.
- **Outcomes**: The person sees results of coping.
- **Disposition**: Some people tend to have positive expectations, others look for information, and still others seek avoidance, and these differences in disposition affect coping.

TRANSTHEORETICAL MODEL

The **Transtheoretical Model** focuses on changes in behavior based on decisions of the individual (rather than outside or social influences) and is used to develop **strategies to promote changes in health behavior**. This model incorporates constructs from other theories and attempts to demonstrate the steps a person goes through in changing a problem behavior and having a positive attitude about change. Change is viewed as a process with many stages:

1. **Precontemplation**: The person is either unaware or under-informed about consequences of a problem behavior and has no intention of changing behavior in the next 6 months.
2. **Contemplation**: The person is aware of costs and benefits of changing behavior and intends to change in the next 6 months but is procrastinating and not ready for action.
3. **Preparation**: The person has a plan and intends to instigate change in the near future (<1 month) and is ready for action plans.
4. **Action**: The person is modifying behavior but it counts as behavior change only if behavior meets a set criterion (such as complete abstinence from drinking).
5. **Maintenance**: The person works to maintain changes and gains confidence that he/she will not relapse.

There are 2 **temporal dimensions** to this process:

- The *distance* of the behavior (from the time the process begins to the time change is made.
- The *duration* of behavior (the time from change to relapse).

The model recognizes that there are **intervening variables**: decisional balance (the costs and benefits of change), self-efficacy (confidence in being able to change), and any other variables, such as social, environmental, psychological, or medical, which may affect behavior and change.

During each stage of the process, people go through 10 **processes of change** as they attempt to modify their behavior:

- **Consciousness raising**: Seeking information.
- **Counterconditioning**: Substituting alternative action for problem behavior, such as using relaxation techniques, positive statements, and desensitization.
- **Dramatic relief**: Expressing feelings (positive and negative) about change of problem behavior and solutions.
- **Environmental reevaluation**: Determining the effect the problem behavior has on others and developing empathy.
- **Helping relationships**: Accepting assistance from other to effectuate change.
- **Reinforcement management**: Accepting reward (from self or others) for changing problem behavior.
- **Self-liberation**: Believing change possible and committing to change.
- **Self-reevaluation**: Reevaluating values in relation to problem behavior.
- **Social liberation**: Becoming aware (emotionally and cognitively) of positive lifestyles and feeling empowered.
- **Stimulus control**: Controlling situations in which problem behavior is triggered.

PATHOPHYSIOLOGIC THEORIES

Pathophysiologic theories are theories by which medical authorities attempt to explain why something occurs. These theories should be based on **functional causes of disease**. While theories are based on perceived facts, these facts are sometimes in error. For example, the prevailing theory for many years was that stomach ulcers were caused by stress, which caused increased production of stomach acid, when, in fact, most ulcers are caused by Helicobacter pylori. Thus, as new information is acquired, pathophysiologic theories may change. In some cases, there may be alternate theories as to causation, and each theory may appear supportable or possible, based on current knowledge. Some theorists believe that schizophrenia is a genetic disorder, while others believe that is a metabolic disorder. The goal of pathophysiologic theories is to serve as a **guide** in the pursuit of a **definitive pathophysiological explanation** for a disease.

BLOOM'S TAXONOMY

THREE TYPES OF LEARNING

Bloom's taxonomy outlines behaviors that are necessary for learning, and this can apply to healthcare. The theory describes 3 types of learning:

- **Cognitive** involves learning and gaining intellectual skills. There are 6 categories to master for effective learning, in order:
  - Knowledge
  - Comprehension
  - Application
  - Analysis
  - Synthesis
  - Evaluation
- **Affective** involves recognizing 5 categories of feelings and values, from simple to complex and is slower to achieve than cognitive learning:
  - Receiving phenomena
  - Responding to phenomena
  - Valuing

278

- o Organizing values
- o Internalizing values
- **Psychomotor** involves mastering motor skills necessary for independence. It consists of 7 categories listed from simple to complex:
  - o Perception
  - o Set
  - o Guided response
  - o Mechanism
  - o Complex overt response
  - o Adaptation
  - o Origination

TEACHING RELATED TO SUCCESSIVE STAGES OF COGNITIVE LEARNING

Teaching can relate to successive stages of cognitive learning in **Bloom's taxonomy**:

1. **Knowledge**: Ask for feedback about teaching points.
2. Ask learner to identify equipment, list steps in procedures, and explain.
3. **Comprehension**: Ask learner to explain principles or procedures in own words: Why are things done this way?
4. Ask learner to summarize purpose of procedures.
5. **Application**: Ask learner to solve problems in different situations: What would happen if...? or How could this problem be solved?
6. Ask learner to demonstrate procedures.
7. **Analysis**: Question learner to determine ability to distinguish fact from inference: What would happen if [this complication] occurred?
8. Ask learner to trouble shoot: How do you deal with this problem?
9. **Synthesis**: Ask learner to integrate knowledge to solve problems: How can issues be resolved?
10. **Evaluating knowledge**: Ask learner questions that demonstrate knowledge by explaining or interpreting: Why is this action important? Ask learner to choose the most effective solution to problems.

USE OF PRINCIPLES OF ADULT LEARNING TO DEVELOP TEACHING STRATEGIES

Adults have a wealth of life and employment experiences. Their attitudes toward education may vary considerably. There are, however, some **principles of adult learning** and typical characteristics of adult learners that an instructor should consider when planning strategies for teaching parents, families, or staff:

- Practical and goal-oriented:
  - o Provide overviews or summaries and examples.
  - o Use collaborative discussions with problem-solving exercises.
  - o Remain organized with the goal in mind.
- Self-directed:
  - o Provide active involvement, asking for input.
  - o Allow different options toward achieving the goal.
  - o Give them responsibilities.
- Knowledgeable:
  - o Show respect for their life experiences and education.

- o Validate their knowledge and ask for feedback.
- o Relate new material to information with which they are familiar.
- Relevancy-oriented:
  - o Explain how information will be applied.
  - o Clearly identify objectives.
- Motivated:
  - o Provide certificates of professional advancement and/or continuing education credit for staff when possible.

VISUAL-AUDITORY-KINESTHETIC MODEL OF COGNITIVE LEARNING

Visual-auditory-kinesthetic model of cognitive learning: Not all people are aware of their preferred learning style. A range of teaching materials and methods that relates to all 3 learning preferences (visual, auditory, kinesthetic) and is appropriate for different ages should be available. Part of assessment for teaching involves choosing the right approach based on observation and feedback. Often presenting learners with different options gives a clue to their preferred learning style. Some people have a combined learning style.

Visual learners learn best by seeing and reading:

- Provide written directions, picture guides, or demonstrate procedures.
- Use charts and diagrams.
- Provide photos, videos.

Auditory learners learn best by listening and talking:

- Explain procedures while demonstrating and have learner repeat.
- Plan extra time to discuss and answer questions.
- Provide audiotapes.

Kinesthetic learners learn best by handling, doing, and practicing.

- Provide hands-on experience throughout teaching.
- Encourage handling of supplies/equipment.
- Allow learner to demonstrate.
- Minimize instructions and allow person to explore equipment and procedures.

EFFECTS OF DEVELOPMENTAL STAGE OF LEARNER ON TEACHING INDEPENDENT CARE

Patients at all **developmental stages** should be independent in care if at all possible, especially for chronic conditions:

1. **Infant/toddler**: Caregivers provide care; instruction encourages bonding and acceptance.
2. **Early childhood**: Children learn by participation, such as role-playing, simple explanation, and teaching dolls. Children can be independent in some procedures by kindergarten.
3. **Childhood**: By 6, children may be independent in care at school, but supplies should be available and school nurse knowledgeable about care. Children should be completely independent in care by 6th grade. Parents and child should be taught together.
4. **Adolescence and young adulthood**: The adolescent may be angry and resistive. Extra time and guidance, including visits with other patients, may help. Parents should allow adolescent to be independent in care.

5. **Middle-aged adult**: Adults may have fears about loss of income, status, sexuality, so individualized teaching, including partners, helps them to cope.
6. **Elderly**: Elderly may face physiological and psychological changes. Teaching should provide coping skills and information in stages to avoid overwhelming them.

EVALUATION OF EFFECTIVENESS OF EDUCATION/TRAINING

Education, like all interventions, must be evaluated for **effectiveness**. Two determinants of effectiveness are measures of behavior modification and compliance rates. **Behavior modification** involves thorough observation and measurement, identifying behavior that needs to be changed and then planning and instituting interventions to modify that behavior. An FNP can use a variety of techniques, including demonstrations of appropriate behavior, reinforcement, and monitoring until new behavior is adopted consistently. This is especially important when longstanding procedures and habits of behavior are changed. **Compliance rates** are often determined by observation, which should be done at intervals and on multiple occasions, but with patients, this may depend on self-reports. Outcome is another measure of compliance; that is, if education is intended to improve patient health and reduce risk factors and that occurs, it is a good indication that there is compliance. Compliance rates are calculated by determining the number of events/procedures and degree of compliance.

EDUCATIONAL MATERIALS FOR NURSE PRACTITIONERS

It is impractical to believe that a family nurse practitioner can produce all educational materials, but careful consideration must be given to a number of issues:

- **Price** ranges from free to hundreds or even thousands of dollars for educational materials, which may be handouts, videos, posters, or entire courses or series of courses available online. The nurse educator must first consider the budget and then look for material within those monetary constraints. Government agencies, such as the CDC, often have posters and handouts as well as PowerPoint presentations and videos available for download online at no cost.
- **Quality** varies considerably as well. The nurse educator should consider the goal and objectives before choosing materials, and the materials should be evaluated to determine if they cover all needed information in a clear and engaging manner.
- **Currency** must be considered as well. If material will soon be outdated because of changes in regulations or procedures, then it will have to be replaced.

EDUCATIONAL WORKSHOPS, LECTURES, DISCUSSION, OR ONE-ON-ONE INSTRUCTION

There are many **approaches to teaching**, and the quality professional must prepare, present, and coordinate a wide range of educational workshops, lectures, discussions, and one-on-one instructions on a variety of topics. Planning time for classes should be made as part of the performance improvement plan while allowing for flexibility to contend with unexpected needs. All types of classes may be needed, depending upon the purpose and material:

- **Educational workshops** are usually conducted with small groups, allowing for maximal participation and are especially good for demonstrations and practice sessions.
- **Lectures** are often used for more academic or detailed information that may include questions and answers but limits discussion. An effective lecture should include some audiovisual support.
- **Discussions** are best with small groups so that people can actively participate. This is good for problem solving.

- **One-on-one instruction** is especially helpful for targeted instruction in procedures for individuals.
- **Computer and internet modules** are good for independent learners.

AUDIENCE SIZE AND AVAILABLE RESOURCES TO DETERMINE APPROPRIATE TEACHING APPROACHES

There are a number of issues related to **audience size** that must be considered when planning presentations for groups of patients:

- **Class participation** is more difficult in a large class because there may not be time for all to speak individually. Breaking the class into small groups or pairs for discussion for part of the class time can increase participation, but there must be a focused purpose to the discussion so that people stay on task.
- In **small groups**, placing chairs in a circle or sitting around a table allows people to look at each other and have more active discussions than if they are sitting in rows.
- **Online "virtual" classes** can vary considerably in size, depending upon the type of presentation and whether or not scores and replies are automated or posted by the instructor. If a large group is taking an online course, setting up a "chat room" can facilitate exchange of ideas.

INTERNAL AND EXTERNAL VALIDITY, GENERALIZABILITY, AND REPLICATION

Many research studies are most concerned with **internal validity**, adequate unbiased data properly collected and analyzed within the population studied, but studies that determine the efficacy of procedures or treatments, for example, should have **external validity** as well; that is, the results should be **generalizable** (true) for similar populations. **Replication** of the study with different subjects, researchers, and under different circumstances should produce similar results. For various reasons, some people may be excluded from a study so that instead of randomized subjects the subjects may be highly selected, so when data is compared with another population, in which there is less or more selection, results may be different. The selection of subjects, in this case, would interfere with external validity. Part of the design of a study should include considerations of whether or not it should have external validity or whether there is value for the institution based solely on internal validation.

QUALITATIVE AND QUANTITATIVE DATA

Both qualitative and quantitative data are used for analysis, but the focus is quite different:

- **Qualitative data**: Data are described verbally or graphically, and the results are subjective, depending upon observers to provide information. Interviews may be used as a tool to gather information, and the researcher's interpretation of data is important. Gathering this type of data can be time-intensive, and it can usually not be generalized to a larger population. This type of information gathering is often useful at the beginning of the design process for data collection.
- **Quantitative data**: Data are described in terms of numbers within a statistical format. This type of information gathering is done after the design of data collection is outlined, usually in later stages. Tools may include surveys, questionnaires, or other methods of obtaining numerical data. The researcher's role is objective.

SELECTION AND INFORMATION BIAS

Selection bias occurs when the method of selecting subjects results in a cohort that is **not representative of the target population** because of inherent error in design. For example, if all patients who develop urinary infections are evaluated per urine culture and sensitivities for microbial resistance, but only those patients with clinically-evident infections are included, a number of patients with sub-clinical infections may be missed, skewing the results. Selection bias is only a concern when participants in studies are specifically chosen. Many surveillance studies do not involve selection of subjects.

Information bias occurs when there are **errors in classification**, so an estimate of association is incorrect. Non-differential misclassification occurs when there is similar misclassification of disease or exposure among both those who are diseased or exposed and those who are not. Differential misclassification occurs when there is a differing misclassification of disease or exposure among both those who are diseased or exposed and those who are not.

POPULATION AND SAMPLING

Defining the **population** is critical to data collection and the criteria must be established early in the process. The population may comprise a particular group of individuals, objects, or events. In some cases, data is gathered on an entire population, such as all cases with a particular disease, all deaths, or all physicians in a particular discipline, usually within a specified time frame. In other cases, **sampling,** using a subset of a population, may be done to measure only part of a given population and to generalize the findings to the larger target population while accurately representing the target population. There are a number of considerations with sampling:

- The sampling must have the **characteristics** of the target population.
- The design of the collection must specify the **size** of the sample, the **location**, and **time period**.
- The **sampling technique** must ensure that the sampling represents the target population accurately.
- The design of the collection must ensure that the sampling will not be **biased**.

TRACKING AND TRENDING

Tracking and trending are central to developing research-supported evidence-based practice and is part of continuous quality improvement. Once processes and outcomes measurements are selected, then at least 1 measure should be **tracked** for a number of periods of time, usually in increments of 4 weeks or quarterly. This tracking can be used to present graphical representation of results that will show **trends**. While trends will show some normal variation, if the trend becomes erratic and measures are inconsistent, this suggests that the processes of care are not consistent or are inadequate. For example, if infections in peripherally inserted central catheter (PICC) lines are tracked and the trend shows wild fluctuations with high levels of infection in 1 period, low in another, and vacillations in a third, then the first step is to ensure that the process is being followed correctly. If the process is stable but the variations persist, then the next course would be to modify the process by looking at best practices.

CONDUCTING LITERATURE SEARCH

Almost all current information can be obtained with an online **search**; however, access to some journals may require membership in organizations or online subscriptions, and these should be included in the nurse practitioner's budget for resources because **research** is critical if the nurse is to stay current and anticipate trends. **Journals** sponsored by national or other organizations:

- The Online Journal of Issues in Nursing (OJIN) (http://www.nursingworld.org/ojin)
- American Journal of Nursing (AJN)
- The Journal for Nurse Practitioners (http://www.npjournal.org/home)

- The Clinical Advisor (http://www.clinicaladvisor.com/content/index.php)
- Journal of the American Academy of Nurse Practitioners (http://www.aanp.org/AANPCMS2/Publications/Journal(JAANP)2)
- The Journal for Nurse Practitioners (http://www.npjournal.org)
- Journal of the American Medical Association (JAMA; http://jama.ama-assn.org/)
- New England Journal of Medicine (Massachusetts Medical Society http://content.nejm.org/).

Government web sites include:

- CDC: http://www.cdc.gov/ncidod/dhqp/index.html
- FDA: http://www.fda.gov

CRITICAL READING OF RESEARCH ARTICLES

There are a number of steps to **critical reading** to evaluate research:

1. **Consider the source** of the material. If it is in the popular press, it may have little validity compared to something published in a juried journal.
2. **Review the author's credentials** to determine if a person is an expert in the field of study.
3. **Determine thesis**, or the central claim of the research. It should be clearly stated.
4. **Examine the organization** of the article, whether it is based on a particular theory, and the type of methodology used.
5. **Review the evidence** to determine how it is used to support the main points. Look for statistical evidence and sample size to determine if the findings have wide applicability.
6. **Evaluate** the overall article to determine if the information seems credible and useful and should be communicated to administration and/or staff.

DATA DEFINITION AND COLLECTION OF DATA

Data definitions must be based on a solid understanding of statistical analysis and epidemiological concepts. Specific issues that must be addressed include:

- The 3 Ss:
  - **Sensitivity**: The data should include all positive cases, taking into account variables, decreasing the number of false negatives.
  - **Specificity**: The data should include only those cases specific to the needs of the measurement and exclude those that may be similar but are a different population, decreasing the number of false positives.
  - **Stratification**: Date should be classified according to subsets, taking variables into consideration.
- 2 Rs:
  - **Recordability**: The tool/indicator should collect and measure the necessary data.
  - **Reliability**: Results should be reproducible.
- UV:
  - **Usability**: The tool or indicator should be easy to utilize and understand.
  - **Validity**: Collection should measure the target adequately, so that the results have predictive value.

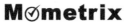

IMPORTANCE OF DATA GATHERING TO DIAGNOSTIC REASONING

The gathering and recording of data are of utmost importance to the **diagnostic evaluation process**. The history and physical section of the patient chart contains a wealth of information (ideally), and should always be taken into consideration when developing a care plan for the patient. Because any number of clinicians can add information to the patient chart (and because all of these clinicians will be reading this information), it is important to record all information clearly and in an organized manner. This can be a daunting task when considering all of the different sources of information, including the patient interview, family member interviews, previous charts, and lab results. By keeping this information clear and concise, the NP can minimize error and can be sure that the differential diagnosis is comprehensive.

POSITIVE PREDICTIVE VALUE AND NEGATIVE PREDICTIVE VALUE

Predictive values are of importance to the clinician because although sensitivity and specificity are used to evaluate the effectiveness of a diagnostic test, they are not particularly clinically relevant. Since a patient's disease state is more or less unknown at admission, these parameters are of no help. This is where the **positive predictive value** (PPV) and **negative predictive value** (NPV) of a test come in. If a patient tests positive for syphilis, what are the chances that the patient actually has syphilis? The chance that this result is correct is the PPV; this is calculated by dividing the number of true positive results by the number of total positive results (true and false positives). NPV, then, is the probability that a patient with a negative result really does not have syphilis. Dividing the number of true negatives by the number of total negatives will result in the NPV.

INCORPORATION OF RESEARCH FINDINGS INTO EVIDENCE-BASED PRACTICE

Incorporating research findings should be central to all work of the nurse practitioner and should be routinely disseminated as part of practice, education and consultation. Any time the nurse gives a presentation or provides written material, **references** should be made to research findings because this provides supporting evidence and lends credence to the information provided. Often research can provide guidance for surveillance or interventions and give valuable insights. References that are used or referred to should always be properly cited so that the work of researchers is credited. If a presentation is given orally, then the nurse should prepare a list of references. Newsletters and e-mail or Internet reports and communications should include research highlights or summaries of current studies of interest, with links to online articles provided when possible to encourage people to read the research for themselves and become more knowledgeable about issues.

OUTCOMES DATA

TYPES

When interpreting outcomes data, one should keep in mind that there are a number of different **types of outcomes data** to be considered, and some data may overlap:

- **Clinical**: This includes symptoms, diagnoses, staging of disease, and indicators of patient health.
- **Physiological**: This includes measures of physical abnormalities, loss of function, and activities of daily living.
- **Psychosocial**: This includes feelings, perceptions, beliefs, functional impairment, and role performance.
- **Integrative**: This includes measures of mortality, longevity, and cost-effectiveness.
- **Perception**: This includes customer perceptions, evaluations, and satisfaction.
- **Organization-wide clinical**: This includes readmissions, adverse reactions, and deaths.

When considering outcomes data, the focus may be on the process or just the outcomes data, and the team analyzing the data should clarify the purpose of reviewing the data and should understand how process and outcomes data interrelate.

INTERPRETATION OF OUTCOMES DATA

Outcomes data provides an effective guide for performance improvement activities because it gives evidence of how well a process succeeds but not necessarily the reason; therefore, outcomes data must be evaluated accordingly. There are inherent problems with outcome data that must be considered when utilizing outcomes for process improvement. First, it is almost impossible to provide sufficient **risk stratification** to provide complete validity to outcomes data, and, second, it is also difficult to accurately attribute the outcomes data to any **1 step in a process** without further study. For example, if outcomes data show a decline in deaths in the emergency department, which recently changed trauma procedures, but doesn't account for the fact that a gang task force has successfully decreased drive-by shootings and killings by 70%, it might be assumed that changes in the emergency department altered the outcome data when, in fact, if the data were adjusted for these external factors, the death rate may have increased.

NP Practice Test

1. An adult patient needs treatment for *Chlamydia trachomatis* urethritis. Which one of the following drugs is useful as a single-dose regimen?

    a. Ceftriaxone intramuscularly.
    b. Levofloxacin.
    c. Azithromycin.
    d. Doxycycline.

2. A patient who gave birth to an infant two months previously seems disengaged and withdrawn. The family nurse practitioner is concerned that the patient may have postpartum depression. Which three of the following symptoms are characteristic of postpartum depression?

    a. Insomnia or hypersomnia.
    b. Disorientation and confusion.
    c. Feeling of worthlessness or inadequacy.
    d. Poor concentration and inability to make decisions.
    e. Delusions associated with the infant.

3. A child with fetal alcohol syndrome (FAS) is likely to exhibit which one of the following findings?

    a. Growth deficiency.
    b. Normal IQ.
    c. Thickened upper lip.
    d. Macrocephaly.

4. To evaluate a child for esotropia, which one of the following is a rapid and convenient diagnostic screening test?

    a. Slit lamp examination.
    b. Corneal light reflex test.
    c. Snellen test.
    d. Fluorescein test.

5. According to Dr. Elisabeth Kübler-Ross, dying patients experience several emotional stages during terminal illness. Which one of these emotions persists throughout all the stages of terminal illness?

    a. Anger.
    b. Hope.
    c. Denial.
    d. Bargaining.

6. A family nurse practitioner is assessing an 11-month-old African-American child who was brought in by his mother for concerns about swelling in both hands and both feet. On examination, the nurse practitioner finds tenderness and obvious swelling of the hands and feet. Vital signs, including temperature and blood pressure, are normal. The most likely diagnosis is:

  a. osteomyelitis.
  b. hand-foot-mouth disease.
  c. glomerulonephritis.
  d. sickle cell disease.

7. A 65-year-old woman complains of urinary incontinence. She is experiencing leakage of urine when she coughs, sneezes, or laughs. This form of urinary incontinence is called:

  a. stress incontinence.
  b. urge incontinence.
  c. overflow incontinence.
  d. functional incontinence.

8. A full-term newborn weighed 7 pounds, 9 ounces at birth. Three days after hospital discharge, the family nurse practitioner is seeing the baby for his first checkup. He now weighs 7 pounds, 4 ounces. This level of weight loss is:

  a. worrisome because it is below birth weight.
  b. Indicative of inadequate nutrition.
  c. A sign of dehydration.
  d. Normal at this age.

9. Which of the following drugs is NOT associated with human teratogenicity?

  a. Valproic acid.
  b. Warfarin.
  c. Phenytoin.
  d. Amoxicillin.

10. The family nurse practitioner is assessing an infant for indications of developmental hip dysplasia utilizing the Ortolani-Barlow maneuver. The maneuver begins by placing the infant on the back and includes the following steps:

  1. Grasp the infant's knees with the thumbs over the inner thighs.
  2. Slowly abduct the infant's hips and observe for equal movement, resistance, or an abnormal "clunk" sound.
  3. Flex the infant's knees and hips to 90 degrees.
  4. Touch the infant's knees together, and then press down on the one femur at a time, observing for dislocation.

Place the steps to this maneuver in sequential order, from first to last:

  a.
  b.
  c.
  d.

11. An adolescent patient presents with severe sore throat, fever, cervical lymphadenopathy, and difficulty opening the mouth. On examination, the family nurse practitioner sees that the uvula is deviated from the midline and there is some bulging of the soft palate near the tonsillar area. What is the most likely diagnosis?

    a. Epiglottitis.
    b. Viral pharyngitis.
    c. Peritonsillar abscess.
    d. Retropharyngeal abscess.

12. Most cases of infectious pharyngitis are caused by:

    a. viruses.
    b. group A streptococcus.
    c. streptococcus pneumoniae.
    d. haemophilus influenzae.

13. A pediatric patient has a tender, boggy lesion on the scalp. There are numerous pustules overlying the lesion. Occipital lymphadenopathy is also present, and there are also three to four small scaly areas of hair loss scattered over the scalp. A Wood's lamp examination shows no fluorescence. What is the most likely diagnosis?

    a. Scalp abscess.
    b. Tinea capitis.
    c. Impetigo.
    d. MRSA infection.

14. Which one of the following is a typical characteristic of *Mycoplasma pneumoniae* infection?

    a. Consolidated infiltrate on chest x-ray.
    b. Headaches.
    c. Hypoxia.
    d. Myositis.

15. Thelarche begins in girls during which Tanner stage?

    a. Stage I.
    b. Stage II.
    c. Stage III.
    d. Stage IV.

16. A nurse practitioner is examining a 55-year-old diabetic man who reports a bilateral pretibial rash. The physical exam reveals a thin epidermis with brown–yellow ulcerated plaques that are oozing blood. What is the most likely diagnosis?

    a. Erythema nodosum.
    b. Myxedema.
    c. Cutaneous Candida albicans infection.
    d. Necrobiosis lipoidica diabeticorum (NLD).

17. Red blood cell (RBC) casts in the urine indicate:

    a. interstitial nephritis.
    b. myoglobinuria.
    c. renal tubular damage.
    d. glomerular disease.

18. Which of the following is NOT a criterion for diagnosis of diabetes mellitus?

    a. Fasting blood glucose > 126 mg/dL.
    b. HgA1c of 6.5%.
    c. Polydipsia and polyuria.
    d. Nonfasting blood glucose > 200 mg/dL.

19. According to federal law, a family nurse practitioner can care for nursing home patients under which of the following conditions?

    a. A physician must be available for emergencies.
    b. Patients must be younger than 80 years of age.
    c. The caseload must not exceed five patients.
    d. All of the above.

20. The public health department has noted a recent increase in cases of West Nile fever, and the family nurse practitioner has begun to see patients with the infection. Which three of the following signs or symptoms does the family nurse practitioner recognize as being typical of West Nile fever?

    a. Alterations of consciousness.
    b. Weakness of facial muscles.
    c. Transient maculopapular rash on the chest, stomach, and back.
    d. Fever, headache, and body aches.
    e. Nausea and vomiting.
    f. Seizures.

21. An African-American woman asks a nurse practitioner about sickle cell disease. She informs the practitioner that she is homozygous for hemoglobin A (AA) and her husband has sickle cell trait (AS). What is the probability that they would have a child with sickle cell disease?

    a. 0%.
    b. 25%.
    c. 50%.
    d. 100%.

22. The percentage of persons with dementia cared for in the home by family members is closest to:

    a. 33%.
    b. 52%.
    c. 65%.
    d. 80%.

23. A family nurse practitioner observes the interaction between a parent and a seven-year-old child. Which three of the following parental behaviors indicate that the parent has an authoritarian parenting style?

    a. Parent issues commands and expects obedience.

    b. Parent communicates little with the child.

    c. Parent shows unconditional love to the child.

    d. Parent sets reasonable limits on behavior.

    e. Parent has rules that are inflexible.

    f. Parent provides little guidance to the child.

24. Which of the following is a HIPAA violation?

    a. Discussing patient treatment information with another provider via e-mail.

    b. Leaving patient charts outside patient exam rooms while they wait to see the provider.

    c. Revealing protected health information with a pharmaceutical representative who needs feedback on his new product.

    d. Releasing health information to the police to aid in an investigation.

25. Which of the following is NOT a cause of secondary hypertension?

    a. Sepsis.

    b. Cocaine use.

    c. Kidney disease.

    d. Oral contraceptive use.

26. An otherwise healthy patient was diagnosed with influenza B within 48 hours of onset of symptoms and was treated with oseltamivir (Tamiflu). Within 24 hours, he reports intermittent heart palpitations. The most likely cause of the palpitations is:

    a. a routine symptom of the flu virus.

    b. high fever.

    c. viral myocarditis.

    d. a side effect of Tamiflu.

27. The family nurse practitioner has noted that a nursing team member has engaged in professional boundary violations. Which three of the following actions may indicate boundary violations?

    a. The nurse accepts a $20 tip from a patient.

    b. The nurse is upset about a family situation and confides in a patient.

    c. The nurse touches a patient's arm when comforting the patient.

    d. The nurse exchanges patients with another nurse in order to care for a favorite patient.

    e. The nurse calls a priest for a patient who wants spiritual support.

28. A three-year-old-boy has had fever of 104 to 105 degrees for six days. While examining the patient, a nurse practitioner notes a strawberry tongue, a maculopapular rash on the trunk, unilateral cervical lymphadenopathy, and nonexudative conjunctivitis. He also has cracked lips and edema of the hands and feet. A physician treated the patient three days prior with antibiotics for a presumed strep infection. What is the most likely diagnosis?

    a. Toxic epidermal necrolysis.

    b. Resistant strep infection.

    c. Kawasaki disease.

    d. Juvenile rheumatoid arthritis.

29. An American elderly person is most likely to be abused by which one of the following?

  a. A sibling.
  b. A spouse.
  c. An adult child.
  d. An unrelated caregiver.

30. Which one of these conditions is associated with the highest suicide rate?

  a. COPD.
  b. Diabetes.
  c. AIDS.
  d. Osteoporosis.

31. An eight-year-old child has had severe nausea and vomiting from enteritis and is at risk for hypokalemia. Which three of the following signs or symptoms are characteristic of hypokalemia?

  a. Bradycardia.
  b. Muscle weakness, cramps, and hyporeflexia.
  c. Renal calculi.
  d. Confusion.
  e. Hypotension.
  f. Lethargy and fatigue.

32. The most common cause of viral pneumonia in adults is:

  a. adenovirus.
  b. RSV.
  c. Haemophilus influenzae.
  d. influenza virus.

33. A family nurse practitioner is evaluating a 21-year-old patient with bilateral eye irritation. He has had several similar episodes in the past, but this one is more severe. The palpebral conjunctivae are edematous and velvety red and the bulbar conjunctivae are injected. No eye discharge is visible. Which one of these other clinical findings would the nurse practitioner expect to see in this case?

  a. Increased intraocular pressure.
  b. Fever.
  c. Myopia.
  d. Pruritus.

34. A 35-year-old male has been an insulin-dependent diabetic for five years and now is unable to urinate. Which of the following would the nurse practitioner most likely suspect?

  a. Atherosclerosis.
  b. Diabetic nephropathy.
  c. Autonomic neuropathy.
  d. Somatic neuropathy.

35. **The most common cause of cancer-related deaths in the 25- to 44-year-olds group is:**

    a. lung cancer.
    b. Hodgkin's lymphoma.
    c. breast cancer.
    d. colon cancer.

36. **An adult patient with iron deficiency anemia asks his family nurse practitioner about foods that are rich in iron. Which one of the following is highest in iron?**

    a. Oranges.
    b. Whole milk.
    c. Beans.
    d. Egg whites.

37. **A 21-month old child has a fever of 103 degrees, fussiness, drooling, and lack of appetite. On exam, the family nurse practitioner notes a red throat with several ulcerations over the tonsillar pillars. What is the most likely diagnosis?**

    a. Herpangina.
    b. Strep pharyngitis.
    c. Gingivostomatitis.
    d. Epiglottitis.

38. **Which of the following is not an etiologic agent of bronchiolitis?**

    a. RSV.
    b. Coronavirus.
    c. Norovirus.
    d. Rhinovirus.

39. **According to Erikson's psychosocial theory, children go through four stages:**

    1. Autonomy versus shame and doubt.
    2. Trust versus mistrust.
    3. Industry versus inferiority.
    4. Initiative versus guilt.

Place the stages (in numbers) in sequential order, from infancy to school age.

    a. Infancy:
    b. Early childhood:
    c. Late childhood:
    d. School age:

40. **A family nurse practitioner has a patient who is habitually at least 30 minutes late for her appointments. She is a 42-year-old Hispanic woman with several health issues. Which of the following statements demonstrates cultural competence on the part of the healthcare provider?**

    a. The provider should not take cultural differences into account in healthcare situations.
    b. Refusing to see the patient unless she arrives on time will teach her a lesson.
    c. Consider that the patient belongs to a culture where being on time is flexible or approximate rather than exact.
    d. Making a reminder call to the patient the day before will solve the problem.

41. Pneumococcal polysaccharide vaccine (PPSV 23, Pneumovax) is:

a. recommended for all adults age 65 or over.
b. administered intradermally.
c. recommended yearly for asplenic patients.
d. not given concurrently with other vaccines.

42. The family nurse practitioner is actively engaged in preventive health maintenance activities. Which two of the following nursing actions are examples of primary prevention?

a. Administering immunizations.
b. Conducting vision screening.
c. Instructing parents about car safety seats.
d. Screening adolescents for scoliosis.
e. Developing rehabilitation activities for a child.

43. The number-one cause of blindness in the elderly is:

a. cataracts.
b. age-related macular degeneration.
c. glaucoma.
d. diabetic retinopathy.

44. A family nurse practitioner is evaluating a three-year-old child with suspected Henoch–Schönlein purpura (HSP). Which one of the following is NOT true about HSP?

a. Patients may complain of joint pain.
b. The purpura is due thrombocytopenia.
c. HSP may be associated with abdominal pain.
d. Microscopic hematuria may be present.

45. Which one of the following is good advice for a patient with gastroesophageal reflux disease (GERD)?

a. Take anticholinergics to speed gastric emptying.
b. Increase fat intake.
c. Raise the head of the bed on two-inch blocks.
d. Eat a high-fiber diet.

46. A family nurse practitioner is instructing a 65-year-old patient on taking psyllium (Metamucil). Which of the following is appropriate advice?

a. Sprinkle psyllium into a half cup of applesauce, and eat the entire serving.
b. Take the psyllium dose mixed in one cup of fluid followed by a second glass of fluid.
c. Psyllium is most effective when taken with a calcium supplement.
d. The onset of action of psyllium is usually within 30 to 45 minutes.

47. What is the treatment of choice for a routine tooth abscess?

a. Extraction of the tooth.
b. Erythromycin.
c. Penicillin VK.
d. Levaquin.

48. A nurse practitioner is seeing an adult patient with a 72-hour history of fever, cough, and runny nose. Her in-clinic flu test is positive for flu type B. She wants a prescription for antibiotics. Which one of the following would be the best thing to tell her?

a. "The virus will just have to run its course. Be patient."
b. "There's just nothing I can do to cure a virus."
c. "Everybody knows antibiotics are not effective for treating the flu."
d. "You must feel miserable and I sympathize with you. Let's discuss some things that will relieve your symptoms."

49. Which of the following statements is true about an infantile umbilical hernia?

a. It will most likely require surgical repair.
b. It will get worse if the baby cries excessively.
c. The baby should wear a band around the abdomen to keep the hernia "in."
d. It will heal on its own because it is less than 2 cm in diameter.

50. The family members of a patient with Alzheimer's disease are having difficulty coping with the patient's repetition of questions and phrases. This phenomenon is known as:

a. perseveration.
b. denial.
c. confabulation.
d. contrivance.

51. A nurse practitioner is instructing a newly diagnosed diabetic on the symptoms of hypoglycemia. Which one of the following is NOT a symptom of hypoglycemia?

a. diaphoresis.
b. tremors.
c. hunger.
d. diplopia.

52. Which of these choices best describes the classic presentation of viral croup in a toddler?

a. Drooling and sitting in a tripod position.
b. Seal-like cough and rhinorrhea.
c. Fever of 104.5 and cough.
d. Oxygen saturation of 92% and severe retractions.

53. A nurse practitioner is performing a breast exam on a 44-year-old woman and detects a painless irregular-shaped mass on the right breast. Which one of these findings is most likely to be associated with breast cancer?

a. Breast lump fixed to muscle or skin.
b. A tender nodule.
c. Nodule that feels rubbery.
d. Lumps in both breasts.

54. A 20-year-old marathon runner is running a race in 100-degree weather, and partway through the race, the runner is unable to continue and complains of severe muscle cramps. His family immediately takes him to see the family nurse practitioner, who finds that the patient is alert, pale, diaphoretic, and slightly dizzy with skin that is cold and clammy. The patient's temperature is 102° F/39° C. Which three of the following initial treatments does the family nurse practitioner employ?

    a. Evaporative cooling.
    b. Alcohol baths.
    c. Benzodiazepines and barbiturates.
    d. Oral rehydration with 0.1% isotonic NaCl solution.
    e. Intravenous (IV) fluids.
    f. Monitor vital signs (VS), temperature, and urinary output.

55. The mechanism of injury in a nursemaid's elbow is usually:

    a. pulling.
    b. twisting.
    c. bending.
    d. compression.

56. A family nurse practitioner is conducting a follow-up visit with a 60-year-old woman who is on Coumadin for a history of deep vein thrombosis originally treated in the hospital. She is in the clinic today for an exam and to have her INR checked. The goal for her INR is:

    a. 1.5 to 2.0.
    b. 2.0 to 3.0.
    c. 3.0 to 4.0.
    d. 4.0 to 4.5.

57. A 42-year-old man wants to quit smoking. He wants to know the symptoms of nicotine withdrawal. All of the following are symptoms EXCEPT:

    a. difficulty sleeping.
    b. tachycardia.
    c. anxiety.
    d. impotence.

58. A 68-year-old patient with osteoarthritis of both knees has been treating his chronic pain with acetaminophen 650 mg four times daily and drinks approximately six to eight alcoholic beverages daily. The patient's diet is poor, leading to a weight loss of 10 pounds in the past three months. The patient's mobility is impaired, causing a decreased activity level. The family nurse practitioner compiles a problem list:

    1.   Chronic pain.
    2.   Risk of hepatotoxicity.
    3.   Impaired physical mobility and activity.
    4.   Risk for imbalanced nutrition.

In which order of priority should the nurse address the patient's problems, from most critical to least critical?

    a.

    b.

    c.

    d.

59. A mother brings her nine-month-old son to see the nurse practitioner for a tight foreskin. What is the best management approach?

    a. Force the foreskin back under direct physician supervision.

    b. Refer the baby to a urologist.

    c. Advise the mother to retract the foreskin little by little at each diaper change until it loosens.

    d. Explain to the mother that a tight foreskin is normal at this age.

60. Which one of the following is a conjugated vaccine?

    a. Inactivated polio vaccine.

    b. Hepatitis B vaccine.

    c. Hib vaccine.

    d. Acellular pertussis vaccine.

61. The rotavirus vaccine is given to children to protect against a potentially severe diarrheal infection. An early version of the vaccine was removed from the market because of its association with:

    a. a high risk of developing the rotavirus infection after vaccination.

    b. a contaminant in the vaccine.

    c. an increased risk of intussusception.

    d. poor development of immunity after vaccination.

62. A family nurse practitioner has given an influenza vaccine to an adult patient. The patient wants to know how long it will take for his body to form antibodies to the virus. The nurse practitioner's answer is:

    a. 4 to 6 weeks.

    b. 72 hours.

    c. 48 hours.

    d. 2 weeks.

63. Due to visual impairment and problems with mobility, an elderly patient is unable to care for himself. In reference to barriers against self-care, these two specific impairments are classified as:

    a. cognitive barriers.

    b. physical barriers.

    c. psychological barriers.

    d. psychosocial barriers.

64. Which of these is NOT associated with infant tooth decay?

    a. Exclusive breastfeeding.

    b. Sleeping with a bottle of formula in the mouth.

    c. Frequent pacifier use.

    d. Presence of only one to four erupted teeth.

65. At what age(s) can one begin to obtain reliable hearing screening results?

    a. Newborn.
    b. Age six months.
    c. Age nine months.
    d. Ages two to three years.

66. Which of the following is true about eye contact in the clinical setting?

    a. Eye contact occurs in generally the same way from one culture to another.
    b. In some cultures, direct eye contact is considered to be rude.
    c. In American culture, avoiding eye contact is usually a signal of respect for the other person.
    d. Avoiding direct eye contact is always a sign of disapproval.

67. A 24-year-old female comes to the clinic with confusion. This patient has a history of a myeloma diagnosis, constipation, intense abdominal pain, and polyuria. Which of the following would the family nurse practitioner most likely suspect?

    a. Diverticulosis.
    b. Hypercalcemia.
    c. Hypocalcemia.
    d. Irritable bowel syndrome.

68. Which of the following is an example of medical negligence?

    a. Delegating a routine task to a trained assistant.
    b. Failure to monitor a patient.
    c. Providing medical advice over the phone.
    d. Referring a patient to a specialist.

69. The family nurse practitioner is examining a five-year-old child. Which three of the following physical skills should the child be able to carry out?

    a. Uses scissors.
    b. Draws shapes such as circles and squares.
    c. Jumps rope.
    d. Roller skates or ice skates.
    e. Rides tricycle or bicycle with training wheels.

70. Which of these statements is true about the nurse practitioner scope of practice?

    a. Nurse practitioners may not prescribe narcotics in most states.
    b. Nurse practitioner scopes of practice vary widely from state to state.
    c. Most states allow nurse practitioners to practice independently.
    d. A nurse practitioner cannot evaluate the psychosocial status of a patient.

71. Scabies is an infestation caused by:

    a. mites.
    b. insects.
    c. ticks.
    d. protozoans.

72. **Which of these is NOT a potential complication of rosacea?**

    a. Folliculitis.
    b. Oral lesions.
    c. Facial pyoderma.
    d. Dry eyes.

73. **Which three of the following are age-associated changes of the cardiovascular system expected in the older adult?**

    a. Heart increases in size.
    b. Adipose tissue accumulates around the heart.
    c. Cardiac output decreases.
    d. Veins become increasingly more elastic.
    e. The heart's sympathetic nervous response to exertion decreases.

74. **A possible complication of gallstones is:**

    a. hepatitis.
    b. gastritis.
    c. acute cholecystitis.
    d. cancer of the gallbladder.

75. **Which of the following is the most appropriate treatment for a single tinea corporis lesion that is less than 2 cm in diameter?**

    a. Topical betamethasone.
    b. Oral griseofulvin.
    c. Topical diphenhydramine.
    d. Topical clotrimazole.

76. **The percentage of patients with Bell's palsy that experience full and spontaneous resolution is closest to:**

    a. 25%.
    b. 50%.
    c. 70%.
    d. 90%.

77. **A key component in the initial overall management of osteoarthritis is:**

    a. nonpharmacologic treatment.
    b. etanercept (Enbrel).
    c. joint replacement surgery.
    d. arthroscopy.

78. **Management of a 34-year-old man with Type 2 diabetes routinely includes all of these EXCEPT:**

    a. referral to an ophthalmologist for periodic retinal exams.
    b. measuring lipid levels periodically.
    c. screen for proteinuria periodically.
    d. measuring HbA1c once yearly.

79. A nurse practitioner is assessing a "suspicious" mole on a 78-year-old man's face. He is concerned about skin cancer. The most common type of skin cancer is:

a. squamous cell carcinoma.

b. melanoma.

c. basal cell carcinoma.

d. mycosis fungoides.

80. A nurse practitioner is performing a Denver II Developmental Screening Test on a toddler. Which of the following is NOT a developmental category screened by the test?

a. Fine motor development.

b. Language development.

c. Gross motor development.

d. Emotional development.

81. A nurse practitioner is counseling a pregnant woman about the risks of smoking during pregnancy. Which one of the following is associated with smoking during pregnancy?

a. Gestational diabetes.

b. Preeclampsia.

c. Low birth weight.

d. Molar pregnancy.

82. Which of the following has a protective effect against the development of neural tube defects during pregnancy?

a. Vitamin B12.

b. Iron sulfate.

c. Folic acid.

d. Vitamin C.

83. A patient has been diagnosed with Alzheimer's disease and is at stage 5: moderate cognitive decline, early dementia. Which four of the following signs or symptoms are typical of stage 5?

a. Patient needs some assistance with personal hygiene.

b. Patient is oriented to self but may be disoriented to place and time.

c. Patient may sometimes forget names of friends and family members.

d. Patient may experience urinary and/or fecal incontinence.

e. Patient may begin to exhibit wandering and sundowning.

f. Patient may forget addresses and telephone numbers.

84. The mother of a nine-year-old girl is concerned that the child is already showing signs of breast development. What would the family nurse practitioner do next?

a. Reassure the mother that breast development at this age is within normal limits.

b. Make a diagnosis of premature breast development.

c. Refer the child to an endocrinologist.

d. Obtain bone age radiographs.

85. During a routine physical exam, a family nurse practitioner notices peripheral edema of both legs in a 48-year-old diabetic woman who also suffers from high blood pressure and depression. Of the following medications, which of the following is most likely causing the edema?

    a. Hydrochlorothiazide.
    b. Fluoxetine (Prozac).
    c. Rosiglitazone (Avandia).
    d. Metformin.

86. The family nurse practitioner is completing a neurologic exam for a patient who is complaining of unexplained weakness and ataxia. The neurologic exam includes:

    1. reflexes.
    2. motor system.
    3. mental status.
    4. cranial nerves.
    5. sensory system.

Place the elements of the neurologic exam (in numbers) in the correct sequence, starting from the first element to the last.

    a.
    b.
    c.
    d.
    e.

87. In general, all of the following should have a preoperative electrocardiogram EXCEPT

    a. men over age 45
    b. patients with known heart disease
    c. patients with a history of costochondritis
    d. patients with hypertension

88. At what age would it be appropriate to stop performing Pap smears on a 53-year-old woman whose previous Pap smears have all been normal? Both she and her husband have been monogamous for 30 years.

    a. 60 years.
    b. 65 years.
    c. 70 years.
    d. She should continue Pap screenings indefinitely.

89. A 66-year-old woman with asthma states she has not received any immunizations since age 14. Aside from her asthma, she is healthy. She asks her nurse practitioner if she currently needs any vaccines. Which one of the following would the nurse practitioner recommend?

    a. FluMist.
    b. Pneumovax.
    c. MMR.
    d. Hib.

90. A family nurse practitioner has diagnosed a 32-year-old woman with influenza A. She wants prophylaxis with oseltamivir (Tamiflu) for her two children, ages 2 months and 2 years. Which of these choices represents the current influenza prophylaxis recommendations?

a. Only the 2-month-old may receive prophylaxis.
b. Only the 2-year-old may receive prophylaxis.
c. Both may receive prophylaxis.
d. Neither may receive prophylaxis.

91. In reference to patient education, which one of these statements is true?

a. Patients usually recall and understand most information given by their provider.
b. Most patients feel their providers overload them with information.
c. When behavioral changes are medically necessary, patients like to be given options for change and then select from the list.
d. Leaning toward the patient while giving instructions does not increase recall.

92. A family nurse practitioner is working in a clinic that sees many Native-American patients. Which of these health conditions has a higher prevalence among Native Americans when compared to other American population groups?

a. Tuberculosis.
b. Hypertension.
c. Coronary artery disease.
d. Obesity.

93. Which one of the following is NOT one of the three fundamental principles of professionalism?

a. Principle of professional appearance.
b. Primacy of patient welfare.
c. Principle of patient autonomy.
d. Principle of social justice.

94. A 42-year-old man has terminal cancer. He will most likely die within one year. He asks his nurse practitioner not to disclose this prognosis to his wife. The nurse practitioner sees his wife as he is walking out of the hospital and she asks him to "tell her the truth" about her husband's condition. The nurse practitioner feels she has a right to know, and he tells her about the grim prognosis. This is a violation of:

a. Patient autonomy.
b. Patient welfare.
c. Patient confidentiality.
d. Professional competence.

95. The family nurse practitioner is conducting a physical examination of a two-year-old child. Which three of the following signs may indicate hearing impairment?

a. The tympanic membranes are slightly red.
b. The child has no speech.
c. The child cannot follow simple age-appropriate commands.
d. The child turns away when addressed by the nurse.
e. The child does not make distinct age-appropriate speech sounds.

96. Which of the following is NOT an area of concern when giving parents anticipatory guidance for a two-year-old?

a. Physical development.
b. Emotional development.
c. Sexual development.
d. Safety issues.

97. A 46-year-old man presents for evaluation of a red rash on both cheeks. This is his third flare-up of the same problem. Some red papules and pustules are visible in the involved areas. On closer inspection, the nurse notices some telangiectasias on his nose and cheeks. There are no comedones present. What is the most likely diagnosis?

a. Lupus erythematosus.
b. Acne.
c. Rosacea.
d. Seborrheic dermatitis.

98. A patient was diagnosed with right temporomandibular joint dysfunction several months ago. She now presents for evaluation of right ear pain. The most likely etiology of her ear pain is:

a. eustachian tube dysfunction.
b. otitis media.
c. otitis externa.
d. referred pain.

99. Which of these conditions most commonly predisposes a patient to recurrent bacterial sinusitis?

a. Immune system deficiency.
b. Allergic rhinitis.
c. GERD.
d. Cigarette smoking.

100. A family nurse practitioner is discussing a treatment plan with an adult patient. The patient is sitting with arms folded across his chest, his legs crossed at the knees, and he is leaning backward. Which type of nonverbal communication is he exhibiting?

a. Body language.
b. Gestures.
c. Facial expressions.
d. Empathy.

101. A family nurse practitioner is caring for a patient who speaks only Vietnamese. A Vietnamese interpreter is present to help. Which of these statements best describes appropriate behavior when using an interpreter?

a. Express two to three ideas at a time before pausing for the interpreter to speak to the patient.
b. Speak clearly and loudly.
c. Face the interpreter when speaking.
d. If the patient gives an unusual response to a question, ask the question in a different way.

102. The assistant at the clinic reports the following vital signs to the nurse practitioner. Which of the following vital signs is abnormal?

    a. 11-year-old male – 90 bpm, 22 resp/min, 100/70 mm Hg.
    b. 13-year-old female – 105 bpm., 22 resp/min, 100/70 mm Hg.
    c. 5-year-old male- 102 bpm, 24 resp/min, 90/65 mm Hg.
    d. 6-year-old female- 100 bpm., 26 resp/min, 90/70mm Hg.

103. According to Peplau's framework for psychodynamic nursing, the nurse carries out a number of different nursing roles. Which nursing roles do the following statements exemplify?

    1. "I heard you yelling at other patients and staff members. Let's talk about what you are feeling and explore other ways to express those feelings."
    2. "BiPAP delivers two different levels of pressure while you sleep. This is where we set those pressures. One pressure is for when you breathe in, and the other pressure is for when you breathe out."
    3. "It's important to take your pulse each morning before you take your digoxin. You must not take the medication if your pulse is lower than 60 because the medicine can slow your heart too much."
    4. "The home health agency can monitor your care when you go home, and the Meals on Wheels program can bring in daily meals until you are able to prepare meals yourself."

Match the statements (in numbers) to the appropriate nursing role.

    a. Teacher:
    b. Counselor:
    c. Technical expert:
    d. Resource person:

104. Which of the following is a "red flag" for patient drug-seeking behavior?

    a. The patient claims allergies to multiple classes of non-narcotic pain medications
    b. The patient is using relaxation techniques under medical supervision for relief of pain
    c. The patient has tried acupuncture
    d. The patient becomes upset when not treated with antibiotics for a virus

105. An adult female with a vaginal discharge presents for evaluation. The nurse practitioner orders a KOH prep on the discharge. The laboratory reports the presence of clue cells. The best treatment for this patient is:

    a. doxycycline.
    b. ceftriaxone.
    c. terconazole.
    d. metronidazole.

106. Fifth disease is caused by:

    a. a parvovirus.
    b. an enterovirus.
    c. a paramyxovirus.
    d. an adenovirus.

107. Which one of the following medications is clearly contraindicated during pregnancy?

a. Amoxicillin.
b. Ondansetron (Zofran).
c. Permethrin 5% cream (Elimite).
d. Isotretinoin (Accutane).

108. The problem-solving process has various components. When identifying a problem, a family nurse practitioner employs the nursing process of:

a. planning.
b. assessment.
c. implementation.
d. evaluation.

109. If two nurse practitioners have incompatible differences in values and patient care beliefs, which type of conflict exists between them?

a. Organizational.
b. Intrapersonal.
c. Interpersonal.
d. Psychological.

110. A nurse practitioner is treating a patient with conjunctivitis. Which of the following microorganisms is related to this condition?

a. Yersinia pestis.
b. Helicobacter pylori.
c. Vibrio cholera.
d. Haemophilus influenzae biogroup aegyptius.

111. When two or more states recognize licensure by other state boards that have equivalent licensing requirements, this is known as:

a. temporary license.
b. licensing by waiver.
c. licensure by examination.
d. reciprocity.

112. A nurse practitioner is reviewing a new patient's medication list. The drug pentoxifylline is present on the list. Which of the following conditions given in the patient's history listed below is being treated with this medication?

a. COPD.
b. CAD.
c. PVD.
d. MS.

113. All of the following are categories of medication errors EXCEPT:

a. wrong patient.
b. incorrect dosage.
c. failure to note patient allergies.
d. surgical removal of wrong body part.

114. A twenty old male has a tender lump area in his left groin. His abdomen is distended and he has been vomiting for the past 24 hours. Which of the following would the nurse practitioner most likely suspect?

a. Ulcerative colitis.
b. Biliary colic.
c. Acute gastroenteritis.
d. Strangulated hernia.

115. A process that analyzes, identifies, and treats potential hazards in a specific setting is known as:

a. risk management.
b. quality assurance.
c. standards of care.
d. patient rights.

116. Which of the following blood therapeutic concentrations is abnormal?

a. Phenobarbital   10-40 mcg/ml.
b. Lithium   0.6-1.2 mEq/L.
c. Digoxin   0.5-1.6 ng/ml.
d. Valproic acid   40-100 mcg/ml.

117. Which of the following blood therapeutic concentrations is abnormal?

a. Digitoxin   9-25 mcg/ml.
b. Vancomycin   5-15 mcg/ml.
c. Primidone   2-14 mcg/ml.
d. Theophylline   10-20 mcg/ml.

118. Which of the following blood therapeutic concentrations is abnormal?

a. Phenytoin   10-20 mcg/ml.
b. Quinidine   2-6 mcg/ml.
c. Haloperidol   5-20 ng/ml.
d. Carbamazepine   5-25 mcg/ml.

119. Five days after a patient hiked through the nearby woods, the patient consulted the family nurse practitioner about a bull's-eye rash (erythema migrans) on the leg. The nurse suspects Lyme disease. Which three additional symptoms are commonly associated with early-stage Lyme disease?

a. Headache.
b. Facial palsy.
c. Myalgia.
d. Enlarged lymph glands near the rash.
e. High fever.
f. Disorientation and confusion.

120. All of the following are true about incident reports EXCEPT:

a. Incident reports can be useful in improving patient care and in identifying risks.
b. Incident reports should be completed accurately.
c. The report form should be copied and placed in the patient record.
d. The report should be filled out following specific documentation guidelines.

121. A 25-year-old patient is having trouble with recurrent conjunctivitis, having had four episodes in the past year. She wears contact lenses. What type of organisms should be strongly suspected as a cause of eye infections in contact lens wearers?

    a. Gram-negative organisms.
    b. Fungi.
    c. Adenoviruses.
    d. Mixed organisms.

122. The family nurse practitioner is evaluating an eight-month-old child whose mother reports a history of frequent vomiting over the past two months. She has mentioned it to other providers, but she has been told the baby would "outgrow it." In looking over his medical record, the nurse notices the patient has also been seen for recurrent episodes of wheezing. However, he is currently not wheezing, is afebrile, and appears healthy. Which of the following is the most likely cause of the vomiting?

    a. Pyloric stenosis.
    b. Gastroesophageal reflux (GER).
    c. Gastroenteritis.
    d. Reactive airway disease.

123. A 30-year-old woman has a body mass index (BMI) of 28. According to her BMI, the patient is:

    a. normal weight.
    b. overweight.
    c. obese.
    d. extremely obese.

124. The percentage of Americans that are overweight (based on BMI) is closest to:

    a. 20%.
    b. 35%.
    c. 50%.
    d. 65%.

125. A four-year-old child presents with a complaint of rust-colored urine. She has no dysuria and no history of urinary tract infections in the past. She has been healthy except for a recent case of impetigo, which has since resolved. Her mother states that the child's eyes looked "a little puffy" this morning, but look fine now. Which of the following is the most likely diagnosis?

    a. UTI.
    b. Kidney stone.
    c. Poststreptococcal glomerulonephritis.
    d. Nephrotic syndrome.

126. An adult patient with persistent sinusitis has failed treatment with amoxicillin, trimethoprim/sulfa, and amoxicillin clavulanate. Which of the following is the best choice for the next round of treatment?

    a. A first-generation cephalosporin.
    b. Clarithromycin.
    c. A fluoroquinolone.
    d. Erythromycin ethylsuccinate.

127. A 38-year-old man developed lower back pain that started two days after lifting up his four-year-old son. He has limited spinal range of motion, but his neurological exam is normal. The nurse practitioner suspects nerve root irritation from a herniated disk. Which of the following would help corroborate the diagnosis?

a. An MRI.
b. Plain lumbosacral radiographs.
c. Testing range of spinal motion.
d. Bend-over test.

128. The parent of a 15-year-old girl is concerned that the girl may be involved in substance abuse. Which four of the following signs or symptoms may be indicative of substance abuse?

a. Abnormal physical changes.
b. Falling grades and school attendance.
c. Periods of moodiness.
d. Repeated unexplained falls and accidents.
e. Constant use of social media.
f. Labile mood and behavior.

129. The family nurse practitioner is discussing avoidance of asthma triggers with an adult patient. Which of these offers the best advice?

a. Vacuum carpets daily to remove allergens.
b. Use ceiling fans throughout the home instead of air conditioning.
c. Maintain home humidity levels over 50%.
d. Encase his mattress and pillows in allergen-blocking covers.

130. Which of these antidepressants is least likely to cause sexual side effects?

a. Bupropion (Wellbutrin).
b. Escitalopram (Lexapro).
c. Amitriptyline (Elavil).
d. Fluoxetine (Prozac).

131. The family nurse practitioner is assessing the development of a five-month-old child. Which four of the following fine and gross motor abilities does the family nurse practitioner expect to observe?

a. Exhibits no head lag when pulled to a sitting position.
b. Uses pincer grasp.
c. Crawls or creeps.
d. Turns from abdomen to back.
e. Uses palmar grasp.
f. Grasps and manipulates objects such as rattles.

132. A 55-year-old woman has swelling of the proximal interphalangeal joints of the first and second digits of both hands. She also complains of prolonged morning stiffness and often experiences excessive fatigue. What is the most likely diagnosis?

a. Gout.
b. Osteoarthritis.
c. Rheumatoid arthritis.
d. Psoriatic arthritis.

133. A 64-year-old man presents with acute onset of redness and severe pain in his right eye. He also complains of blurred vision, headache, nausea, and seeing halos around lights. After examining the patient and taking a history, what is the next course of action?

a. Reassure the patient and prescribe antibiotic eye drops for conjunctivitis.
b. Apply tetracaine drops to relieve pain.
c. Perform a fluorescein test to check for a corneal abrasion.
d. Arrange for immediate referral to an ophthalmologist.

134. A 6-month-old infant has been diagnosed and hospitalized with pertussis. The infant is not in daycare. The only known sick contact is a 12-year-old sibling who has had a cough for 3 weeks. Which of the following represents the best option for chemoprophylaxis in this case?

a. Treat all household contacts and other close contacts with erythromycin.
b. Treat only the sibling who has the cough and the sick infant.
c. Treat all household and other close contacts with either azithromycin or clarithromycin.
d. If all other close contacts are current on their immunizations, there is no need for prophylaxis.

135. A nine-month-old Caucasian child has been seen in the clinic for frequent respiratory infections and frequent bouts with loose stools. Stool cultures and ova and parasites have been negative. During her routine physical examination, the nurse practitioner discovers that in the past four months her growth parameters have dropped from the 60th percentile to the 10th percentile for weight and from the 75th percentile to the 25th percentile for height. What is the best thing to do next?

a. Order thyroid function tests.
b. Order a sweat chloride test.
c. Admit the child to the hospital to see if she gains weight when fed appropriately.
d. Evaluate for tuberculosis.

136. A family nurse practitioner is evaluating a newborn infant for a Moro reflex. Of the following, which is the best way to elicit the reflex?

a. Gently stroke the perioral area with a finger.
b. Turn the newborn's head to one side, and observe his arm movements.
c. Apply firm pressure to the palm of the baby's hand.
d. Clap hands loudly and suddenly.

137. The family nurse practitioner is providing guidance to nurses caring for preschoolers after a bus accident resulted in the hospitalization of six children. Which four of the following nursing management techniques should the family nurse practitioner recommend?

a. Encourage parents to stay with their children.
b. Allow the child to make choices when possible.
c. Explain all procedures to the child.
d. Encourage the child to discuss fears.
e. Encourage peer interaction.
f. Provide a night light.

138. Which of the following is useful as a rescue medication in the treatment of asthma?

a. Corticosteroid inhaler.
b. Leukotriene inhibitor.
c. Anti-allergic medications.
d. Short-acting beta-2 agonist.

139. Which of the following is most likely to be the first symptom of tuberculosis?

a. Chest pain.
b. Cough productive of bloody sputum.
c. Mild cough with nonbloody mucoid sputum.
d. Shortness of breath.

140. An 11-month-old baby recently completed a course of oral antibiotics for otitis media. She now presents with a beefy red rash in the diaper area. The rash is surrounded by small satellite lesions and has not responded to diaper rash ointments. What is the best way to manage this rash?

a. Prescribe topical nystatin cream.
b. Advise the parents to apply talcum powder at each diaper change.
c. Prescribe mupirocin ointment.
d. Prescribe oral fluconazole.

141. The family nurse practitioner is examining a 16-year-old male patient who is active in sports. Which three of the following teaching topics are important as part of injury prevention education?

a. Protective gear.
b. Bicycle, skateboard, and automobile safety.
c. Sexuality.
d. Drinking and driving.
e. Social media safeguards.
f. Study habits.

142. A 10-year-old girl has a two-week history of a mucocele inside her lower lip. There is no pain or bleeding. What is the next course of action?

a. Manually rupture the lesion and let the contents flow out.
b. Cauterize the lesion with silver nitrate.
c. Advise the parents that spontaneous rupture will occur.
d. Refer immediately to an oral surgeon.

143. Which one of the following is true about primary enuresis in children?

a. A physical etiology, such as a UTI, is found in about 20% of children.
b. Bed wetting is more common in boys than girls.
c. The patient should take imipramine.
d. It is crucial to perform a renal ultrasound as soon as possible.

144. A four-year-old child presents with a four-day history of cough and nasal congestion. He had a temperature of 100.8 for the initial 24 hours only. Today, his nasal mucus is thicker and yellow. What is the most likely diagnosis?

a. Allergic rhinitis.
b. Sinusitis.
c. Viral upper respiratory infection (URI).
d. Foreign body in the nose.

145. A 21-year-old asymptomatic woman has a positive purified protein derivative (*PPD*) test result of 13 mm. What is the next step in managing this patient?

a. Chest x-ray.
b. Chest x-ray and six to nine months of treatment with isoniazid (INH).
c. Sputum culture.
d. Repeat the PPD in three months.

146. Which of the following patients is at increased risk for recurrent otitis media?

a. A teenager on the school swimming team.
b. A child with narrow ear canals.
c. A child with cleft palate.
d. An infant with blocked tear ducts.

147. All of the following are associated with childhood exposure to cigarette smoke EXCEPT:

a. colic.
b. bacterial conjunctivitis.
c. SIDS.
d. wheezing.

148. The family nurse practitioner is carrying out an assessment of a two-week-old newborn and observes indications of developmental delay. Which two of the following signs indicate the need for a complete medical and developmental evaluation?

a. Infant sucks poorly and feeds very slowly.
b. Respiratory rate at rest is 45 beats per minute.
c. Limbs are loose and floppy.
d. Infant exhibits occasional jitteriness.
e. Infant frequently moves arms and legs.

149. Which of these illnesses is most frequently reported by patients who have recently traveled overseas?

a. Hepatitis A.
b. Traveler's diarrhea.
c. Malaria.
d. Amoebiasis.

150. Which of the following types of patients is most likely to be interested in using alternative medical therapies?

a. Patients older than age 65.
b. Men.
c. Women.
d. High school and college students.

151. The parents of a 17-year-old child who was involved in an auto accident have been told that their child died. The parents repeatedly say, "This can't be true!" and appear unable to believe that their child is dead, refusing to allow the child's body to be removed. Which two of the following responses are most therapeutic?

a. "I'm so sorry for your loss."
b. "I'm afraid that nothing can bring your child back."
c. "It is almost unbelievable."
d. "You must accept that your child has died."
e. "Take the time you need to be with your child."

152. A two-year old child has viral diarrhea. Several other children in his daycare have the same illness. He is not vomiting and is eating well. His mother asks for treatment recommendations. What should be done next?

a. Advise his mother to keep the child well hydrated.
b. Recommend Imodium AD.
c. Prescribe Levsin.
d. Tell the mother to stop solid foods for now.

153. A 72-year-old man complains of cramping pain in both calves after walking. The pain disappears after resting. His condition is most likely:

a. restless legs syndrome.
b. multiple sclerosis.
c. intermittent claudication.
d. normal for his age.

154. Which one of the following about the erythrocyte sedimentation rate (ESR) is true?

a. It measures the rate red blood cells fall in an upright tube of anticoagulated blood in a 30-minute period.
b. It is a specific test for inflammation.
c. It is an acute phase reactant.
d. The faster the red blood cells fall, the higher the sedimentation rate.

155. A young and inexperienced mother brings in her 6-month-old infant for evaluation of vomiting and diarrhea. Because he has been vomiting his formula, the baby's mother has been giving him nothing but plain water for the past 24 hours. The infant suddenly has a seizure in the clinic. Of the following choices, he is most likely suffering from:

a. hyponatremia.
b. sepsis.
c. idiopathic epilepsy.
d. carotenemia.

156. A 65-year-old client states that he has received no immunizations since childhood. The client had chickenpox when he was eight years old. Which four immunizations should the family nurse practitioner recommend?

a. Tetanus, diphtheria, and pertussis (Tdap).
b. Varicella (chickenpox).
c. Influenza.
d. Herpes zoster (shingles).
e. Pneumococcal vaccine (PCV13 and PPSV23).
f. Measles, mumps, and rubella (MMR).

157. The Adams forward bend test is used to:

a. screen for scoliosis.
b. test for a herniated disk.
c. assess cerebellar function.
d. assess for spinal arthritis.

158. Contributory negligence occurs when:

a. the healthcare provider willfully disregards the safety of the patient.
b. the healthcare provider fails to provide appropriate standard of care.
c. the patient contributes to his own negative outcome.
d. a percentage of negligence is assigned to each party involved.

159. A patient weighs 64 kilograms and is 1.6 meters tall. What is her body mass index (BMI)?

a. 22.
b. 25.
c. 28.
d. 30.

160. A mother tells her family nurse practitioner that her two-year-old child refuses almost all solid foods. She states, "All he'll take is whole milk." This child is most at risk for:

a. hemolytic anemia.
b. developing milk allergy.
c. gastroesophageal reflux.
d. iron deficiency anemia.

161. A 79-year-old multiparous woman complains of a pulling sensation in her vagina and bloody spotting on her underwear. She has also started to have some mild urinary incontinence. As the nurse practitioner prepares to examine the area, she notices a rather large ulcerated soft tissue mass at the vaginal introitus. What is the most likely diagnosis?

a. Urethral prolapse.
b. Uterine prolapse.
c. Vaginal neoplasm.
d. Pelvic hernia.

162. Which of the following is NOT a symptom of retinal detachment?

a. Eye pain.
b. Flashes of light.
c. Floaters.
d. Loss of central vision.

163. Which of the following hernias is most likely to be acquired?

a. Indirect inguinal hernia.
b. Direct inguinal hernia.
c. Infant umbilical hernia.
d. Hiatal hernia in a child.

164. An elderly, immobile patient in a nursing home has an area of dark purple, boggy skin that is intact in the sacral area. The skin is still intact. What is the most likely explanation for this condition?

a. Stage I Pressure Ulcer.
b. Stage II Pressure Ulcer.
c. Suspected Deep Tissue Injury.
d. Unstageable Pressure Ulcer.

165. All of the following are grounds for nursing malpractice EXCEPT:

a. failure to report a change in a patient's condition.
b. neglecting to monitor a patient properly.
c. administering a medication not ordered by the physician.
d. failure to maintain continuing education requirements.

166. An adolescent complains of acute left ear pain. The ear hurts with manipulation of the external ear. On examination, the ear canal is red, swollen, and very tender. The nurse practitioner also notices flaky debris in the ear canal. Which of the following is the most appropriate treatment?

a. Antipyrine/benzocaine ear drops (Auralgan).
b. Combination antibiotic and corticosteroid ear drops.
c. Ibuprofen and warm compresses to the ear.
d. Oral antibiotics.

167. A patient is receiving citalopram (Celexa) for depression. Which three of the following adverse effects are commonly associated with citalopram?

a. Sedation and lethargy.
b. Orthostatic hypotension.
c. Agitation, anxiety, and insomnia.
d. Heart block.
e. GI distress.
f. Increased sex drive.

168. The family nurse practitioner is performing a developmental exam on a child. He is able to use a pincer grasp, pull up to stand, and he understands the word "no." His age is closest to:

a. 4 months.
b. 5 months.
c. 6 months.
d. 9 months.

169. An obviously distressed 14-year-old boy has recently noticed that one of his breasts has grown larger than the other and is also somewhat tender. His mother seems equally concerned. What is the best management course to follow?

a. Treat for mastitis.
b. Offer reassurance that this is temporary and benign.
c. Check testosterone levels.
d. Refer him to an endocrinologist.

170. Which of the following is the best way to stop a nosebleed?

a. Apply an ice pack to the forehead.
b. Apply pressure on the bridge of the nose.
c. Pinch nostrils shut and apply pressure for 10 continuous minutes.
d. Have the patient relax and tilt his head back.

171. An 81-year-old woman complains of darkening of the skin right above her ankles, itching, thinning of the skin, and progressive irritation. Her ankles swell intermittently. What is the most likely diagnosis?

a. Venous stasis dermatitis.
b. Zinc deficiency.
c. Atopic dermatitis.
d. Id reaction.

172. A known asthmatic has a peak flow meter reading that is 78% of his personal best. This measurement is in the:

a. normal zone.
b. green zone.
c. yellow zone.
d. red zone.

173. In reference to adult CPR, the currently recommended ratio of chest compressions to breaths is:

a. 15:2.
b. 10:2.
c. dependent on the age of the patient.
d. 30:2.

174. Which of the following is the best prophylactic treatment for traveler's diarrhea in an adult?

 a. Amoxicillin.
 b. Ciprofloxacin.
 c. Trimethoprim/sulfa.
 d. Doxycycline.

175. Which of the following is the treatment of choice for an adult female with gonococcal cervicitis?

 a. Intramuscular penicillin.
 b. Intramuscularly ceftriaxone.
 c. Oral doxycycline.
 d. Oral cefixime.

176. A nurse practitioner is examining a 12-year-old female patient and notes in the chart that her Tanner stage is B-2, Ph-2. This means she has:

 a. breast buds and a light growth of long pubic hair, mainly on the labia.
 b. breast and areola enlargement without a differentiation of the contours and dark, coarse pubic hair connecting over the mons pubis.
 c. no breast enlargement and no pubic hair.
 d. breast enlargement with protrusion of the areola from the breast and thick, coarse pubic hair completely covering the mons pubis.

177. A new mother expresses concern over the tiny white bumps on her newborn's nose and chin. The best explanation for her is:

 a. she can usually remove these by applying some pressure and pinching the bumps.
 b. she will need a referral to Dermatology for further evaluation of this.
 c. there is a special cream the nurse practitioner can prescribe to help resolve this.
 d. this is due to plugged pores in the skin and it will go away on its own.

178. A 52-year-old female was having irregular periods for approximately one year followed by a full year of no bleeding. Which of the following lab results could confirm that she has reached menopause?

 a. High normal levels of estradiol of 350 pg/mL or higher.
 b. FSH levels consistently elevated to 30 mIU/mL or higher.
 c. Elevated progesterone level of 90 ng/mL or higher.
 d. Elevated testosterone level of 80 ng/dL or higher.

179. A 44-year-old male is being seen by the nurse practitioner as a new patient to establish care. His blood pressure reading is 142/92. He is not aware of his blood pressure ever being elevated in the past and he has not had any subjective symptoms of hypertension. The most appropriate action is to:

 a. start him on a low dose of an ACE inhibitor or diuretic and advise him to monitor and record his blood pressure daily.
 b. start him on a low dose of a beta blocker and advise him to monitor and record his blood pressure daily.
 c. provide him with information on how to lower his blood pressure through diet and exercise and advise him to monitor and record his blood pressure daily.
 d. refer him to the ED for treatment of malignant hypertension.

180. Which of the following is NOT a reliable test to check for dehydration in an elderly patient?

a. Hypotension.
b. Tenting of skin.
c. Elevated heart rate.
d. Dizziness or confusion.

181. A 67-year-old male presents to the clinic with complaints of vision changes causing some yellowish discoloration in his visual field. He has a past medical history of hypertension, coronary artery disease, and congestive heart failure. He is currently taking lisinopril, metoprolol, digoxin, and Plavix. Which of these medications is most likely causing his symptoms?

a. Plavix.
b. Metoprolol.
c. Digoxin.
d. Lisinopril.

182. Which of the following drugs would be least likely to help with bradykinesia associated with Parkinson's disease?

a. Amantadine.
b. Anticholinergics.
c. Levodopa.
d. MAOIs.

183. A 3-year-old male is brought to the pediatrician's office for evaluation of sore throat. The nurse practitioner enters the exam room and sees the patient sitting on the exam table leaning forward and drooling. His vital signs are as follows: temperature 102.2, pulse 146, respiratory rate 34, and O2 saturation 91%. The next appropriate step would be to:

a. let the parents know he most likely has a viral illness and to treat symptomatically.
b. perform a throat swab to check for strep throat.
c. give the child some cool water or a popsicle.
d. have a staff member contact emergency services to arrange transport to the closest ED and gather supplies to assist in maintaining the patient's airway.

184. A nurse practitioner is riding in the elevator with a co-worker at the end of shift, along with a few hospital visitors. The co-worker is complaining about the very demanding family members of one of the patients she cared for today. The most appropriate response is to:

a. quietly let her know she should not be discussing patient care in a public place.
b. try to lighten the mood and make her feel better after a hard shift.
c. tell her about some difficult patients she had during her shift, also.
d. say nothing, but report the conversation to the Risk Management Department at the hospital.

185. Using the patient-centered medical home model of healthcare delivery, the main person coordinating the patient's care is:

a. the primary care provider.
b. the lead nurse within the primary care office.
c. an assigned social worker.
d. the patient coordinates their own care.

186. The purpose of quality improvement is to:

a. improve employee satisfaction.
b. monitor the leadership skills of the administration of a healthcare facility.
c. implement specific changes in healthcare which have a measurable improvement for a specific group of patients.
d. provide specific training and education opportunities to employees to ensure the quality of the care provided is reaching high standards.

187. A nurse practitioner works in the ER at a local children's hospital. At her child's soccer game, another mother asks how the daughter of a mutual friend is doing who was brought into the ER the day before with a broken arm. The most appropriate response is:

a. the daughter is doing well and will be seeing Orthopedics.
b. deny having seen the child.
c. tell her the child was seen, but that her care cannot be discussed with anyone else.
d. explain to her that you are not able to discuss the care or prognosis of any patients.

188. What is the difference between palliative care and hospice care?

a. Palliative care can be started at the time of diagnosis during treatment and hospice care is started when the patient is not going to survive the illness and the end of life is nearing.
b. Palliative care is for inpatient end of life care and hospice care is performed in the home.
c. Palliative care can be provided by a patient's primary care provider and hospice care is provided by a certified hospice care agency.
d. Palliative care specializes in only the different forms of therapy that a patient needs and hospice care specializes in end of life comfort care.

189. The fastest growing emerging cultural population in the United States is:

a. Hispanic.
b. Asian.
c. Middle Eastern.
d. Eastern European.

190. A dressing change is being performed on a patient and his family is present bedside. They are devout, practicing Muslims. Knowing this, it is important to:

a. keep as much of the patient's skin covered at all times during the dressing change.
b. try not to talk while touching the patient.
c. ask everyone to leave the room except for the male head of the family.
d. explain what is being done to the female head of the family only.

191. A teenage Vietnamese girl is interested in starting oral contraceptive pills, but is concerned that her parents will find out and be disappointed because of their cultural beliefs. This is because:

a. the Vietnamese culture does not believe in birth control of any kind.
b. the Vietnamese culture believes that men should be responsible for birth control.
c. the Vietnamese culture is firmly against premarital sex, and they may ostracize her for this.
d. the Vietnamese culture believes that OCPs can cause handicapped babies.

192. When communicating with a non-English speaking patient and her family, it is best to:

a. have another family member interpret if possible.

b. improvise with using pictures and video to teach.

c. hold most of the conversation through an online translating program.

d. arrange to have an interpreter familiar with medical terminology present.

193. When teaching a patient who has a hearing impairment, it is important to:

a. face them directly so the face and lips are clearly visible to them.

b. give them educational materials in print to take home and read on their own.

c. have the patient be the only person receiving educational material so they can feel more involved in their treatment plan.

d. discuss the treatment plan with the parents so that they can communicate with the patient in the way that best suits her needs.

194. A 10-year-old child with muscular dystrophy has been treated as an inpatient for pneumonia. The discharge plan is being prepared and the nurse practitioner is reviewing the treatments he will need at home. While doing the teaching for the patient and his family, it is important that:

a. they know that home health and respiratory therapy will be coming in daily for evaluations and nebulizer treatments, so they will not need to worry about how to do these.

b. the primary focus be on the parents because it is not as important that the child understand his treatment.

c. give all of the educational material in writing rather than reviewing it in person to save time.

d. the patient be included to help him maintain some independence in his treatment.

195. A 52-year-old female presents to the clinic with a bad sore throat and low-grade fever. She tests positive for strep pharyngitis. Her past medical history includes hyperlipidemia and a past history of SVT with her last episode being 1 year ago. She is currently taking atorvastatin and atenolol. Which of the following antibiotics would be contraindicated for this patient?

a. Amoxicillin.

b. Cefdinir.

c. Azithromycin.

d. Penicillin.

196. Which of the following medications is most likely to cause pupil dilation, photophobia, and blurred vision?

a. Warfarin (Coumadin).

b. Diphenhydramine (Benadryl).

c. Oseltamivir (Tamiflu).

d. Ketorolac (Toradol).

197. A 39-year-old female is started on levothyroxine for hypothyroidism. When should she return for lab work to check the effectiveness of the dosage of her medication?

a. 6 to 8 weeks.

b. 4 weeks.

c. 2 weeks.

d. 1 week.

198. A 50-year-old female presents to the clinic with complaints of epigastric abdominal pain, right shoulder pain, nausea, vomiting, and decreased appetite. Of the following differential diagnoses, which would be the most like diagnosis?

a. Peptic ulcer disease.
b. Pancreatitis.
c. Acute cholecystitis.
d. Urinary tract infection.

199. When interpreting pulmonary function test results, the expected FEV1 value for a patient with severe COPD (stage 3) would be:

a. 0-10% below normal.
b. 10-15% below normal.
c. 15-30% below normal.
d. 30-50% below normal.

200. A 55-year-old male is being seen as a new patient to establish in a family practice. He has no known chronic medical problems and does not take any medications. He tells the nurse practitioner that he was told several years before that he had "borderline diabetes." He has baseline labs checked while in the office and his hemoglobin A1C is 6.2%. This is interpreted as:

a. a normal blood sugar level.
b. prediabetes that can be initially treated through lifestyle changes, diet, and exercise.
c. diabetes that will require oral medication to control.
d. severe diabetes that will require insulin to control.

Answer Key and Explanations

1. C: Only azithromycin has shown effectiveness when taken as a single dose for treatment of chlamydial urethritis. Levofloxacin and doxycycline are also effective treatment choices, but would have to be taken for seven days. Ceftriaxone (Rocephin) is not effective in this case.

2. A, C, and **D:** A patient who has given birth within the previous two to three months and seems disengaged and withdrawn may be exhibiting signs of postpartum depression. Characteristic symptoms include:

- Insomnia or hypersomnia.
- Feeling of worthlessness or inadequacy.
- Poor concentration and ability to make decisions.
- Lack of interest and pleasure.
- Recurrent thoughts of death.
- Lack of energy and constant fatigue.
- Marked change in appetite.
- Consistently sad or depressed mood.

Postpartum psychosis often begins early and is more acute and dangerous and can include disorientation, confusion, hallucinations, and delusions associated with the infant.

3. A: FAS is caused by alcohol consumption during pregnancy. Pregnant women should be counseled against drinking any amount of alcohol because there is no known "safe" amount to drink. Pregnant women should abstain from alcohol during all trimesters. Alcohol has a wide range of permanent effects on children, particularly on the nervous system. Some common characteristics include abnormal facial features (thin upper lip and smooth philtrum), microcephaly, growth deficiency, hyperactivity, learning disabilities, and low IQ.

4. B: Corneal reflex tests are useful to diagnose strabismus (e.g., esotropia). To perform the test, shine a light directly onto both corneas at the same time with the patient looking straight at the light source. In patients with strabismus, the light reflected on the cornea appears off-center in the affected eye. Note that corneal light reflex tests may not detect an intermittent strabismus.

5. B: The five emotional stages of dying are hope, denial, isolation, anger, and bargaining. The hope of a cure (even if slim) persists throughout all the other stages of terminal illness. Isolation and denial help handle the shock of approaching death. After this, the patient experiences anger followed by bargaining.

6. D: Dactylitis (hand-foot syndrome) is often the first manifestation of sickle cell disease in an infant or toddler. Swelling and pain are usually symmetric and result from ischemia of small bones. Bone marrow is expanding and compromising circulation to the bones of the hands and feet. X rays are not helpful in the acute phase, but they eventually show bone destruction and repair. Management includes hydration and pain control. Patients who present with dactylitis before 24 months of age often go on to have a severe course of sickle cell disease.

7. A: Stress incontinence refers to leakage of urine by performance of an activity that puts pressure on the bladder. These activities include laughing, sneezing, lifting something heavy, or coughing. Urge incontinence is present when a patient develops a sudden, strong urge to urinate and begins passing urine before making it to the bathroom. Patients who have functional incontinence have a physical or mental disability that prevents normal urination even though the urinary tract is normal. Examples are Parkinson's disease, dementia, and severe depression.

8. D: Most babies lose several ounces during the first week of life. They usually get back to birth weight and start gaining weight by two weeks of age. Breastfed babies may take a little longer to get back to birth weight. A weight loss of between 5% and 10% in the first week is within normal range.

9. D: Valproic acid (Depakene, Depakote) is an anticonvulsant associated with an elevated risk of neural tube defects, such as spina bifida and meningocele, among others. Phenytoin (Dilantin) affects the developing fetus and may cause such defects as cleft lip, cleft palate, mental deficiency, and hypoplastic fingers and nails. Warfarin (Coumadin), a common anticoagulant, is known to cause nasal deformities, brain abnormalities, and stillbirth. Of the answer choices given for this question, only amoxicillin is not known as a teratogen.

10. The infant is placed on the back for the Ortolani-Barlow maneuver. Steps to the maneuver include:

    a. 1. Grasp the infant's knees with the thumbs over the inner thighs.
    b. 3. Flex the infant's knees and hips to 90 degrees.
    c. 4. Touch the infant's knees together, and then press down on the one femur at a time, observing for dislocation.
    d. 2. Slowly abduct the infant's hips and observe for unequal movement, resistance, or an abnormal "clunk" sound.

11. C: Peritonsillar abscesses are typical in teens. Symptoms include sore throat, fever, and difficulty swallowing and opening the mouth (trismus). In fact, the exam may be difficult due to trismus. The abscess causes bulging of the soft palate in the tonsillar area. Cultures usually grow group A strep and mixed anaerobes. Retropharyngeal abscesses occur most frequently in children under five years of age and are less common in older patients whose retropharyngeal nodes have involuted. Epiglottitis also causes sore throat and fever, but it is accompanied by respiratory distress and typically occurs in younger children.

12. A: Viruses cause over 62% of infectious pharyngitis. The remaining answer choices are bacterial agents. Contrary to what patients often believe, group A strep pharyngitis is significantly less common than viral pharyngitis.

13. B: This patient has tinea capitis. The boggy lesion on the scalp is a kerion, which is often mistaken for an abscess. Itchy, scaly areas on the scalp and scattered areas of hair loss are common, as are swollen occipital lymph nodes. Most cases of tinea capitis in the United States are caused by *Trichophyton tonsurans,* which does not fluoresce on Wood's lamp examination. While impetigo can occur on the scalp, it is not associated with hair loss. All clinical information provided in this clinical scenario points to tinea capitis, making all other choices incorrect.

14. B: Constitutional symptoms such as malaise and headaches are typical with *Mycoplasma* infection. The expected norm for chest x-ray findings is diffuse infiltrates as opposed to a consolidated infiltrate. Myalgias and myositis are more common with viral pneumonia. Hypoxia is also atypical for pneumonia due to *Mycoplasma*.

15. B: Breast bud development (thelarche) starts during Tanner stage II. Stage I represents preadolescent girls who have not yet developed secondary sex characteristics. Stages III and IV are more advanced stages of sexual development. Stage V is the highest level of sexual development and is equivalent to an adult in sexual characteristics.

16. D: NLD is characterized by collagen degeneration, granulomatous reaction, fat deposits, and thickened blood vessel walls. The specific cause is unknown, but several theories hint at peripheral blood vessel disease, vasculitis, or trauma. Erythema nodosum usually also occurs on the pretibial areas, but consists of tender red subcutaneous nodules. Myxedema is a nonpitting edema associated with hypothyroidism. Candida infections most commonly occur in warm, moist skin folds.

17. D: Urinary casts may be composed of red blood cells, white blood cells, or renal cells. To perform a test for casts, the patient provides a midstream clean-catch urine specimen. RBC casts indicate bleeding into the renal tubule, commonly seen in glomerular diseases such as lupus nephritis, IgA nephropathy, and Wegener's granulomatosis. With renal tubular damage, renal tubular epithelial cell casts are present in the urine. Neither UTIs nor interstitial nephritis is associated with RBC casts.

18. B: A fasting blood glucose > 126 mg/dL, polydipsia/polyuria, and a nonfasting blood glucose of > 200 mg/dL are all criteria for diagnosing diabetes. HgA1c is useful for periodic assessment of average glucose levels. It is not recommended for diagnostic purposes.

19. A: A nurse practitioner can care for nursing home patients as long as a physician is available in case of emergency. There are no age restrictions for a FNP's patient population, nor is there a caseload limit.

20. C, D, and **E**: West Nile infections are classified as viremia, West Nile fever, or West Nile encephalitis/meningitis, depending on the severity of symptoms. West Nile fever is characterized by fever, headache and body aches, nausea and vomiting, eye pain (occasional), swollen lymph glands (occasional), and maculopapular skin rash on the chest, stomach, and back (occasional). West Nile fever affects about 20% of those who become infected, with symptoms lasting from a few days to several weeks.

21. A: None of their children will have sickle cell disease. For this couple, with each pregnancy, there is a 50% probability of having a child with sickle cell trait and a 50% probability of having a child who is homozygous (AA), but a 0% chance that the child will have sickle cell disease.

22. D: The percentage of patients with dementia that are cared for in the home by family members is about 80%.

23. A, B, and **E**: An authoritarian parent is highly controlling and tends to show little warmth. Authoritarian behavior includes:

- Issuing commands and expecting obedience without question.
- Communicating little with the child outside of giving orders.
- Maintaining inflexible rules.
- Permitting little independence on the child's part.

This parenting style results in a child with poor negotiation skills and an inability to initiate independent activities or achieve autonomy. Additionally, the child may become unassertive and withdrawn. During adolescence, girls often become passive and dependent and boys may become rebellious and aggressive.

24. C: It is not a HIPAA violation to communicate with another provider via email. It is permissible by law to release health information to the police, but the practitioner should verify the identity of the police officer. It is acceptable to leave charts outside patient rooms, but care should be done that PHI is not in open view.

25. A: Most people with high blood pressure have primary hypertension, meaning that there is no known cause. Secondary hypertension refers to high blood pressure with a known cause. Cocaine use, renal disease, and oral contraceptive use are all causes of secondary hypertension. Sepsis is associated with hypotension rather than hypertension.

26. D: Tamiflu (oseltamivir) is indicated for the treatment of uncomplicated illness due to influenza. To be effective, it must be started within 48 hours of onset of symptoms. Nausea, vomiting, and diarrhea are all common side effects of Tamiflu. Heart palpitations are not a symptom routinely associated with influenza.

27. A, B, and **D:** The following actions may indicate boundary violations:

- Accepting a $20 tip from a patient. The nurse should not accept personal gifts for professional services.
- Confiding to a patient about a family situation. Personal situations should only be shared very judiciously for therapeutic purposes, such as telling a patient who struggles with quitting cigarettes about a similar successful struggle.
- Exchanging patients in order to care for a favorite patient. It's always a warning sign if a nurse begins to show favoritism or wants to avoid a patient.

28. C: High fever for more than five days, cervical lymphadenopathy, nonexudative pharyngitis, red strawberry tongue, and maculopapular rash are hallmarks of Kawasaki disease. The fact that the illness did not respond to antibiotics and duration of fever makes the diagnosis of strep infection unlikely. This group of symptoms is not characteristic of either toxic epidermal necrolysis or juvenile rheumatoid arthritis.

29. B: A spouse is most likely to perpetrate abuse. The abuse may be either active or passive. Spouses feel most trapped in their situations of being caregivers and feel no hope of escape. A day-shift unrelated caregiver, by contrast, can leave and "decompress" after her shift.

30. C: The risk of suicide is over 60 times greater than normal in people with AIDS. In patients with chronic lung disease, the risk is 10 times greater. Comparatively speaking, diabetes and osteoporosis do not have high suicide rates.

31. B, E, and **F:** Hypokalemia is a risk factor for those with severe nausea and vomiting as well as those on nasogastric suctioning. Symptoms of hypokalemia include muscle weakness, cramps, and hyporeflexia as well as hypotension, lethargy, and fatigue. Although this child has diarrhea, hypokalemia can lead to abdominal distention and constipation. Hypokalemia can eventually impair kidney function and result in polyuria and polydipsia. Electrocardiogram (ECG) changes characteristic of hypokalemia include premature ventricular contractions (PVCs), a prolonged QT interval, depressed ST segment, and flat or inverted T-waves.

32. D: Influenza virus is the most common cause of viral pneumonia in adults. Respiratory syncytial virus may be associated with pneumonia in children. *Haemophilus influenzae* is a bacterium, not a virus.

33. D: This patient has allergic conjunctivitis, which is associated with pruritus. Causes are allergens or environmental agents. Allergic conjunctivitis is not associated with increased intracranial pressure, fever, or myopia.

34. C: Autonomic neuropathy can cause inability to urinate. The autonomic system innervates many organs including the bladder and urinary tract. As the nerves become damaged, in this case due to diabetes, the nerves of the bladder can't respond to pressure normally when the bladder fills.

35. C: Breast cancer causes the most cancer-related deaths in the 25- to 44-year age range. Lung cancer is the overall leading cause in patients of all ages. Hodgkin's disease occurs commonly in the 15- to 34-year age group and over age 60. The incidence of colon cancer peaks between 60 to 75 years of age. It is the second leading cause of cancer death in Western countries.

36. C: Iron-rich foods include leafy green vegetables, beans, egg yolks, fish, and poultry. Oranges are rich in vitamin C. Milk is rich in calcium and is typically not fortified with iron.

37. A: Herpangina is a viral illness caused by Coxsackie virus. Symptoms include fever, fussiness, throat pain, and drooling. In the early stages, vesicles appear on the tonsillar pillars. The vesicles subsequently ulcerate. Strep pharyngitis is uncommon at this age and is not associated with ulcerations. Gingivostomatitis, also viral, is associated with inflamed, bleeding gums, and mucosal ulcers over the anterior oral cavity. Epiglottitis is a severe, life-threatening bacterial infection associated with respiratory distress.

38. C: Norovirus (also called Norwalk-like virus) causes gastroenteritis. RSV, coronavirus, and rhinovirus have all been shown to cause bronchiolitis. Rhinovirus has recently been implicated in severe bronchiolitis illness. Human metapneumovirus is also an etiologic agent. In fact, the list of pathogens is growing.

39. According to Erikson's psychosocial theory, children go through four stages, followed by four additional stages leading through adolescence to old age. Childhood development impacts later adult development. Stages of childhood include the following:

    a. Infancy (birth to 1 year): 2. Trust versus mistrust.
    b. Early childhood (1 to 3 years): 1. Autonomy versus shame and doubt.
    c. Late childhood (3 to 6 years): 4. Initiative versus guilt.
    d. School age (6 to 12 years): 3. Industry versus inferiority.

40. C: People can have different concepts of time based on their cultures. Americans have more exacting standards for being on time. Hispanics (and others as well), often have a flexible interpretation of time and are more likely to be more approximate with their timelines. Providers should take cultural differences into account in healthcare settings.

41. A: Pneumovax is recommended for all patients 65 years and over. It can be administered with other vaccines but must be injected using a separate syringe at a different injection site. It should never be injected intradermally.

42. A and C: Preventive health maintenance activities may focus on primary prevention, secondary prevention, and tertiary prevention. Primary prevention occurs before illness or injury and attempts to prevent it. Primary prevention includes administering immunizations and instructing parents about car safety seats. Secondary prevention aims to lessen the severity of an illness through early diagnosis and treatment. Examples of secondary prevention include conducting vision screening and screening adolescents for scoliosis. Tertiary prevention aims to prevent deterioration and maintain optimum function. Tertiary prevention measures would include developing rehabilitation activities for a child.

43. B: About one in three people over age 65 has some form of visual impairment. The number-one cause of loss of vision in this age group is age-related macular degeneration.

44. B: HSP is a type of vasculitis seen mostly in children. Patients with HSP often complain of abdominal pain. GI bleeding may also be present as well as joint pains. Patients should also be monitored for renal involvement by checking for hematuria. Purpura typically occurs on the buttocks and lower legs. Patients with HSP do not have thrombocytopenia, but may in fact have thrombocytosis.

45. D: A high-fiber diet is good advice for patients with GERD. Anticholinergic drugs are to be avoided, as they delay gastric emptying and thus would be counterproductive to the management of GERD. Excessive fat intake also delays gastric emptying, and it increases acid secretion in the stomach. Elevating the head of the bed helps prevent the flow of acid into the lower esophagus during sleep; however, the recommendation for elevation is 6 to 8 inches.

46. B: Bulk-forming laxatives such as psyllium (Metamucil) should be taken with a glass of water or other suitable liquid, immediately followed by a second glass. If not taken with enough fluid, it may cause choking or impaction of psyllium in the gastrointestinal tract. It is not necessary to take it with a calcium supplement.

47. C: The treatment of choice for an uncomplicated tooth abscess is penicillin VK. Erythromycin may also be used if the patient is allergic to penicillin. Extraction of the tooth is not necessary.

48. D: It is important maintain therapeutic communication with patients. Answers A, B, and C are nontherapeutic statements because of their defensive nature. Answer A has a punitive tone, implying a punishment of waiting an extra hour for attention. Answer B implies that the patient's problem is not worth the doctor's time. The correct answer, D, is therapeutic because it does not have a negative tone and it reinforces validation of the patient's feelings.

49. D: Umbilical hernias that are less than 2 cm in diameter will heal on their own. It is normal for an umbilical hernia to pouch out when intra-abdominal pressure increases, such as when the baby crying. This does not cause harm and will not cause enlargement of the abdominal wall defect that is present. Wrapping a band around the abdomen will not heal the hernia.

50. A: Perseveration is a repetitive, involuntary pathologic verbal or motor response to stimuli. It occurs in patients with organic mental disorders such as Alzheimer's disease and other forms of dementia. Repeating the same questions over and over is an example of perseveration. Contrivance refers to development of a clever scheme. By confabulating, a person makes up a plausible story or experience to compensate for memory lapses.

51. D: Symptoms of hypoglycemia include hunger, diaphoresis, light-headedness, tremors, nervousness, irritability, sleepiness, and confusion. Diplopia is not a symptom of low blood sugar.

52. B: Croup, also known as viral laryngotracheobronchitis, is associated with subglottic swelling, URI symptoms, and mild to moderate fever. The parainfluenza virus is a common cause. Routine croup is characterized by normal oxygen saturation and mild, if any, retractions. The hallmark is a barking or seal-like cough. On the other hand, fever of 104.5, tripod position, and drooling are signs of a life-threatening acute airway obstructive bacterial infection known as epiglottitis.

53. A: Breast cancer masses tend to be unilateral, firm, painless and irregular in shape. As the disease progresses, there may be redness and retraction of the nipple or the skin overlying the mass. A rubbery, smooth consistency is characteristic of a fibroadenoma, which is most common in women in their twenties and thirties.

54. A, D, and **F**: The patient's symptoms are consistent with heat exhaustion. The initial treatment for heat exhaustion is evaporative cooling. Alcohol baths are no longer recommended, and ice immersion is reserved for severe cases of heat stroke. Oral rehydration with 0.1% isotonic NaCl solution is given, usually at the rate of four ounces every 15 to 20 minutes, although IV fluids may be given in severe cases or if oral rehydration does not bring about a positive response. The patient's VS, temperature, and urinary output must be carefully monitored.

55. A: Nursemaid's elbow (radial head subluxation) is common in toddlers, usually 1 to 4 years of age. When taking a history of the mechanism, it usually reveals that a parent suddenly pulled the child up by the arm as he started to fall. When the nursemaid's elbow is successfully reduced, the radial head relocates into its ligament. The clinician can usually feel a "pop" as it goes back into place.

56. B: Most anticoagulant treatment is directed toward a goal *international normalized ratio* (INR) of 2 to 3. An INR over 3 increases risk of bleeding. Specifically for DVT, a goal of 2.0 to 3.0 drastically reduces the chances of bleeding when compared to having a higher INR without a reduction in effectiveness.

57. B: Nicotine withdrawal is associated with bradycardia rather than tachycardia. Answers A, C, and D are all symptoms of nicotine withdrawal. Additional symptoms include poor concentration, irritability, depression, restlessness, and weight gain.

58. The order of priority in which the nurse should address the patient's problems, from most critical to least critical, is as follows:

    a. 2. Risk of hepatotoxicity: Risks markedly increase when drinking more than three alcoholic beverages daily combined with acetaminophen.
    b. 1. Chronic pain: Better methods of pain control should be explored.
    c. 4. Risk for imbalanced nutrition: Excessive drinking often interferes with nutrition. This patient may benefit from nutritional counseling.
    d. 3. Impaired physical mobility and activity: Physical therapy and better pain control may help to improve mobility.

59. D: The penile foreskin serves a protective function for the glans penis. During the first 12 months of age, nearly all uncircumcised boys will have foreskin that tightly adheres to the glans. By 3 years of age, 90% will retract spontaneously. For some boys, it is normal to achieve retraction by age 5 or 6 years of age. Never forcibly retract the foreskin, as it is painful and may cause infection, phimosis, or paraphimosis.

60. C: Of all the choices given, only Hib (*Haemophilus influenzae*) vaccine is a conjugated vaccine. A conjugated vaccine is made from an altered organism that has been combined with a protein. Conjugation heightens the immune response to the vaccine.

61. C: Rotavirus has long been recognized as a cause of substantial morbidity in pediatric patients from infancy to age five years. An earlier version of the vaccine was taken off the market because of an associated incidence of intussusception, an obstructive condition in which one section of intestine "telescopes" into an adjacent section. Since the introduction of the current vaccine, intussusception rates have not increased beyond the expected range for this age group.

62. D: Antibodies to the killed influenza viruses used to prepare the vaccine form in approximately 2 weeks. The other answer choices are obviously incorrect.

63. B: Physical barriers are impediments that result from inadequate functioning of one or more systems of the body. These include vision, hearing, and mobility. In the case of this patient, his eyesight is impaired and he has limited mobility. Other barriers are psychological (such as emotional instability) and cognitive (such as dementia).

64. C: Frequent pacifier use is not associated with an increased risk of infant tooth decay. Decay may occur when an infant sleeps with a bottle of formula in his mouth and occurs regardless of the number of teeth present. Even babies who are exclusively breastfed can develop dental caries.

65. A: Reliable hearing screening results can be obtained as early as the newborn period.

66. B: Eye contact utilization varies from one culture to another. In some cultures, direct eye contact is considered rude, while in others, it is the desired norm. Observation of eye contact behaviors through experience working with different cultures can help the nurse practitioner appreciate differences in eye contact customs.

67. B: Hypercalcemia can cause polyuria, severe abdominal pain, and confusion. The acronym CRAB is part of the criteria to help diagnose myeloma (calcium elevation, renal insufficiency, anemia, and bone disease). More than 25% of patients with a diagnosis of multiple myeloma will experience hypercalcemia.

68. B: Failure to monitor a patient is an example of medical negligence. Delegating routine tasks to a trained assistant, giving sound medical advice over the telephone, and referring a patient to a specialist are all appropriate actions.

69. A, B, and **E**: During the preschool years (ages three to six), the child should be able to carry out a number of physical skills:

- Uses scissors to cut.
- Draws shapes such as circles and squares.
- Rides tricycle or bicycle with training wheels.
- Ties own shoes.
- Buttons clothes.
- Brushes teeth and washes hands.
- Climbs well with good coordination of arms and legs.
- Learns letters and numbers and may recognize some words and have rudimentary reading skills.

70. B: Nurse practitioner scopes of practice do vary widely from state to state. Contrary to the statements in the answer choices, nurse practitioners may prescribe narcotics in most states and can also perform evaluations of psychosocial status.

71. A: Scabies is caused by the mite *Sarcoptes scabiei*. Mites are in the arachnid family and have eight legs. Insects have six. Ticks and protozoans are not etiologic factors in scabies infestation.

72. B: Rosacea is a chronic dermatosis. Characteristic features include facial redness, papules, and rhinophyma (hyperplasia of nasal tissue). It is commonly found on the cheeks, chin, forehead, and nose. Complications are dry eyes, deep painful facial nodules (pyoderma faciale), folliculitis, and blepharitis.

73. B, C, and **E**: Age-associated changes of the cardiovascular system expected in the older adult include

- Adipose tissue accumulates about the heart.
- Cardiac output decreases.
- The veins become decreasingly elastic.
- The heart's sympathetic nervous response to exertion decreases.
- Mitochondrial DNA in the cardiac muscle is damaged.
- Specialized conduction cells decrease in number.

In a healthy individual, the heart does not increase in size but does so in response to hypertension and heart failure.

74. C: Approximately 30% of patients who have gallstones experience biliary colic, and about 10% will develop acute cholecystitis. Less common (< 1%) complications are gallbladder hydrops, small bowel obstruction, pancreatitis, and gallbladder perforation.

75. D: Because the lesion is localized, topical antifungal treatment is sufficient. In cases where lesions are generalized, oral antifungal therapy is appropriate and more practical. Topical corticosteroids, such as betamethasone, only suppress itching and inflammation. Topical diphenhydramine is not an antifungal medication, but rather an anti-itch product.

76. C: Over two-thirds of Bell's palsy patients recover completely and spontaneously. Approximately 15% have only mild sequelae.

77. A: Key components of overall management of osteoarthritis are nonpharmacological including exercise, physical therapy, thermal therapy, and weight loss if indicated. Joint replacement surgery and arthroscopy may eventually be needed, but not initially. Etanercept (Enbrel) is indicated for treatment of rheumatoid arthritis.

78. D: Hemoglobin A1c is typically measured every three to six months, depending on the desired tightness of glycemic control. Diabetics should also receive retinal exams at least once yearly to screen for retinopathy. In addition, urine should be tested for protein. If protein is negative, a screen for microalbuminuria would also be appropriate. Lipid measurement and control are routine in the management of Type 2 diabetes.

79. C: Basal cell carcinoma accounts for approximately 60% of primary skin cancers, while squamous cell carcinoma comprises 20%. Although most skin cancer deaths are from malignant melanoma, it is relatively rare and accounts for only 1% of skin cancers. Mycosis fungoides is a cutaneous T-cell lymphoma that initially appears in the skin but involves the whole reticuloendothelial system.

80. D: Developmental categories of Denver II are gross motor, fine motor, language, and personal/social. The test evaluates development in children from ages one month to six years.

81. C: Tobacco use in pregnancy is associated with numerous adverse outcomes. Maternal smoking accounts for over 20% of low-birth-weight infants. Other associated problems are placenta previa, preterm birth, placental abruption, and an increased risk of miscarriage.

82. C: Neural tube defects (NTDs) are congenital malformations caused by failure of neural tube closure during embryologic development. The neural tube forms the brain, spinal cord, and other central nervous system tissues. Folic acid protects against development of NTD. According to the Centers for Disease Control, all women who may potentially become pregnant should take folic acid daily.

83. A, B, C, and **F**: Alzheimer's disease is characterized by stages ranging from 1 to 7, with no apparent symptoms at stage 1 and severe cognitive decline and dementia at stage 7. Stage 5, moderate cognitive decline, early dementia, is characterized by

- Needing some assistance with personal hygiene and other activities of daily living.
- Being oriented to self but sometimes being disoriented to place and time.
- Sometimes forgetting names of friends or family.
- Being frustrated at lapses in memory and withdrawing and becoming increasingly self-absorbed.

84. A: Normal breast development may start as early as 8 years of age or as late as age 13 years. The girl in this clinical scenario is not, therefore, developing breasts prematurely and does not need medical evaluation.

85. C: Numerous medications are known to cause the side effect of peripheral edema. Rosiglitazone, an insulin sensitizer, can cause peripheral edema as in this patient. Neither SSRIs (Paxil and others) metformin, nor thiazide diuretics (hydrochlorothiazide) are associated with this side effect.

86. The neurologic exam is conducted following a logical sequence that proceeds from the top down:

a. 3. Mental status: Various instruments may be used, depending on the patient's age and condition.
b. 4. Cranial nerves: Cranial nerves I through XII.
c. 2. Motor system: Includes evaluation of muscles and cerebellar function.
d. 5. Sensory system: Includes assessment of the spinothalamic tract and posterior column tract.
e. 1. Reflexes: Includes assessment of the stretch or deep tendon reflexes and the superficial cutaneous reflexes.

87. C: The majority of experts agree that routine preoperative electrocardiograms should be conducted on all men over age 45, patients with a history of heart disease, and patients with hypertension. Costochondritis is an inflammation of the anterior chest wall and is not associated with an abnormal ECG.

88. C: The patient in this clinical scenario is low risk. The incidence of an abnormal Pap test is low in women who have been screened at 65 years of age. According to the American Cancer Society, the recommendation for stopping is 70 years.

89. B: Of the choices given, only Pneumovax is appropriate. It is recommended for all persons over 65. FluMist is given to healthy patients under age 50. People born before 1957 are considered immune and do not need MMR. Hib vaccine is given to children under 6 years of age.

Mometrix

90. B: Only the 2-year-old may receive prophylaxis with Tamiflu. Oseltamivir (Tamiflu) is generally not recommended in children under 12 months of age.

91. C: Patients appreciate the opportunity to make choices from a list of viable options when they are available. Contrary to what many believe, patients often feel they have not received enough information rather than too much. Leaning toward patients has been shown to improve recall. Patients often do not understand or recall information, making it important to use techniques that help improve patient recall such as moving closer to the patient and increasing eye contact.

92. D: Of the choices given, obesity has a higher prevalence among Native Americans. Other conditions that are more prevalent in Native Americans when compared to other populations are diabetes, alcoholism, and suicide.

93. A: The principle of professional appearance is not one of the fundamental principles of professionalism. The true principles are as follows: primacy of patient welfare (serving the interest of the patient and not doing harm), patient autonomy (empowering patients to make informed treatment decisions), and social justice (eliminating discrimination in healthcare).

94. C: Disclosing this information would be a violation of patient confidentiality. The desire not to disclose protected information is the patient's prerogative, even if his wife asks for disclosure.

95. B, C, and **E**: Indications of possible hearing impairment in a two-year-old child include the following:

- The child has no speech. Although language acquisition varies, at two years old, a child should say some words, such as "No."
- The child cannot follow simple age-appropriate commands, such as "Show me your toy." Children's comprehension usually precedes language production.
- The child does not make distinct age-appropriate speech sounds. Children should make a wide range of sounds even before they begin speaking in words.

96. C: Family nurse practitioners often give anticipatory guidance to children and parents. Because children move from one developmental phase to another, parents need guidance on what to expect in certain areas of concern. Common areas for discussion for two-year-olds are growth and development, nutrition, emotional development, and safety. As children grow older, sports, exercise, sexual development, and warnings about drug abuse become important.

97. C: Rosacea is a chronic skin problem that is common in middle age. Most people with rosacea develop a cyclic pattern of disease. It may be confused with acne, but unlike acne, patients with rosacea do not develop comedones. Telangiectasia is common on the cheeks and nose with rosacea. The classic lupus malar rash is butterfly shaped and involves the cheeks and bridge of the nose. Seborrheic dermatitis appears on the face, upper chest, and any other areas of oily skin. There are often flaky, greasy white, or yellow scales present.

98. D: Temporomandibular dysfunction is a common cause of referred ear pain, making the other choices unlikely.

99. B: All of the choices given predispose patients to recurrent sinus infections. However, allergic rhinitis is the most common one of those listed. Allergic rhinitis is seen in approximately 60% of patients with recurrent sinusitis.

100. A: This patient is exhibiting body language that poses a barrier to communication with the provider by him appearing disinterested. Gestures are performed with hands or with the head as in nodding in agreement or waving hands to mimic an activity. Facial expressions show emotions such as happiness or fear. Empathy is not a type of nonverbal communication.

101. D: It is sometimes necessary to use an interpreter in a clinical setting. The interpreter should be medically trained. The provider should address the patient directly, as if the interpreter was not there. Use a normal voice volume and try to employ simple language, expressing one concept at a time. Place chairs in a triangular configuration and face the patient while speaking.

102. B: HR and Respirations are slightly increased. BP is decreased from normal for this age range. Normal pedi heart rate: 1-3 yrs: 70-110; 3-6 yrs: 65-110; 6-12 yrs: 60-95; >12 yrs: 55-85. Normal pedi respiratory rate: 1-3 yrs: 20-30; 3-6 yrs: 20-25; 6-12 yrs:14-22; >12 yrs: 12-18.

103. According to Peplau's framework for psychodynamic nursing, the nurse carries out a number of different nursing roles:

a. Teacher: 3. "It's important to take your pulse each morning before you take your digoxin. You must not take the medication if your pulse is lower than 60 because the medicine can slow your heart too much."
b. Counselor: 1. "I heard you yelling at other patients and staff members. Let's talk about what you are feeling and explore other ways to express those feelings."
c. Technical expert: 2. "BiPAP delivers two different levels of pressure while you sleep. This is where we set those pressures. One pressure is for when you breathe in, and the other pressure is for when you breathe out."
d. Resource person: 4. "The home health agency can monitor your care when you go home, and the Meals on Wheels program can bring in daily meals until you are able to prepare meals yourself."

104. A: Drug-seeking patients often claim "allergies" to various pain medications and claim that only one specific narcotic works for their pain. In addition, drug seekers usually hop from one doctor to another to get the drugs they want. The term "drug seeker" applies to a person who is trying to obtain narcotics. The term is not usually used to refer to patients who want antibiotics.

105. D: This patient has bacterial vaginosis. A KOH prep characteristically reveals a fishy odor and clue cells. The treatment is metronidazole. Doxycycline is used to treat Chlamydia. Terconazole is used to treat vaginal candidiasis and ceftriaxone is used to treat gonococcal infections.

106. A: Fifth disease is primarily a disease of children. It produces the so-called slapped cheek rash and is caused by parvovirus B19. The other answer choices are incorrect.

107. D: Accutane (an acne drug) is a known teratogen that belongs to pregnancy category X. In fact, it is best not taken by women of childbearing age unless acne is extremely severe and unresponsive to other therapies. It is associated with a high potential for fetal injury. Healthcare providers perform a pregnancy test on the patient before starting Accutane and will likely continue doing pregnancy tests monthly prior to prescription renewal.

108. B: By identifying a problem, the nurse practitioner is employing the process of assessment. Planning involves the process of determining an action plan. Implementation carries out the plan, and evaluation involves examining and appraising the plan of action.

109. C: Interpersonal conflict exists between one person and another, whereas intrapersonal conflict is an internal conflict involving only one person.

110. D: *Haemophilus influenzae* biogroup *aegyptius* is related to conjunctivitis. *Yersinia pestis* is linked to Plague, *Helicobacter pylori* is linked to peptic ulcers, and *vibrio cholera* is linked to Cholera.

111. D: Licensure by examination is required when a state does not grant licensure by reciprocity and a candidate must pass an examination in that state. A temporary license allows a nurse to practice while the license is pending. Licensure by waiver occurs if the candidate meets or exceeds some licensure requirements. These requirements can be waived, but the nurse must be able to demonstrate other requirements.

112. C: Pentoxifylline is a hemorheological agent that helps blood viscosity. This drug is used for symptomatic PVD. It is contraindicated in patients with a sensitivity to caffeine or theophylline.

113. D: While surgically removing the wrong body part is an egregious error, it does not involve a medication-related error.

114. D: A hernia is the most likely indicated in this case. The tender lump in the groin cannot be explained by any of the other diagnoses listed. Moderate or more pain in a hernia is not normal and should make the case to consider strangulation in conjunction with the other symptoms. The patient may be febrile, have nausea/vomiting, and systemic symptoms of sepsis.

115. A: This process is known as risk management. Quality assurance is an evaluation of medical services, their results, and how they compare to the accepted standards. Patient rights are a form of nursing intervention involving healthcare rights.

116. C: The normal range for Digoxin is 0.7-1.4 ng/ml.

117. C: The normal range for Primidone is 4-12 mcg/ml.

118. D: The normal range for Carbamazepine is 10-20 mcg/ml.

119. A, C, and **D**: Other symptoms that are typical of early-stage Lyme disease include headache, myalgia, and enlarged lymph glands near the rash. Typically, the first erythema migrans is at the site of the tick bite. As the disease progresses, multiple rash sites may appear as well as more pronounced signs of infection, such as fever and facial palsy. Arthritic and neurological symptoms may occur as the disease disseminates.

120. C: Answer choices A, B, and D are all correct. The incident report form should not be copied nor placed in the patient's record.

121. A: The nurse practitioner should strongly suspect gram-negative organisms as the cause of conjunctivitis in contact lens wearers. Topical gentamicin or tobramycin would therefore be a good choice for treatment. In people who do not wear contact lenses, bacterial conjunctivitis is most commonly caused by either *Staphylococcus aureus* or *Streptococcus pneumoniae*.

122. B: GER is a common cause of vomiting in infants. It may also be associated with episodes of recurrent wheezing. This patient is too old to be presenting with pyloric stenosis, which typically manifests itself with recurrent vomiting within three to five weeks after birth and is rare in babies over three months of age. Viral gastroenteritis is self-limited and does not last two months. Reactive airway disease is associated with wheezing but not with vomiting.

123. B: To determine BMI, divide the patient's weight in kilograms by their height in meters squared. A BMI greater than 25 is overweight. If the BMI is more than 30, the patient is considered obese. Morbidly obese patients have BMIs over 35.

124. D: An estimated 65% of Americans are overweight and about 35% are obese.

125. C: The patient in this clinical scenario has post-streptococcal glomerulonephritis (PSGN). The source of the strep infection was the impetigo. Children often present with periorbital edema because of a loss of protein in the urine. A diagnosis of UTI is not likely, given the symptoms of painless hematuria and edema. Painless hematuria requires investigation. Kidney stones are associated with intermittent severe colicky pain.

126. C: A fluoroquinolone such as levofloxacin is a good choice of antibiotic considering there was treatment failure with first-line drugs. First-generation cephalosporins and erythromycin are not recommended because they do not provide adequate coverage of major pathogens. In addition, clarithromycin may not provide coverage for resistant *Streptococcus pneumoniae*.

127. A: Of the choices given, an MRI is the best choice. A herniated disk will not show up on a plain radiograph. Bend-over tests screen for scoliosis. Loss of range of motion is nonspecific.

128. A, B, D, and **F**: Periods of moodiness and constant use of social media are fairly typical behavior associated with adolescents. However, signs or symptoms that may be indicative of substance abuse include abnormal physical changes (dental problems, skin color, rash, hair loss, and nasal discharge), falling grades and school attendance because of lack of motivation and inability to concentrate, repeated unexplained falls and accidents (including burns), and labile mood and behavior. The adolescent may have difficulty setting goals, act irresponsibly, and may feel hopeless and depressed. Appetite and sleep habits may change.

129. D: Placing allergen-blocking covers on the mattress and pillows are a good way to decrease asthma triggers. Frequent vacuuming and use of ceiling fans actually help spread allergen particles into the air. Home humidity levels should ideally be less than 50%.

130. A: Tricyclic antidepressants such as amitriptyline and SSRIs such as citalopram are often associated with sexual dysfunction. Of the choices given, bupropion is least likely to cause sexual side effects.

131. A, D, E, and **F**: Fine and gross motor abilities that are typical of a five-month-old child include

- Exhibits no head lag when pulled to a sitting position.
- Turns from abdomen to back and then from back to abdomen by six months.
- Uses a palmar rather than a pincer grasp. Able to pick up items.
- Grasps and manipulates objects such as rattles.
- Mouths objects, including pulling feet to mouth.
- Supports much of own weight if held in a standing position.

132. C: This patient is showing signs and symptoms of rheumatoid arthritis: proximal interphalangeal joint involvement of the hands, symmetrical swelling, fatigue, and prolonged morning stiffness. Symptoms of osteoarthritis usually develop gradually. Joints of the hips, back, base of the thumb and neck are often affected in osteoarthritis. Psoriatic arthritis occurs in patients who have psoriasis. In this type of arthritis, joints are less symmetrically involved. Gout most often involves the joints of the feet.

133. D: The patient in this scenario has symptoms of acute glaucoma. This is a medical emergency. The only correct answer is to refer the patient immediately to an ophthalmologist.

134. C: All household and close contacts should be treated with azithromycin or clarithromycin, which each have fewer side effects and are associated with better patient compliance with once-daily dosing. The medication is taken by close contacts and household members regardless of immunization status. This helps limit the transmission of infection to others.

135. B: This clinical scenario raises strong suspicion for cystic fibrosis. CF is more common in Caucasians and is associated with frequent respiratory infections and digestive problems such as diarrhea and greasy stools (high fat content). These finding are not characteristic of either thyroid disorders or tuberculosis. Performing a sweat chloride test will aid in the diagnosis of CF.

136. D: A newborn infant exhibits the Moro reflex in response to a loud noise such as a hand clap. This reflex is also known as the startle reflex. Stimulation of the perioral area elicits the rooting reflex. The tonic neck reflex occurs when the newborn's head is turned to one side and he assumes a "fencing posture."

137. A, B, C, and **F**: The family nurse practitioner should recommend the following nursing management techniques for nurses caring for preschoolers:

- Encourage parents to stay with children: Children often have separation anxiety and fear of abandonment.
- Allow the child to make choices when possible: Children may feel totally out of control and fearful.
- Explain all procedures to the child in age-appropriate terms: Children often have a poor understanding of medical procedures and may fear that tubes are permanent or that they will lose body parts.
- Provide a night light: Children often fear the dark or monsters, especially in a strange environment.

138. D: A short-acting beta-2 agonist, such as albuterol or levalbuterol, is appropriate for use as a rescue medication. Corticosteroid inhalers, leukotriene inhibitors, and anti-allergic medications are useful for long-term control.

139. C: An initial symptom of tuberculosis is a mild cough productive of nonbloody mucoid sputum. Bloody sputum production, chest pain, and breathing difficulty are all late symptoms.

140. A: The infant has a candida diaper rash, which is usually treated with nystatin cream. The use of talcum powder is no longer recommended due to the risk of aspiration of particles by the infant and because it was not shown to be effective in decreasing moisture in the diaper area. Oral fluconazole is not first-line treatment for cutaneous candidiasis. Mupirocin is useful in the treatment of localized bacterial skin infections.

141. A, B, and **D**: Although all of these topics are important, those that are specific to injury prevention education for a 16-year-old patient include:

- Protective gear.
- Bicycle, skateboard, and automobile safety.
- Drinking and driving.

Some injury prevention topics may be specific to the adolescent's environment. For example, farm safety measures should be covered for an adolescent living in a rural area but are not generally necessary for adolescents in urban areas. Other topics that should be covered for adolescents include sleep, school performance, peer interactions, discipline, and future planning.

142. C: Mucoceles are usually caused by trauma to the inner lining of the lip. They rupture easily and spontaneously. Most patients with mucoceles are under age 20 years. Unroofing or aspirating the lesion is associated with recurrences. If the patient has frequent recurrences, refer them to an oral surgeon.

143. B: Enuresis is more common in boys than girls. UTI is not a common cause of nocturnal enuresis. A renal ultrasound is usually not necessary. Imipramine has a success rate of less than 50%.

144. C: This child most likely has a viral URI. Allergic rhinitis and nasal foreign bodies are not associated with fever. In addition, nasal foreign bodies cause unilateral nasal discharge. The yellow color of the mucus is not significant. Symptoms of four days' duration are highly unlikely to be caused by sinusitis, which is uncommon at this age anyway.

145. B: A chest x-ray is recommended for asymptomatic patients with a positive PPD to rule out the slight possibility of an active TB infection. Treatment with INH decreases the progression of latent TB to active TB infection. Nine months is the optimal duration of treatment. A sputum culture is done if there are findings of old TB on chest x-ray.

146. C: Children with a cleft palate are at increased risk for recurrent otitis media. Children with clefts are more likely to develop fluid behind the tympanic membrane. Usually the fluid drains through the Eustachian tube, but the tube is often distorted by the cleft and interferes with proper drainage. During surgical repair of the cleft, surgeons usually insert ventilator tubes in the eardrum to allow fluid to drain.

147. B: Colic, sudden infant death syndrome (SIDS), and wheezing are all associated with cigarette smoke exposure. Bacterial conjunctivitis is not associated with exposure to smoking.

148. A and C: Indications of developmental delay should trigger a complete medical and developmental evaluation to determine the cause. Indications include

- Infant sucks poorly and feeds very slowly.
- Limbs are loose and floppy.
- Eyes don't blink in response to bright light and do not follow a nearby object moving from one side to the other.
- Movement of arms and legs is restricted or stiff.
- Lower jaw constantly trembles.
- Child does not respond to loud sounds.

149. B: About 50% of people who travel abroad become ill while traveling. The most common illness is traveler's diarrhea. The other illnesses listed as answer choices are less frequent.

150. C: Of all the choices given, women are most likely to be interested in using alternative medicine therapies.

151. A and E: Denial is not uncommon, especially with the unexpected death of a child. The most therapeutic responses are "I'm so sorry for your loss" and "Take the time you need to be with your child." Although the family nurse practitioner should not reinforce the denial, the nurse should also avoid arguing or forcing the parents to acknowledge the death until they are ready. Parents may need some quiet time with the deceased to come to terms with their feelings and to accept that their child has died.

152. A: The mainstay of treatment for viral diarrhea in children is to maintain adequate hydration. If the child with diarrhea is not vomiting, there is no need to stop feeding solid foods. Antidiarrheal and antispasmodic medications are not recommended for children.

153. C: Intermittent claudication is an aching, cramping, or burning in the legs due to poor circulation in the arteries. It often occurs with walking and disappears with rest. It is not normal and can be due to atherosclerosis or vasospasm. Restless legs syndrome is a neurologic disorder associated with an unpleasant sensation in the legs and with a compulsion to move the legs. Multiple sclerosis is also a neurologic disorder.

154. C: The ESR is an acute phase reactant. An elevated ESR is indicative of inflammation, but it is not specific for any disorder. In performing the test, red blood cells are allowed to settle in a tube of unclotted blood. At the end of one hour, the distance the cells have fallen is measured. Inflammation produces a change in blood proteins, causing red blood cells to aggregate and become heavier than normal and therefore take longer to form sediment at the bottom of the tube.

155. A: As in this case, an infant given free water is at risk for developing hyponatremia. Low levels of sodium are associated with seizures. Infants who need hydration should be given an oral electrolyte solution or intravenous fluids rather than plain water.

156. A, C, D, and **E:** A 65-year-old client who states that he has received no immunizations since childhood and had chickenpox as a child should receive the following immunizations:

- Tdap: The Tdap immunization one time and then Td boosters every 10 years.
- Influenza: The flu immunization every year before flu season.
- Herpes zoster: The shingles immunization one time.
- Pneumococcal: A series of two different injections.

Depending on risk factors, some adults may receive recommendations to receive the hepatitis A and B immunizations as well.

157. A: The Adams forward bend test is used to screen for scoliosis. The test is performed by asking the patient to bend forward 90 degrees at the waist, as if to touch his toes. The examiner looks for asymmetry of the trunk (an asymmetric thoracic prominence on one side). The test has its limitations in that it cannot detect the exact severity of scoliosis, nor can it detect lower spine curvatures.

158. C: Contributory negligence occurs when the patient contributes to his own negative outcome.

159. B: To calculate BMI, divide the weight in kilograms by the height in meters squared. In this example, BMI = 64 divided by (1.6 x 1.6) = 64/2.54 = 25.

160. D: A child subsisting on a diet of mostly whole milk is at risk for developing iron deficiency anemia. Whole milk is not iron fortified. Because he is not eating any solid foods, there are no other sources of iron in his diet.

161. B: The patient in this clinical scenario has a prolapsed uterus. The uterus is the only organ that can fall into the vagina. Depending on duration and severity, the uterus can become ulcerated and result in bleeding. This is often the result of child bearing and weakening of the pelvic tissues as a woman ages. It is common for urinary incontinence to exist in these cases.

162. A: Retinal detachment is typically not associated with eye pain. The patient complains of seeing floaters, flashes of light, and loss of the central portion of vision.

163. B: Direct inguinal hernias are generally acquired due to heavy lifting, straining, or coughing. Indirect inguinal hernias, hiatal hernias in children, and umbilical hernias in infants are congenital.

164. C: The National Pressure Ulcer Advisory Panel developed a staging system to ensure that definitions for pressure ulcers were standardized. Stage I: Nonblanchable erythema: Intact, reddened area that does not blanch. Area remains intact but the physical appearance is altered. Stage II: Partial thickness: Destruction of the epidermis and/or dermis. This type of injury may be an intact blister, ruptured blister, or an open ulcer if it has a pinkish or a reddish wound bed. Stage III: Full thickness skin loss. Muscle, tendons, and bones have not been injured. Stage IV: Full thickness tissue loss: Damage has progressed to bone, muscle, or tendons. Unstageable/Unclassified Injury is present and involves full thickness, but cannot be staged until slough is removed. Suspected Deep Tissue Injury Discolored skin that is still intact but has been damaged. Area may feel boggy and appear deeper than stage I.

165. D: A nurse can be sued for malpractice for various reasons including failure to report a change in a patient's condition, failure to answer calls from a patient, neglecting to monitor a patient, administering the wrong medication, and administering a treatment not ordered by the physician. All nurses should maintain continuing education requirements, but failing to do so is not grounds for a malpractice suit.

166. B: This patient has otitis externa. Topical treatment with combination antibiotic and corticosteroid drops has been shown to be very effective. Because the inflammation is localized, systemic antibiotics are rarely indicated. Antipyrine/benzocaine drops are ineffective. Ibuprofen may help with pain, but by itself, it is not the best answer.

167. A, C, and **E**: Citalopram (Celexa) is a selective serotonin reuptake inhibitor (SSRI) that is used to treat depression. Common adverse effects include:

- Sedation and lethargy.
- Agitation, anxiety, and insomnia.
- GI distress: nausea, dry mouth, diarrhea, constipation, and anorexia.
- Vision disturbances: blurring, tunnel vision, dry eyes, and pain.
- Decreased sex drive, impotence, and erectile dysfunction.

Citalopram may cause suicidal ideation, especially in those younger than 18, and its use may result in a life-threatening interaction if taken with a monoamine oxidase (MAO) inhibitor. Citalopram is in Food and Drug Administration (FDA) pregnancy category C and can pass into breast milk.

168. D: The developmental milestones are closest to those of a 9-month-old. Infants that are 8 to 10 months old are able to use a pincer grasp, pull up to stand, and walk holding onto furniture, and recognize the word "no."

169. B: Breast development in adolescent boys can be very distressing. These patients are often teased at school. However, it is a temporary and benign condition due to hormonal imbalances of estrogen and testosterone during puberty. It affects 40 to 60% of male teens. No treatment, workups, or referrals are needed.

170. C: Routine nosebleeds often originate from Kiesselbach's plexus over the anterior nasal septum. To stop a nosebleed, pinch the nostrils shut and apply continuous pressure for 10 minutes. Applying pressure to the nasal bridge, tilting the head back, and applying ice packs to the forehead are common mistakes people make when treating nosebleeds.

171. A: Venous stasis dermatitis is an inflammatory skin disease that occurs in the lower extremities of middle-aged and elderly patients. It is caused by venous insufficiency that occurs when venous valves become incompetent.

172. C: Peak flow is a useful measure of asthma control. Peak flow meters measure the air flow out of the lungs as a patient blows forcefully into the device. Measurements between 80 to 100% of personal best are in the green zone, indicating good control. Measurements at 50 to 79% are in the yellow zone, a caution indicating some loss of asthma control. Adjustments may need to be made with medications. The red zone is a reading less than 50% of personal best and indicates a need for immediate medical attention.

173. D: The recommended ratio of chest compressions to breaths in adult CPR is 30:2. The same ratio applies to children.

174. B: Ciprofloxacin may be used safely and effectively for prophylaxis of traveler's diarrhea. Increased resistance has limited the effectiveness of trimethoprim-sulfa and doxycycline.

175. B: The treatment of choice for gonococcal cervicitis is intramuscular ceftriaxone in combination with oral azithromycin. Oral cefixime may be substituted if ceftriaxone is not available.

176. A: The Tanner stages are used to classify the physical symptoms of male and female adolescents as they progress through puberty. In females, the breasts and distribution of pubic hair are assessed, while in males the distribution of pubic hair and genital development are assessed. In females, the classifications range from B-1 when there is no breast development up to B-5 when the breasts have completed full development. Pubic hair is assessed on a scale of Ph-1 when there is none present up to Ph-5 when there is an inverse triangle of hair present that extends to the medial thighs.

177. D: Milia are very common and occur when flakes of skin become trapped within pores. It is most common in newborns and occurs most often on the nose and chin. It is important to not pick or pinch these lesions because this could damage the tissue or lead to a skin infection. The lesions usually resolve on their own within a few weeks.

178 B: When a woman has gone a full year without any menstrual bleeding and her FSH levels are consistently elevated at 30 mIU/mL or higher, she is considered to have reached menopause. Estrogen and progesterone levels will be low in a woman who has reached menopause. A normal testosterone level for a woman is 15-70 ng/dL. A thorough history should also be taken to identify other symptoms of menopause, such as hot flashes, sleep disturbances, vaginal dryness, and mood changes.

179. C: Hypertension is diagnosed after 3 readings of a blood pressure higher than 140/90. The most appropriate action in this case is to provide the patient with information about his blood pressure and the conservative measures he can take at home to help lower it without the use of medications. This includes watching his diet to decrease sodium intake, increase his activity level to include a regular exercise program, and monitor and record his blood pressure daily. This blood pressure log should be brought to his next appointment to review the readings and then determine whether he needs to start on an anti-hypertensive medication.

180. B: Skin will tent when pinched due to dehydration, but in the elderly patient this can also occur because of decreased elasticity of the skin. As the skin ages, the elastic connective tissue underneath loses its ability return to normal after it is pinched. It can take up to 30 seconds for elderly skin to return to its normal appearance even in a well-hydrated patient. The other choices listed are more reliable at identifying dehydration in the elderly patient than assessing skin turgor.

181. C: One of the earliest signs of digoxin toxicity is a yellowish discoloration in vision, especially while looking at light. This is called xanthopsia. A digoxin level should be checked regularly in patients who are taking this medication. The normal range is 0.5-2 ng/mL.

182. B: Anticholinergic drugs can help with some of the rigidity seen with Parkinson's, but they do little to help with the bradykinesia. The side effects seen with this class of drugs can be more severe in elderly populations. The other medications listed are helpful with all of the symptoms of Parkinson's disease.

183. D: The symptoms described are consistent with epiglottitis, a medical emergency. Airway compromise is the biggest risk with this illness. Epiglottitis is treated in the hospital and usually requires intubation to maintain the airway.

184. A: It is important to be aware of the conversations co-workers are having, especially in a public place. HIPAA regulations prohibit conversations in a public space regarding a patient. It would be appropriate to subtly remind co-workers of this if it occurs.

185. A: The patient-centered medical home model utilizes the primary care provider as the main person coordinating all care for the patient. This way, specific specialties or other medical care that is needed can be delegated by one person.

186. C: Quality improvement is instrumental in improving the way healthcare services are provided, while continually measuring the effect those changes have on the health status of the patients served. This is often measured through patient satisfaction information.

187. D: HIPAA regulations state that the care of a patient cannot be discussed to anyone without appropriate permission. This includes confirming or denying that the patient was seen at a specific healthcare facility. Most people understand this once it is explained to them.

188. A: Palliative care is often utilized to offer a patient the extra care of therapy they need when faced with a chronic illness. Some palliative care patients will "graduate" from this and others may need to transition to hospice care as their chronic disease progresses.

189. B: The Asian population has been the fastest growing in the United States since 2000. There are approximately 21 million people of Asian descent living in the U.S. today.

190. B: It is respectful to not speak while touching a person who practices the Muslim faith. Any explanations of what is being done, such as a dressing change, should be communicated before the procedure is performed and this should be explained to the patient and family.

191. D: In the Vietnamese culture, there are specific feelings regarding birth control. Oral contraceptive pills are thought of as a "hot" medication that may cause a newborn baby to be handicapped. They also believe the IUD can cause cancer and personality changes. Termination of a pregnancy is considered very dangerous because the spirit of the fetus may stay with the family to cause them problems.

192. D: Whenever possible, have an interpreter present in these types of situations who has undergone some training in medical terminology. Using a family member is not ensuring that any medical training or terms will be correctly translated. Online software may not be accurate and there is no way to verify that the terms and concepts are being interpreted appropriately.

193. A: Having a patient with a hearing impairment offers the opportunity to utilize different forms of teaching. Some of these patients may have some degree of hearing acuity left, but most have learned to adapt and read lips. It is important to be aware of any distracting background noises and to face the patient directly so that the face and mouth are clearly visible. Remember not to turn away when talking or cover the mouth with the hand as that will make it difficult for the patient.

194. D: Education should be done with the patient and the family. The patient should try to maintain as much independence as possible and be informed as to what treatments will need to be continued at home. Including the patient in the teaching process can also increase compliance to the treatment plan.

195. C: Azithromycin is very effective at treating Group A strep pharyngitis; however, it has been linked to an increased risk of cardiac dysrhythmias. This would make azithromycin contraindicated for this particular patient with a history of SVT. Azithromycin, and other macrolide antibiotics, increase the risk of developing QT prolongation. There have also been reported cases of torsades de pointes and ventricular dysrhythmias while taking azithromycin.

196. B: Benadryl can cause anticholinergic side effects, such as pupil dilation, photophobia, and blurred vision. This is most likely due to relaxation of the ciliary muscle and the decrease in accommodation of the eyes. Other medications that commonly cause anticholinergic side effects include antipsychotics, medications used to treat the symptoms of Parkinson's disease, and antispasmodics.

197. A: It usually takes approximately 6 to 8 weeks for the TSH to show changes in levels following when medication is started or after adjusting the dosage of medication. The TSH still remains the most reliable lab test for diagnosing or monitoring thyroid disease. If labs need to be performed before 6 to 8 weeks, the free T_4 and total T_3 levels can be checked. This should still be followed up with a check of the TSH at the appropriate time, though.

198. C: Abdominal pain with nausea and vomiting can occur with any of these choices. Only acute cholecystitis, however, also presents with right shoulder pain. This is called referred pain. Right shoulder pain occurs with gallbladder disease because of its proximity to the phrenic nerve. The phrenic nerve runs down each side of the next to the diaphragm in the upper abdomen. The gallbladder is close to this and can cause nerve impulses, such as pain, to pass through the phrenic nerve and refer pain to the right shoulder, or between the shoulders.

199. D: The FEV1 value that is associated with severe, or stage 3, COPD is 30-50% below normal. The FEV1 is the forced expiratory volume which measures the amount of air a person can forcibly exhale in 1 second. The worse the degree of COPD, the lower the FEV1 will be. This is also helpful to monitor in order to track the progression of COPD and the rate at which the disease has worsened.

200. B: Prediabetes is diagnosed when the hemoglobin A1C is between 5.7% and 6.4%. It is usually managed with lifestyle changes to include diet and exercise. A hemoglobin A1C less than 5.7% is normal, but patients with a strong family history of type 2 diabetes should be made aware of some of the steps they can take to help decrease their risk of diabetes. Diabetes is diagnosed when the hemoglobin A1C is greater than 6.4%.

How to Overcome Test Anxiety

Just the thought of taking a test is enough to make most people a little nervous. A test is an important event that can have a long-term impact on your future, so it's important to take it seriously and it's natural to feel anxious about performing well. But just because anxiety is normal, that doesn't mean that it's helpful in test taking, or that you should simply accept it as part of your life. Anxiety can have a variety of effects. These effects can be mild, like making you feel slightly nervous, or severe, like blocking your ability to focus or remember even a simple detail.

If you experience test anxiety—whether severe or mild—it's important to know how to beat it. To discover this, first you need to understand what causes test anxiety.

Causes of Test Anxiety

While we often think of anxiety as an uncontrollable emotional state, it can actually be caused by simple, practical things. One of the most common causes of test anxiety is that a person does not feel adequately prepared for their test. This feeling can be the result of many different issues such as poor study habits or lack of organization, but the most common culprit is time management. Starting to study too late, failing to organize your study time to cover all of the material, or being distracted while you study will mean that you're not well prepared for the test. This may lead to cramming the night before, which will cause you to be physically and mentally exhausted for the test. Poor time management also contributes to feelings of stress, fear, and hopelessness as you realize you are not well prepared but don't know what to do about it.

Other times, test anxiety is not related to your preparation for the test but comes from unresolved fear. This may be a past failure on a test, or poor performance on tests in general. It may come from comparing yourself to others who seem to be performing better or from the stress of living up to expectations. Anxiety may be driven by fears of the future—how failure on this test would affect your educational and career goals. These fears are often completely irrational, but they can still negatively impact your test performance.

> **Review Video: 3 Reasons You Have Test Anxiety**
> Visit mometrix.com/academy and enter code: 428468

Elements of Test Anxiety

As mentioned earlier, test anxiety is considered to be an emotional state, but it has physical and mental components as well. Sometimes you may not even realize that you are suffering from test anxiety until you notice the physical symptoms. These can include trembling hands, rapid heartbeat, sweating, nausea, and tense muscles. Extreme anxiety may lead to fainting or vomiting. Obviously, any of these symptoms can have a negative impact on testing. It is important to recognize them as soon as they begin to occur so that you can address the problem before it damages your performance.

> **Review Video: 3 Ways to Tell You Have Test Anxiety**
> Visit mometrix.com/academy and enter code: 927847

The mental components of test anxiety include trouble focusing and inability to remember learned information. During a test, your mind is on high alert, which can help you recall information and stay focused for an extended period of time. However, anxiety interferes with your mind's natural processes, causing you to blank out, even on the questions you know well. The strain of testing during anxiety makes it difficult to stay focused, especially on a test that may take several hours. Extreme anxiety can take a huge mental toll, making it difficult not only to recall test information but even to understand the test questions or pull your thoughts together.

> **Review Video: How Test Anxiety Affects Memory**
> Visit mometrix.com/academy and enter code: 609003

Effects of Test Anxiety

Test anxiety is like a disease—if left untreated, it will get progressively worse. Anxiety leads to poor performance, and this reinforces the feelings of fear and failure, which in turn lead to poor performances on subsequent tests. It can grow from a mild nervousness to a crippling condition. If allowed to progress, test anxiety can have a big impact on your schooling, and consequently on your future.

Test anxiety can spread to other parts of your life. Anxiety on tests can become anxiety in any stressful situation, and blanking on a test can turn into panicking in a job situation. But fortunately, you don't have to let anxiety rule your testing and determine your grades. There are a number of relatively simple steps you can take to move past anxiety and function normally on a test and in the rest of life.

> **Review Video: How Test Anxiety Impacts Your Grades**
> Visit mometrix.com/academy and enter code: 939819

Physical Steps for Beating Test Anxiety

While test anxiety is a serious problem, the good news is that it can be overcome. It doesn't have to control your ability to think and remember information. While it may take time, you can begin taking steps today to beat anxiety.

Just as your first hint that you may be struggling with anxiety comes from the physical symptoms, the first step to treating it is also physical. Rest is crucial for having a clear, strong mind. If you are tired, it is much easier to give in to anxiety. But if you establish good sleep habits, your body and mind will be ready to perform optimally, without the strain of exhaustion. Additionally, sleeping well helps you to retain information better, so you're more likely to recall the answers when you see the test questions.

Getting good sleep means more than going to bed on time. It's important to allow your brain time to relax. Take study breaks from time to time so it doesn't get overworked, and don't study right before bed. Take time to rest your mind before trying to rest your body, or you may find it difficult to fall asleep.

Review Video: The Importance of Sleep for Your Brain
Visit mometrix.com/academy and enter code: 319338

Along with sleep, other aspects of physical health are important in preparing for a test. Good nutrition is vital for good brain function. Sugary foods and drinks may give a burst of energy but this burst is followed by a crash, both physically and emotionally. Instead, fuel your body with protein and vitamin-rich foods.

Also, drink plenty of water. Dehydration can lead to headaches and exhaustion, especially if your brain is already under stress from the rigors of the test. Particularly if your test is a long one, drink water during the breaks. And if possible, take an energy-boosting snack to eat between sections.

Review Video: How Diet Can Affect your Mood
Visit mometrix.com/academy and enter code: 624317

Along with sleep and diet, a third important part of physical health is exercise. Maintaining a steady workout schedule is helpful, but even taking 5-minute study breaks to walk can help get your blood pumping faster and clear your head. Exercise also releases endorphins, which contribute to a positive feeling and can help combat test anxiety.

When you nurture your physical health, you are also contributing to your mental health. If your body is healthy, your mind is much more likely to be healthy as well. So take time to rest, nourish your body with healthy food and water, and get moving as much as possible. Taking these physical steps will make you stronger and more able to take the mental steps necessary to overcome test anxiety.

Review Video: How to Stay Healthy and Prevent Test Anxiety
Visit mometrix.com/academy and enter code: 877894

Mental Steps for Beating Test Anxiety

Working on the mental side of test anxiety can be more challenging, but as with the physical side, there are clear steps you can take to overcome it. As mentioned earlier, test anxiety often stems from lack of preparation, so the obvious solution is to prepare for the test. Effective studying may be the most important weapon you have for beating test anxiety, but you can and should employ several other mental tools to combat fear.

First, boost your confidence by reminding yourself of past success—tests or projects that you aced. If you're putting as much effort into preparing for this test as you did for those, there's no reason you should expect to fail here. Work hard to prepare; then trust your preparation.

Second, surround yourself with encouraging people. It can be helpful to find a study group, but be sure that the people you're around will encourage a positive attitude. If you spend time with others who are anxious or cynical, this will only contribute to your own anxiety. Look for others who are motivated to study hard from a desire to succeed, not from a fear of failure.

Third, reward yourself. A test is physically and mentally tiring, even without anxiety, and it can be helpful to have something to look forward to. Plan an activity following the test, regardless of the outcome, such as going to a movie or getting ice cream.

When you are taking the test, if you find yourself beginning to feel anxious, remind yourself that you know the material. Visualize successfully completing the test. Then take a few deep, relaxing breaths and return to it. Work through the questions carefully but with confidence, knowing that you are capable of succeeding.

Developing a healthy mental approach to test taking will also aid in other areas of life. Test anxiety affects more than just the actual test—it can be damaging to your mental health and even contribute to depression. It's important to beat test anxiety before it becomes a problem for more than testing.

Review Video: <u>Test Anxiety and Depression</u>
Visit mometrix.com/academy and enter code: 904704

Study Strategy

Being prepared for the test is necessary to combat anxiety, but what does being prepared look like? You may study for hours on end and still not feel prepared. What you need is a strategy for test prep. The next few pages outline our recommended steps to help you plan out and conquer the challenge of preparation.

STEP 1: SCOPE OUT THE TEST

Learn everything you can about the format (multiple choice, essay, etc.) and what will be on the test. Gather any study materials, course outlines, or sample exams that may be available. Not only will this help you to prepare, but knowing what to expect can help to alleviate test anxiety.

STEP 2: MAP OUT THE MATERIAL

Look through the textbook or study guide and make note of how many chapters or sections it has. Then divide these over the time you have. For example, if a book has 15 chapters and you have five days to study, you need to cover three chapters each day. Even better, if you have the time, leave an extra day at the end for overall review after you have gone through the material in depth.

If time is limited, you may need to prioritize the material. Look through it and make note of which sections you think you already have a good grasp on, and which need review. While you are studying, skim quickly through the familiar sections and take more time on the challenging parts. Write out your plan so you don't get lost as you go. Having a written plan also helps you feel more in control of the study, so anxiety is less likely to arise from feeling overwhelmed at the amount to cover.

STEP 3: GATHER YOUR TOOLS

Decide what study method works best for you. Do you prefer to highlight in the book as you study and then go back over the highlighted portions? Or do you type out notes of the important information? Or is it helpful to make flashcards that you can carry with you? Assemble the pens, index cards, highlighters, post-it notes, and any other materials you may need so you won't be distracted by getting up to find things while you study.

If you're having a hard time retaining the information or organizing your notes, experiment with different methods. For example, try color-coding by subject with colored pens, highlighters, or post-it notes. If you learn better by hearing, try recording yourself reading your notes so you can listen while in the car, working out, or simply sitting at your desk. Ask a friend to quiz you from your flashcards, or try teaching someone the material to solidify it in your mind.

STEP 4: CREATE YOUR ENVIRONMENT

It's important to avoid distractions while you study. This includes both the obvious distractions like visitors and the subtle distractions like an uncomfortable chair (or a too-comfortable couch that makes you want to fall asleep). Set up the best study environment possible: good lighting and a comfortable work area. If background music helps you focus, you may want to turn it on, but otherwise keep the room quiet. If you are using a computer to take notes, be sure you don't have any other windows open, especially applications like social media, games, or anything else that could distract you. Silence your phone and turn off notifications. Be sure to keep water close by so you stay hydrated while you study (but avoid unhealthy drinks and snacks).

Also, take into account the best time of day to study. Are you freshest first thing in the morning? Try to set aside some time then to work through the material. Is your mind clearer in the afternoon or evening? Schedule your study session then. Another method is to study at the same time of day that you will take the test, so that your brain gets used to working on the material at that time and will be ready to focus at test time.

STEP 5: STUDY!

Once you have done all the study preparation, it's time to settle into the actual studying. Sit down, take a few moments to settle your mind so you can focus, and begin to follow your study plan. Don't give in to distractions or let yourself procrastinate. This is your time to prepare so you'll be ready to fearlessly approach the test. Make the most of the time and stay focused.

Of course, you don't want to burn out. If you study too long you may find that you're not retaining the information very well. Take regular study breaks. For example, taking five minutes out of every hour to walk briskly, breathing deeply and swinging your arms, can help your mind stay fresh.

As you get to the end of each chapter or section, it's a good idea to do a quick review. Remind yourself of what you learned and work on any difficult parts. When you feel that you've mastered the material, move on to the next part. At the end of your study session, briefly skim through your notes again.

But while review is helpful, cramming last minute is NOT. If at all possible, work ahead so that you won't need to fit all your study into the last day. Cramming overloads your brain with more information than it can process and retain, and your tired mind may struggle to recall even previously learned information when it is overwhelmed with last-minute study. Also, the urgent nature of cramming and the stress placed on your brain contribute to anxiety. You'll be more likely to go to the test feeling unprepared and having trouble thinking clearly.

So don't cram, and don't stay up late before the test, even just to review your notes at a leisurely pace. Your brain needs rest more than it needs to go over the information again. In fact, plan to finish your studies by noon or early afternoon the day before the test. Give your brain the rest of the day to relax or focus on other things, and get a good night's sleep. Then you will be fresh for the test and better able to recall what you've studied.

STEP 6: TAKE A PRACTICE TEST

Many courses offer sample tests, either online or in the study materials. This is an excellent resource to check whether you have mastered the material, as well as to prepare for the test format and environment.

Check the test format ahead of time: the number of questions, the type (multiple choice, free response, etc.), and the time limit. Then create a plan for working through them. For example, if you have 30 minutes to take a 60-question test, your limit is 30 seconds per question. Spend less time on the questions you know well so that you can take more time on the difficult ones.

If you have time to take several practice tests, take the first one open book, with no time limit. Work through the questions at your own pace and make sure you fully understand them. Gradually work up to taking a test under test conditions: sit at a desk with all study materials put away and set a timer. Pace yourself to make sure you finish the test with time to spare and go back to check your answers if you have time.

After each test, check your answers. On the questions you missed, be sure you understand why you missed them. Did you misread the question (tests can use tricky wording)? Did you forget the information? Or was it something you hadn't learned? Go back and study any shaky areas that the practice tests reveal.

Taking these tests not only helps with your grade, but also aids in combating test anxiety. If you're already used to the test conditions, you're less likely to worry about it, and working through tests until you're scoring well gives you a confidence boost. Go through the practice tests until you feel comfortable, and then you can go into the test knowing that you're ready for it.

Test Tips

On test day, you should be confident, knowing that you've prepared well and are ready to answer the questions. But aside from preparation, there are several test day strategies you can employ to maximize your performance.

First, as stated before, get a good night's sleep the night before the test (and for several nights before that, if possible). Go into the test with a fresh, alert mind rather than staying up late to study.

Try not to change too much about your normal routine on the day of the test. It's important to eat a nutritious breakfast, but if you normally don't eat breakfast at all, consider eating just a protein bar. If you're a coffee drinker, go ahead and have your normal coffee. Just make sure you time it so that the caffeine doesn't wear off right in the middle of your test. Avoid sugary beverages, and drink enough water to stay hydrated but not so much that you need a restroom break 10 minutes into the test. If your test isn't first thing in the morning, consider going for a walk or doing a light workout before the test to get your blood flowing.

Allow yourself enough time to get ready, and leave for the test with plenty of time to spare so you won't have the anxiety of scrambling to arrive in time. Another reason to be early is to select a good seat. It's helpful to sit away from doors and windows, which can be distracting. Find a good seat, get out your supplies, and settle your mind before the test begins.

When the test begins, start by going over the instructions carefully, even if you already know what to expect. Make sure you avoid any careless mistakes by following the directions.

Then begin working through the questions, pacing yourself as you've practiced. If you're not sure on an answer, don't spend too much time on it, and don't let it shake your confidence. Either skip it and come back later, or eliminate as many wrong answers as possible and guess among the remaining ones. Don't dwell on these questions as you continue—put them out of your mind and focus on what lies ahead.

Be sure to read all of the answer choices, even if you're sure the first one is the right answer. Sometimes you'll find a better one if you keep reading. But don't second-guess yourself if you do immediately know the answer. Your gut instinct is usually right. Don't let test anxiety rob you of the information you know.

If you have time at the end of the test (and if the test format allows), go back and review your answers. Be cautious about changing any, since your first instinct tends to be correct, but make sure you didn't misread any of the questions or accidentally mark the wrong answer choice. Look over any you skipped and make an educated guess.

At the end, leave the test feeling confident. You've done your best, so don't waste time worrying about your performance or wishing you could change anything. Instead, celebrate the successful completion of this test. And finally, use this test to learn how to deal with anxiety even better next time.

Important Qualification

Not all anxiety is created equal. If your test anxiety is causing major issues in your life beyond the classroom or testing center, or if you are experiencing troubling physical symptoms related to your anxiety, it may be a sign of a serious physiological or psychological condition. If this sounds like your situation, we strongly encourage you to seek professional help.

Thank You

We at Mometrix would like to extend our heartfelt thanks to you, our friend and patron, for allowing us to play a part in your journey. It is a privilege to serve people from all walks of life who are unified in their commitment to building the best future they can for themselves.

The preparation you devote to these important testing milestones may be the most valuable educational opportunity you have for making a real difference in your life. We encourage you to put your heart into it—that feeling of succeeding, overcoming, and yes, conquering will be well worth the hours you've invested.

We want to hear your story, your struggles and your successes, and if you see any opportunities for us to improve our materials so we can help others even more effectively in the future, please share that with us as well. **The team at Mometrix would be absolutely thrilled to hear from you!** So please, send us an email (support@mometrix.com) and let's stay in touch.

> **If you'd like some additional help, check out these other resources we offer for your exam:**
> **http://mometrixflashcards.com/NP**

Additional Bonus Material

Due to our efforts to try to keep this book to a manageable length, we've created a link that will give you access to all of your additional bonus material.

Please visit https://www.mometrix.com/bonus948/npfamily to access the information.

95334516R00203